AF733172

Early Pathologic Diagnosis of Gynecologic Cancer Including a Clinician's View

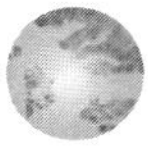

Early Pathologic Diagnosis of Gynecologic Cancer Including a Clinician's View

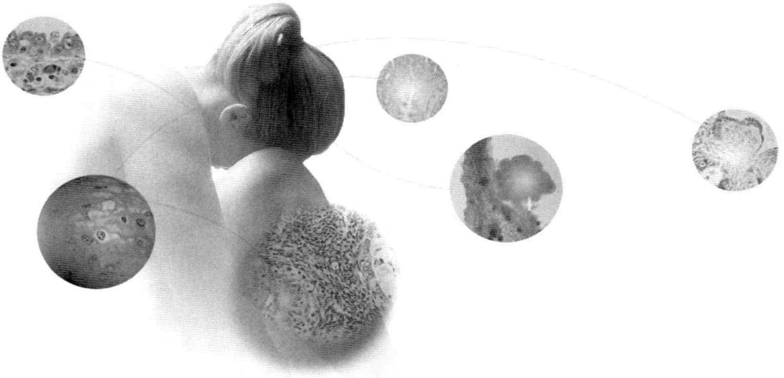

Editor

Liane Deligdisch

Mount Sinai School of Medicine, USA

Co-editor

Albert Altchek

Mount Sinai School of Medicine & Lenox Hill Hospital, USA

Co-authors

Peter Schlosshauer

Maoxin Wu

Mount Sinai School of Medicine, USA

Frédérique Penault-Llorca

Clermont-Ferrand Medical School, France

World Scientific

NEW JERSEY • LONDON • SINGAPORE • BEIJING • SHANGHAI • HONG KONG • TAIPEI • CHENNAI

Published by

World Scientific Publishing Co. Pte. Ltd.
5 Toh Tuck Link, Singapore 596224
USA office: 27 Warren Street, Suite 401-402, Hackensack, NJ 07601
UK office: 57 Shelton Street, Covent Garden, London WC2H 9HE

British Library Cataloguing-in-Publication Data
A catalogue record for this book is available from the British Library.

EARLY PATHOLOGIC DIAGNOSIS OF GYNECOLOGIC CANCER INCLUDING A CLINICIAN'S VIEW

Copyright © 2009 by World Scientific Publishing Co. Pte. Ltd.

All rights reserved. This book, or parts thereof, may not be reproduced in any form or by any means, electronic or mechanical, including photocopying, recording or any information storage and retrieval system now known or to be invented, without written permission from the Publisher.

For photocopying of material in this volume, please pay a copying fee through the Copyright Clearance Center, Inc., 222 Rosewood Drive, Danvers, MA 01923, USA. In this case permission to photocopy is not required from the publisher.

ISBN-13 978-981-281-895-9
ISBN-10 981-281-895-2

Typeset by Stallion Press
Email: enquiries@stallionpress.com

Printed in Singapore by Mainland Press Pte Ltd

CONTENTS

Contributors ix

Preface xi

Chapter 1 EARLY DIAGNOSIS OF VULVAR CANCER **1**
Peter Schlosshauer

Introduction 1
Normal Anatomy and Histology 2
Clinical Identification of Early Vulvar Neoplasms 3
Processing of a Surgical Specimen for Pathologic Evaluation 4
Non-Neoplastic Epithelial Disorders 6
Pre-Malignant Squamous Epithelial Lesions 11
Invasive Carcinoma 18
References 43

Chapter 2 EARLY DIAGNOSIS OF CERVICAL AND VAGINAL CANCER **47**
Peter Schlosshauer

Introduction 47

	Normal Anatomy, Histology and Physiologic Changes	48
	Clinical Identification of Early Vaginal and Cervical Neoplasms	52
	Processing of a Surgical Specimen for Pathologic Evaluation	54
	Benign Disorders	56
	Human Papilloma Virus (HPV): Life Cycle and Role in Tumorigenesis	62
	Premalignant Epithelial Lesions	65
	Invasive Carcinoma of the Cervix	79
	Carcinoma of the Vagina	97
	Other Malignant Tumors of the Vagina and Cervix	101
	Ancillary Studies	101
	HPV-Vaccine	107
	References	109
Chapter 3	**EARLY DIAGNOSIS OF CERVICAL, VAGINAL AND VULVAR CANCER: A CLINICIAN'S VIEW** *Albert Altchek*	**115**
	Cervical Cancer	115
	Vaginal and Vulvar Cancer	129
	References	144
Chapter 4	**EARLY DIAGNOSIS OF ENDOMETRIAL CANCER** *Liane Deligdisch*	**149**
	Introduction	149
	Precursors of Endometrial Carcinoma	150
	Classification of Endometrial Carcinoma	157
	Early Endometrial Carcinoma	160
	Pathology of Endometrial Carcinoma	163

	Histologic Patterns of Endometrial Carcinomas	165
	Molecular Biology of Endometrial Carcinoma	168
	Conclusions	170
	References	172
Chapter 5	**EARLY DIAGNOSIS OF OVARIAN CANCER** *Liane Deligdisch*	**175**
	Introduction	175
	Risk Factors, Genetic Risk	176
	Ovarian Dysplasia	177
	Prophylactic Oophorectemy and the Ovary at Risk	183
	Stage I Ovarian Carcinoma	188
	Conclusions	195
	References	195
Chapter 6	**EARLY DIAGNOSIS OF OVARIAN AND ENDOMETRIAL CANCER: A CLINICIAN'S VIEW** *Albert Altchek*	**199**
	Ovarian Cancer	199
	Endometrial Cancer	212
	References	224
Chapter 7	**CYTOLOGY FOR EARLY DIAGNOSIS OF GYNECOLOGIC CANCER** *Maoxin Wu*	**229**
	Introduction	229
	Cervical, Vaginal and Vulvar Neoplasms	234
	Endometrial Neoplasia	253
	Ovarian Neoplasia	256
	Summary	261
	References	261

Chapter 8 MOLECULAR AND BIOLOGICAL DIAGNOSIS OF EARLY GYNECOLOGIC CANCERS **267**
Frederique Penault-Llorca

Ovarian Cancer 267
Cervical Cancer 274
Endometrial Cancer 280
References 282

Index **285**

CONTRIBUTORS

Albert Altchek, MD, FACOG, FACS
Clinical Professor with Tenure of Obstetrics
Gynecology and Reproductive Science
Attending Obstetrician-Gynecologist
Chief of Pediatric and Adolescent Gynecology
The Mount Sinai School of Medicine and Hospital
One Gustave L. Levy Place
New York, NY 10029, USA
Attending Obstetrician-Gynecologist Lenox Hill Hospital

Liane Deligdisch, MD, FCAP
Professor of Pathology
Professor of Obstetrics-Gynecology and Reproductive Science
Attending Pathologist and Obstetrician-Gynecologist
The Mount Sinai School of Medicine and Hospital
One Gustave L. Levy Place
New York, NY 10029, USA
Member of the French National Academy of Medicine, Paris, France

Frederique Penault-Llorca, MD, PhD
Professor of Pathology
Medical School Clermont-Ferrand
Director of Pathology
Institute Jean Perrin, Clermont-Ferrand, France

Peter Schlosshauer, MD, FCAP
Assistant Professor
Attending Pathologist
The Mount Sinai School of Medicine and Hospital
One Gustave L. Levy Place
New York, NY 10029, USA

Maoxin Wu, MD, PhD
Associate Professor of Pathology
Director of Cytopathology
The Mount Sinai School of Medicine and Hospital
One Gustave L. Levy Place
New York, NY 10029, USA

PREFACE

It is common knowledge that early diagnosis and, if possible, prevention, represent one main goal for improving the outcome of neoplastic diseases. The high morbidity and mortality due to gynecologic cancer represents a major issue in women's health, calling for much needed efforts to achieve an early diagnosis. A quite unique success story in gynecologic pathology is that of the spectacular decline of the incidence of invasive cervical cancer in those areas of the world where precancerous lesions are identified and removed before they become overtly cancerous, due to an organized system of early detection. The earliest descriptions of cervical precancerous lesions were based on microscopic analysis of histological tissue sections and of cytologic smears. They were followed by virologic studies that identified the causal agent (HPV), and recently, by a vaccine aimed at the worldwide prevention of this common and still highly lethal cancer. This sequence of events highlights a significant aspect of "translational medicine" encompassing basic science discoveries, histologic and cytologic descriptions, "translated" into clinical-surgical management and prevention.

Unfortunately not all gynecologic cancers can be handled as successfully. Ovarian cancer, while not the most common is still the most lethal gynecologic malignancy, despite recent progress. Early diagnosis of the majority of ovarian cancers is rare and an organized system of early detection and prevention, as for cervical cancer, does not exist at the present time. This book is presenting the early stages and precursor lesions of gynecologic cancer in a multidisciplinary approach. The subjects are treated from the point of view of different specialties, such as pathology (including computerized image analysis), molecular biology and clinical gynecology. The authors also express their personal insights, based on their individual professional experience, original research and recent scientific progress. The various subjects are presented in a relatively concise manner, offering the reader a diversity of approaches as well as an update of our knowledge at the present time, in the hope that better understanding of disease inception and spread will lead to improved therapeutic and preventive efficiency.

Acknowledgments: We thank Angelica Mares, MD, for her research and editorial assistance and Mr. Joseph Samet for photographical assistance.

Liane Deligdisch, MD
Professor of Pathology
Professor of Obstetrics-Gynecology
and Reproductive Science
The Mount Sinai School of Medicine
and the Mount Sinai Medical Center
New York, USA

CHAPTER 1

EARLY DIAGNOSIS OF VULVAR CANCER

Peter Schlosshauer

INTRODUCTION

Surgery on vulvar malignancies has become more conservative over the past several decades. A radical vulvectomy with removal of bilateral inguinal lymph nodes *en bloc*, a mutilating procedure fraught with high complication rates still performed in the 1980s, has become a rarity in today's practice. This may be partially due to the fact that tumors tend to be diagnosed at earlier stages, thanks to better patient education and improved healthcare. While a more conservative surgical approach is desirable for the patient, therapeutic efficacy should not be compromised. Because of the close proximity of important structures in the vulvar region, space is often very limited for the surgeon to achieve wide enough margins around the lesion. This chapter will specifically address the issues arising in the context of diagnosing and evaluating early stage vulvar malignancies and their precursor lesions. The current concepts of carcinogenic mechanisms of vulvar neoplasms are also reviewed.

Since a major part of the vulva is composed of skin, virtually any dermatologic disorder may be encountered on the vulva. For lesions unrelated to vulvar malignancies, including benign tumors and the manifestations of a generalized dermatologic or medical condition, the reader is referred to textbooks of gynecologic pathology, dermatopathology or dermatology.

NORMAL ANATOMY AND HISTOLOGY

The vulva is synonymous with the external female genitalia and includes the mons pubis anteriorly, the labia majora laterally, the labia minora medially, the clitoris at the anterior junction of the labia minora, the fourchette at the posterior junction of the labia minora, and the perineum extending posteriorly between the fourchette and the anus. The introitus (or vestibule) is the space limited by the labia minora laterally, the clitoris anteriorly, the fourchette posteriorly, and is separated from the vagina by the hymenal ring. Important structures related to the introitus are the vagina, the urethra, the paraurethral (Skene) glands and their ducts, and the major vestibular (Bartholin) glands, which are drained posterolaterally to the hymenal ring. In addition, there are minor vestibular glands around the external base of the hymenal ring. In the adult, the mons pubis, the labia majora and part of the perineum carry hair-bearing skin with adnexal structures, underlaid by ample adipose tissue.

While the clitoris and the lateral aspects of the labia minora are covered by keratinizing squamous epithelium, the introitus is lined by non-keratinizing squamous epithelium. Except for sebaceous glands, the labia minora do not carry any skin adnexal structures. The body of the clitoris consists of the richly vascularized corpora cavernosa and abundant nerve fibers. The mucinous Skene glands open into the introitus via a transitional-type epithelium lined duct. The Bartholin gland is composed of acini lined by columnar mucinous epithelium. Its duct typically displays mucinous epithelium proximally, transitional-type epithelium in its middle portion, and squamous epithelium close to the orifice. The lymphatic drainage of the vulva occurs generally to the ipsilateral femoral and inguinal lymph nodes.

However, lymph from the midline portions of the vulva may drain to both sides. In addition, there is a minor lymphatic drainage pathway from the clitoris via the urethral lymphatics to the interiliac, external iliac and obturator lymph nodes.

The rare occurrence of vulvar tumors that resemble lesions frequently found in the mammary gland has led to the theory that ectopic breast tissue may be encountered in the vulva as a result of incomplete regression of an embryologic "milk line". Alternatively, such lesions may be derived from "mammary-like glands" that have eccrine and apocrine features and are a normal constituent of vulvar and perianal skin.

CLINICAL IDENTIFICATION OF EARLY VULVAR NEOPLASMS

The key to early diagnosis of a vulvar malignancy is of course clinical recognition of a suspicious lesion. Since it is not uncommon for patients to delay seeking medical attention, the first step to earlier diagnosis is improved patient education. Similar to breast self-examination, patients should be encouraged to self-examine the vulva regularly. The use of a mirror is helpful. Informed women will know to look for changes in skin color or thickness and the appearance of open sores or wart-like growths, and not to delay a visit to the gynecologist if a new lesion is noticed.

The understanding of the risk factors for developing vulvar neoplastic disease will increase the physician's index of suspicion. These include a previous history of genital human papilloma virus (HPV) infection, cervical or vaginal intraepithelial neoplasia, lichen sclerosus, squamous hyperplasia, and chronic granulomatous diseases of the vulva. In recent years, immunosuppression due to HIV infection, status post organ transplantation, or chemotherapy has emerged as a major risk factor for intraepithelial or invasive neoplastic disease, especially in young women. Up to 50% of patients with vulvar neoplastic disease are asymptomatic. Also, symptoms may not be reported due to embarrassment or denial. Therefore, on routine annual gynecologic check-up visits, a careful anamnestic exploration always includes a question regarding changes or discomfort in the vulvar region. Common early symptoms include chronic vulvar pruritus or pain ("vulvodynia"), ulceration and bleeding, dysuria and "vaginal" discharge. Any of these complaints should alert the physician to the possibility of an underlying malignancy and prompt a thorough clinical examination, including the inspection and palpation of the vulva and inguinal lymph nodes. Biopsies should be taken liberally of any visible vulvar lesion. Symptomatic treatment or application of topical ointments for any condition without a defined working diagnosis is not recommended. The use of a colposcope and/or application of toluidine blue or 5% acetic acid (which on the vulva, as opposed to the cervix, may need to be applied for several minutes in order to visualize a dysplastic lesion!) may be helpful to identify a subtle lesion and choose the site for biopsy. Generally, it is preferable not to excise the entire lesion if no previous histopathologic diagnosis is available. It must be kept in mind that in the event of an invasive carcinoma, optimal results are achieved with an at least 1.0 cm disease free margin. Also, if there is stromal invasion of more than 1.0 mm in depth, inguinal lymph node dissection is recommended. Thus, an optimal treatment strategy should be developed based on biopsy results. Biopsies should be taken from areas that appear clinically most suspicious for invasion, avoiding necrotic areas. The biopsy should be deep enough and include underlying connective tissue to allow the evaluation of invasion, if present. The periphery of a lesion may show only *in situ* disease. Often, multiple biopsies are indicated, especially in multifocal disease.

PROCESSING OF A SURGICAL SPECIMEN FOR PATHOLOGIC EVALUATION

For optimal pathologic evaluation, a good collaboration between pathologist and surgeon is crucial. After obtaining a biopsy specimen, communication of pertinent clinical information to the pathologist is of utmost importance. While this is true for all surgical pathology, in the case of vulvar biopsies, it is essential for the pathologist to know whether the "lesion" appeared clinically as an exophytic papillary structure, a pigmented spot, an ulcer, or something else. An accurately oriented specimen is necessary for correct identification of resection margins, in case they are involved by the pathologic process. Commonly, a stitch is attached to the specimen by the surgeon indicating a certain clockface position. For optimal preservation of orientation, and to prevent distortion during fixation, the resected specimen may be pinned onto cardboard before placed into 10% formalin. Additional information may be indicated on the cardboard, preferably with pencil, since other types of ink may be washed out by the formalin. The more clinical information is given to the pathologist, the more useful the rendered diagnosis will be.

Most surgical specimens resected from the vulva will fall into one of three categories:

1. An incisional biopsy represents lesional tissue removed without the intention to completely excise the lesion. These are typically small tissue fragments, a few millimeters in greatest dimension. When embedding the specimen into the paraffin block, care must be taken to orient the tissue such that a perpendicular section of the epidermis and underlying tissue will be seen on the slide. Incorrect embedding may not only compromise diagnostic accuracy, but can even destroy the tissue for further analysis. On incisional biopsies the pathologist is asked to give a mere diagnosis as to what kind of lesion is present (e.g. reactive versus neoplastic). If malignant, the report should also include a statement whether stromal invasion and/or lymphvascular involvement can be identified. Accurate evaluation of the size of the lesion and/or depth of invasion is not possible on incisional biopsies. The assessment of margins is less of an issue, since it is understood that the lesion was not completely excised. However, if the pathologist is not sure whether the specimen was meant to be an incisional or an excisional biopsy, it is prudent to ink the specimen and report on the status of the surgical resection margins anyway.
2. An excisional biopsy is taken with the intention to completely remove the lesion and achieve clear resection margins. These

specimens usually have the shape of an ellipse with a visible central lesion. Since the evaluation of margins is a required part of the pathologic evaluation, an excisional biopsy should always be inked. According to the surgeon's indication for orientation, opposite resection margins can be inked in different colors (e.g. medial = black, lateral = red). For optimal assessment of the margins, it is recommended to cut off the tips of the elliptically shaped specimen, bivalve them longitudinally and submit them in separate cassettes. Then the remainder of the specimen is serially sectioned transversely and entirely submitted. Again, care must be taken to embed the sections "on edge" to allow optimal evaluation of the full thickness of the specimen.

3. After the diagnosis of a malignancy has been made, a radical procedure (wide resection, radical vulvectomy/hemivulvectomy) results in a larger specimen including inguinal lymph nodes. Correct orientation is still critical, but may be more easily recognizable from the specimen. Additional margins, e.g. vaginal and/or urethral margins, may need to be evaluated. Usually representative sections are sufficient to obtain the necessary pathologic information.

NON-NEOPLASTIC EPITHELIAL DISORDERS

Vulvar Dermatoses

Although the vulvar dermatoses lichen sclerosus (formerly known as lichen sclerosus et atrophicus) and squamous hyperplasia are not thought to be direct precursors of neoplastic lesions, they may be seen in association with vulvar carcinoma, especially with the human papillomavirus (HPV) unrelated keratinizing squamous cell carcinoma. Whether these associated dermatoses are due to similar stimuli that give rise to the cancer, or a reaction to the neoplastic process, is unclear. Regardless, the presence of these dermatoses should alert both clinician and pathologist to the possibility of an associated malignancy and prompt careful examination, close follow-up, and thorough pathological work-up of resected specimens. In addition, both lesions may clinically mimic a neoplastic process and are therefore frequently biopsied. Lichen sclerosus and squamous cell hyperplasia may coexist ("mixed dystrophy") and often present with vulvar pruritus. Visible lesions may be described as "leukoplakia" (literally "white plaque"), a term that is greatly appreciated by the pathologist as a piece of clinical information, but does not designate a specific histopathologic diagnosis.

Neither lichen sclerosus nor squamous hyperplasia are causally related to HPV infection.

Lichen Sclerosus

This disorder affects primarily postmenopausal women, but can be seen at any age, including children. Grossly, the epidermis is thinned, whitish and may show varying degrees of shrinkage leading to effacement of the labia minora, constriction of the introitus or clitoral phimosis ("kraurosis vulvae"). While it may affect the entire vulva including the perineum and perianal region, the vagina is not usually involved. Histologically, the fully developed lichen sclerosus is characterized by a thinned atrophic layer of viable squamous epithelium, marked hyper- and parakeratosis, flattening of the rete ridges at the dermoepidermal junction, a hyalinized hypocellular zone underneath the squamous epithelium, and a band-like chronic inflammatory infiltrate deep to the hypocellular zone (Fig. 1). In earlier stages, not all of these features may be present. Not infrequently, only the squamous epithelium will be obtained during the biopsy procedure, with no dermis available for evaluation. In such cases, the finding of a strip of hyperkeratotic squamous epithelium in which the layer of hyperkeratosis is thicker than the remaining viable epithelium is highly suggestive of the diagnosis of lichen sclerosus.

The etiology of lichen sclerosus remains unclear. Immunologic, genetic, hormonal, infectious and local reactive factors have been implicated. Vulvar lichen sclerosus is not associated with HPV infection, although HPV-positivity has been reported in a subset of penile lichen sclerosus cases.[1] There is an increased incidence of

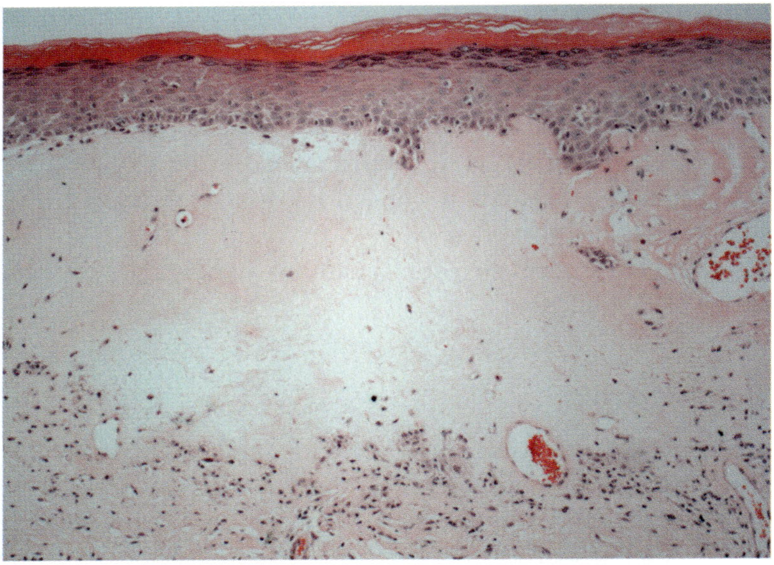

Fig. 1 Lichen sclerosus. The epidermis is atrophic and hyperkeratotic. Rete ridges are effaced. There is a hypocellular subepidermal layer and a sparse chronic inflammatory infiltrate underneath. Hematoxylin/eosin, original magnification 100×.

p53 mutations in vulvar lichen sclerosus compared to the adjacent normal skin.[2] Similar findings have been reported in the differentiated subtype of vulvar intraepithelial neoplasia (VIN), which is often associated with lichen sclerosus, suggesting that *p53* mutations may be an early event in the carcinogenesis of non-HPV related vulvar squamous cell carcinoma. As stated above, lichen sclerosus is not considered a direct precursor of neoplastic disease, but histological evidence of lichen sclerosus is seen in approximately 61% of cases with invasive squamous cell carcinoma. Conversely, up to 21% of patients with symptomatic lichen sclerosus develop squamous cell carcinoma within a mean of four years.[3,4] A recent study suggests that cases of lichen sclerosus that subsequently develop squamous cell carcinoma display a higher Mib-1 labeling index than those that do not develop carcinoma.[5]

Squamous Hyperplasia/Lichen Simplex Chronicus

Formerly known as hyperplastic vulvar dystrophy, squamous hyperplasia is thought to be a non-specific reactive process due to a variety of irritants. Clinically, the involved area may appear whitish or reddened, excoriated due to scratching, but unlike lichen sclerosus, there is no shrinkage of the skin. Histologically, squamous hyperplasia shows somewhat opposite features as lichen sclerosus, including a thickening of the viable epithelium (acanthosis) and elongation of the rete ridges. There is a prominent granular cell layer and variable degrees of hyper-and parakeratosis. Intercellular bridges may be prominent due to edema (spongiosis). Of note, there is no significant cytologic atypia, and mitotic activity is confined to the basal cell layer (Fig. 2). If associated with a lymphocytic superficial dermal inflammatory

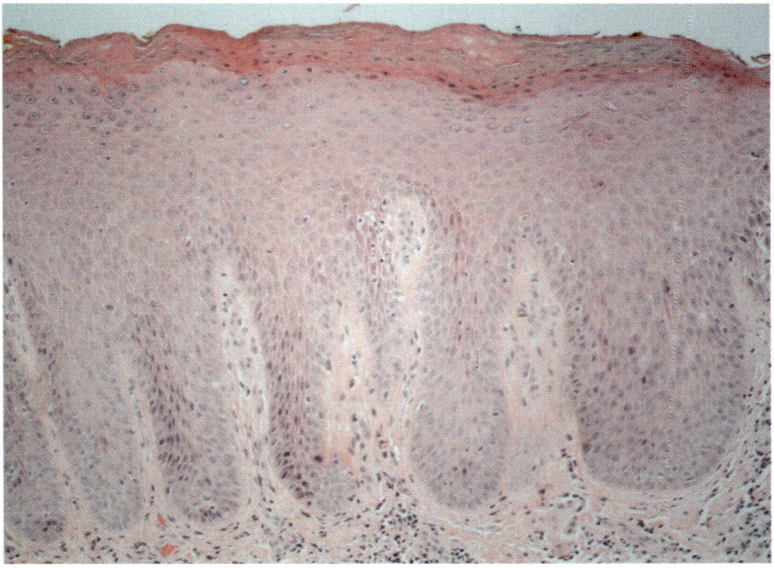

Fig. 2 Squamous hyperplasia/Lichen simplex chronicus. The epidermis is thickened and shows hyper- and parakeratosis. Rete ridges are elongated. There is a chronic inflammatory infiltrate within the superficial dermis. Hematoxylin/eosin, original magnification 100×.

infiltrate, it is also called lichen simplex chronicus (LSC). There is no dermal sclerosis. The differential diagnosis includes vulvar intraepithelial neoplasia (VIN), fungal infections, and other dermatoses like psoriasis or lichen planus, which need to be excluded in order to establish the diagnosis of squamous hyperplasia. Similar to lichen sclerosus, squamous hyperplasia is seen in association with over 50% of vulvar squamous cell carcinomas.

Condylomata Acuminata

Warts caused by human papillomavirus (HPV) types 6 and 11 are generally considered an infectious, sexually transmitted disease, and not a direct precursor lesion of neoplasia. However, epidemiologic analyses suggest that the long-term risk of developing invasive vulvar carcinoma is increased as much as 10-fold in patients hospitalized for anogenital condylomata acuminata.[6]

More than 100 genetically distinct HPV types have been identified, most of which target a very specific epithelial region. On the vulva, HPV 6 and 11 are the most frequently encountered types, which give rise to sessile or papillary growths, known as condylomata acuminata. There are usually multiple lesions covering the vulvar skin to varying degrees. Moreover, they may be present in the vagina, cervix, urethra or perianal region. Most patients present in the third and fourth decade of life. Up to 50% of women with vulvar condylomata acuminata also have cervical HPV infections. The natural course of the disease is often very protracted, and it may take years until immunity is acquired and the warts are shed. For a more detailed discussion of the biology of HPV infections, the reader is referred to chapter 2, pp. 62–63.

Histologically, a condyloma acuminatum is characterized by a relatively thin fibrovascular core, surrounded by a thickened (acanthotic) epithelium. The pathognomonic criterion on routine light microscopy is the presence of koilocytes. These are squamous cells with an abnormal (hyperchromatic, enlarged, irregularly shaped) nucleus and a surrounding cytoplasmic clearing ("halo"), which are considered HPV-specific cytopathic changes. Multinucleation is frequent; however, an occasional binucleated cell is non-specific, unless it displays the nuclear atypia required to classify it as a koilocyte. Likewise, a clear cytoplasm is not to be interpreted as a koilocytotic halo unless it is accompanied by an atypical nucleus. Koilocytotic changes tend to be more subtle on the vulva than they are on the cervix. Often, they are most obvious at the base of clefts between two adjacent papillary projections (Fig. 3). Mitotic figures are rare, not atypical, and confined to the basal or parabasal cell layers. Condylomata may display varying degrees of hyper-and parakeratosis, although the mere finding of parakeratosis is non-specific.

Rarely, vulvar condylomata acuminata may progress to VIN and invasive squamous cell carcinoma,[7] especially if they are associated with high risk HPV types. The so-called "giant condyloma" (Buschke-Löwenstein) is now considered a well differentiated verrucous squamous cell carcinoma that is locally invasive, rarely if ever metastasizes and may be associated with HPV, including the "low-risk" type 6.[8]

PRE-MALIGNANT SQUAMOUS EPITHELIAL LESIONS

In analogy to precursor lesions of the uterine cervix, intraepithelial premalignant squamous cell lesions of the vulva have been termed vulvar intraepithelial neoplasia (VIN). Over the past few decades, a dramatic increase in incidence of VIN has been observed, especially in women younger than 50 years of age. As a result the peak age for VIN has shifted from the seventh decade (in the 1970s) to the fifth decade.[9] Up to 50% of patients with VIN have an associated cervical or vaginal neoplastic lesion. Clinically, VIN typically presents as single or multiple raised skin lesions that may involve any area of the vulva. In the perianal region, the term anal or perianal intraepithelial neoplasia is also used (AIN or PAIN, respectively). It may cause pruritus. The color may range from whitish over red, grey, to darkly pigmented. The term "bowenoid papulosis" refers to multiple pigmented papular lesions, while "erythroplasia of Queyrat" describes a reddish lesion involving the epithelium of the introitus. Both

(a)

(b)

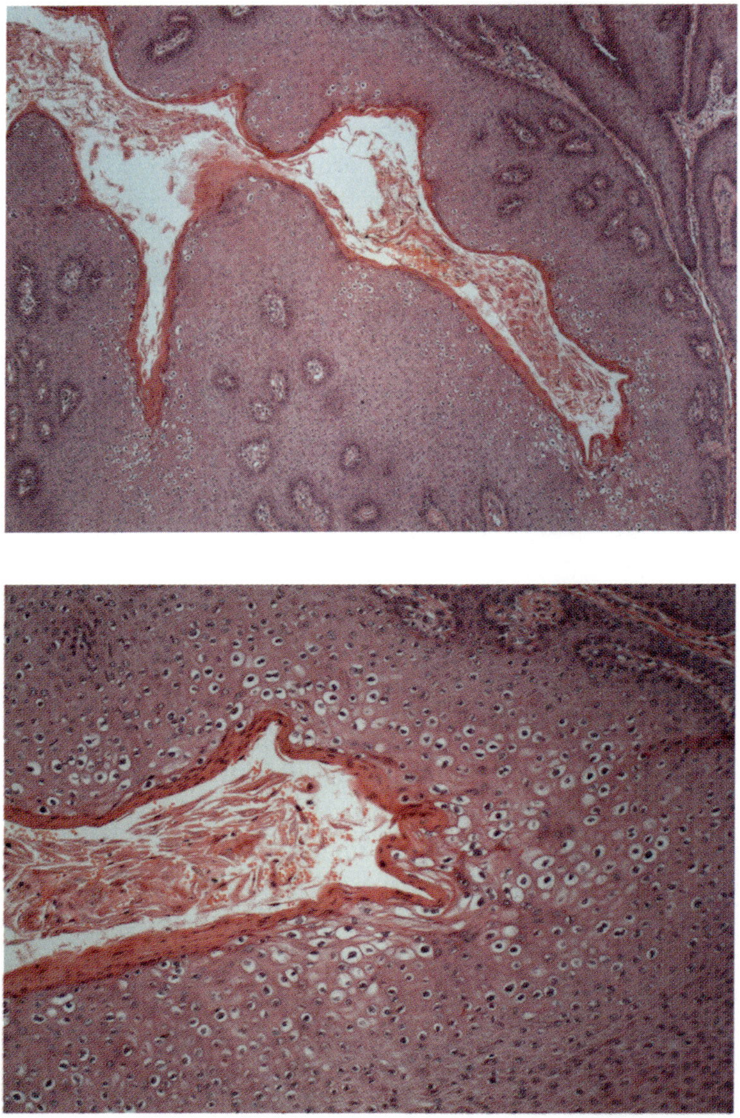

Fig. 3 Condyloma acuminatum. (a) The lesion has a papillary architecture. The epithelium contains numerous koilocytes, especially at the base of clefts. Hematoxylin/eosin, original magnification 40×. (b) Higher magnification of an area containing koilocytes, which are characterized by an atypical nucleus surrounded by a clear cytoplasmic space ("halo"). Hematoxylin/eosin, original magnification 100×.

terms designate variants in clinical presentation of VIN; histopathologically, they do not represent distinct entities.

Two types of VIN are distinguished. The "usual" (also known as "classic", "bowenoid" or "undifferentiated") VIN comprises approximately 80% of all diagnosed VIN cases. It is HPV-associated (mostly types 16 and 18), occurs in a younger age group (third and fourth decades) and is often multifocal. These lesions are characterized by a lack of normal maturation as cells migrate from the basement membrane toward the surface. This is manifested by a persistently high nuclear/cytoplasmic ratio, cellular crowding, mitotic activity (including atypical mitotic figures) distant from the basement membrane, and the failure of the cell body to assume an orientation parallel to the skin surface. Acanthosis, hyper- and parakeratosis are also frequent features. Morphologically, basaloid, warty or mixed features are distinguished. Basaloid VIN is composed of relatively small cells with high nuclear/cytoplasmic ratio, hyperchromatic nuclei and coarse chromatin pattern (Fig. 4). Warty (condylomatous) VIN has larger cells with greater nuclear pleomorphism, clumped chromatin, frequent multinucleated cells and, especially towards the surface, koilocytotic changes (Fig. 5). Intermediate or mixed basaloid/warty lesions are frequent. Usual VIN is considered the precursor lesion of the HPV-associated basaloid and warty/condylomatous types of invasive vulvar squamous cell carcinoma.

The second VIN type is known as "differentiated" or "simplex" VIN. It is composed of cells that appear relatively mature with ample cytoplasm but enlarged atypical nuclei containing prominent nucleoli populating the basal and parabasal cell layers. An important diagnostic feature is the presence of dyskeratotic cells in the parabasal cell layer and keratin pearl formation within rete ridges (Fig. 6(a) and (b)). Differentiated VIN is typically unifocal, occurs in the postmenopausal age group, and is frequently seen in patients with a history of lichen sclerosus.[10,11] On immunohistochemistry, p53 overexpression has been reported in the basal and parabasal layer of differentiated VIN, which may be useful to support the diagnosis (Fig. 6(c)).[12] Ki-67 expression is confined to the basal cell layer in differentiated VIN (Fig. 6(d)). This is in contrast to normal vulvar epidermis, in which

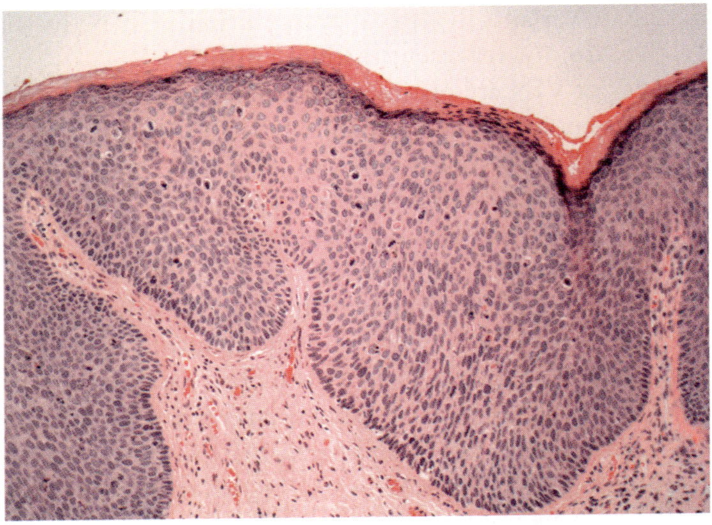

Fig. 4 High grade VIN, basaloid type. The lesion is composed of cells with a high nuclear/cytoplasmic ratio. Numerous mitotic figures are present throughout the entire thickness of the epithelium. Hematoxylin/eosin, original magnification 100×.

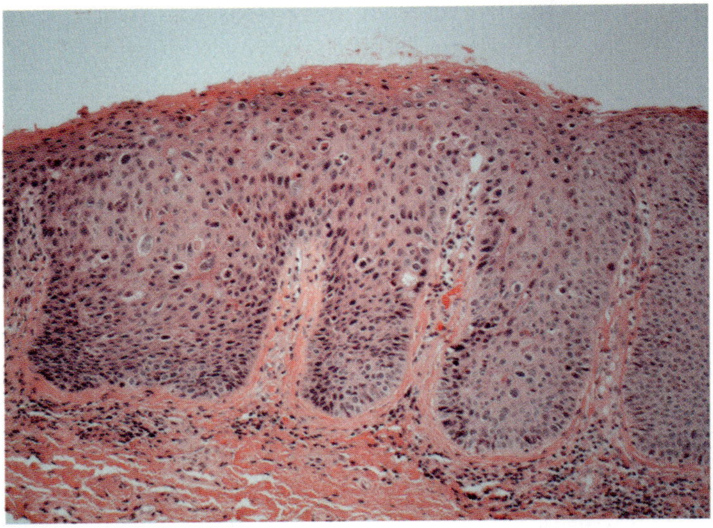

Fig. 5 High grade VIN, warty (condylomatous) type. Cells have ample cytoplasm and koilocytotic features. Hematoxylin/eosin, original magnification 100×.

(a)

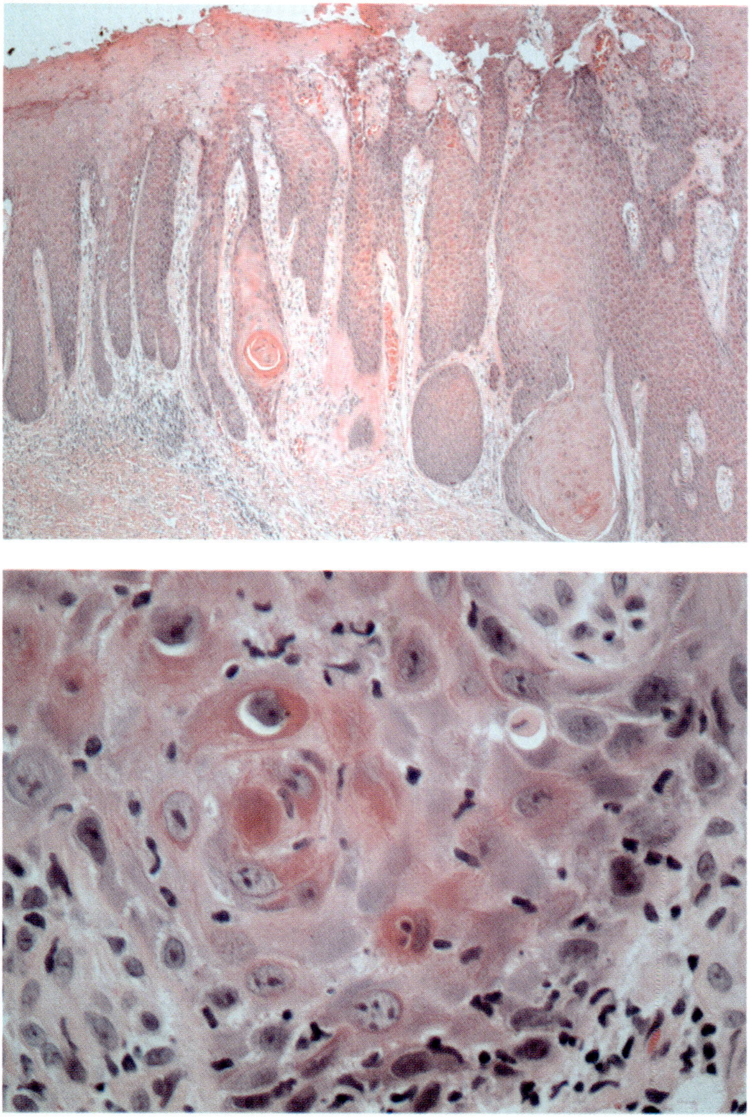

(b)

Fig. 6 Differentiated (simplex) VIN. (a) The epithelium is markedly thickened and appears relatively mature. Note keratin pearl formation in rete ridges. Hematoxylin/eosin, original magnification 40×. (b) High magnification shows nuclear atypia with prominent nucleoli, and dyskeratosis of individual cells. Hematoxylin/eosin, original magnification 400×.

(c)

(d)

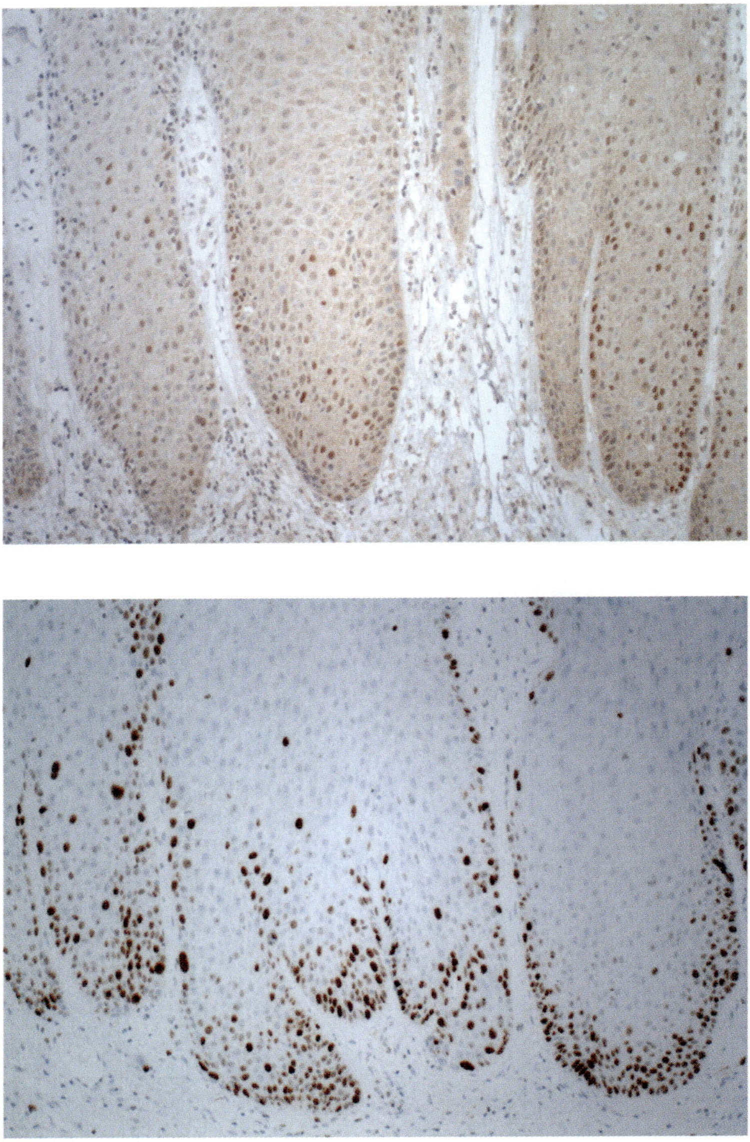

Fig. 6 (*Continued*) (c) Immunohistochemical stain for p53. Nuclear positivity is seen in basal and parabasal cells. Orginal magnification 100×. (d) Immunohistochemical stain for Ki-67 (MIB-1). Nuclear positivity is present in basal cells. Original magnification 100×.

the basal cell layer is typically negative and the parabasal cell layer positive for Ki-67.[13] Increased expression of p53 and Ki-67 may herald transformation to invasive carcinoma.[14] Differentiated VIN is HPV-negative and hence does not overexpress p16.

Differentiated VIN is thought to be the direct precursor of invasive HPV-unrelated keratinizing squamous cell carcinoma. Its risk of progression to invasive carcinoma is probably even higher than that for "usual" high grade VIN. Although the majority of vulvar carcinomas are HPV-unrelated, differentiated VIN is relatively rarely diagnosed, especially when not (yet) associated with an adjacent invasive carcinoma. Possible reasons for this phenomenon include that differentiated VIN may often remain unrecognized by the pathologist because of the more subtle morphologic changes, and that the progression time to invasive carcinoma may be rather short.

While differentiated VIN is not further graded, usual VIN was originally subdivided into mild (VIN 1, confined to lower third), moderate (VIN 2, involving lower and middle third), and severe (VIN 3, involving lower, middle and upper third of the epithelium) dysplasia. The term carcinoma *in situ* is applied to those lesions with no evidence of maturation at all throughout the full thickness of the epithelium. However, this is a purely academic distinction that has no clinical implications. For practical purposes, lesions classified as VIN 2 and 3 or carcinoma *in situ* are grouped together as high grade dysplasia.

Lesions that qualify for a diagnosis of VIN 1 are quite rare, and some authors even question the existence of such an entity. The International Society for the Study of Vulvar Disease (ISSVD) has recommended applying the term VIN to high grade (i.e. VIN 2 and 3, carcinoma *in situ*) lesions only without further grading, and discontinuing the use of the term VIN 1, the rationale being that "VIN 1" lesions and condylomata are manifestations of a viral infection rather than immediate precursors of invasive squamous cell carcinoma.[15] However, a subset of vulvar "low grade" lesions does contain high risk HPV types, and these are morphologically indistinguishable from the low risk HPV-associated lesions.[16,17] Discussion of the grading of

VIN, its appropriate terminology, and how this terminology reflects the biologic behavior of the lesions is ongoing.

High grade VIN can spontaneously regress, especially in young women. However, beyond 30 years of age, the potential to become invasive is great enough that surgical treatment is preferred.[18] In contrast to the cervix, cytologic smears do not appear to be a practical tool to detect precursor lesions of vulvar carcinoma.[19]

INVASIVE CARCINOMA

Squamous Cell Carcinoma

Epidemiology, Etiology and Pathogenesis

Squamous cell carcinoma of the vulva represents approximately 3%–5% of all female genital carcinomas. Eighty-six percent of all vulvar carcinomas are of squamous cell origin. A 20% increase in the incidence of invasive vulvar carcinoma has been observed in the USA over the past three decades. While invasive vulvar carcinoma is rare below the age of 30, the incidence continues to increase continuously thereafter without reaching a peak. Unlike VIN, no significant shift to a younger population has been observed in recent years.[9] Not only is there this disparity between the incidence patterns of *in situ* and invasive vulvar carcinoma, but they also differ from the respective incidence patterns of cervical *in situ* and invasive carcinoma. These epidemiologic data suggest that a variety of as yet unidentified factors contribute to the progression from VIN to invasive vulvar carcinoma, and that these factors are different from those implicated in the majority of cervical carcinomas.

It is now well recognized that two types of vulvar squamous cell carcinoma can be distinguished based on epidemiology, pathogenesis and clinical presentation. The first group, comprising about one third of all vulvar squamous cell carcinomas, presents at a mean age of 55 years. Patients are often smokers. Tumors are positive for HPV DNA, mostly types 16 and 18. Histologically, these tumors are typically of the basaloid or warty types and often have associated "usual" VIN. The carcinogenetic mechanism is thought to be similar to that in

HPV-associated squamous cell carcinoma of the uterine cervix and involves integration of the viral DNA into the host cell genome,[20] and inactivation of the p53 and retinoblastoma tumor suppressor proteins by the viral proteins E6 and E7, respectively (see chapter 2, pp. 62–65). Immunosuppressed patients are at increased risk to acquire HPV-related vulvar disease, including invasive squamous cell carcinoma. However, unlike cervical carcinoma, invasive vulvar carcinoma is not (yet) recognized as an AIDS-defining illness in HIV positive patients. The progression from *in situ* to invasive carcinoma appears to be associated with a reduction in the number of intraepithelial CD1a-positive antigen presenting dendritic cells in both HIV-positive and HIV-negative patients, further supporting a role of the immune system in the carcinogenic process.[21,22] With the advent of HPV vaccines, a decrease in the incidence of these carcinomas is anticipated over the next decades.

Patients of the second group present at a mean age of 77 years. They tend to be non-smokers, and often have an associated vulvar dermatosis (lichen sclerosus or squamous hyperplasia).[11] If there is VIN, it is of the differentiated (simplex) type. These tumors are HPV-negative and tend to be well differentiated and keratinizing. Mutations of the p53 tumor suppressor gene are thought to be an important event in the early pathogenesis of these HPV-unrelated tumors, since they are frequently found in lichen sclerosus, differentiated (simplex) VIN, and well differentiated keratinizing squamous cell carcinoma.[23]

In addition, chronic granulomatous diseases of the vulva, especially granuloma inguinale, have been associated with an increased risk for developing vulvar carcinoma. Our knowledge about molecular genetic events in the pathogenesis of vulvar carcinoma is still very fragmentary. Apart from the alterations mentioned above, mutations in the PTEN tumor suppressor gene have been reported in both *in situ* and invasive squamous cell carcinoma of the vulva, suggesting a role in its early carcinogenesis.[24] Other genes implicated in the development of vulvar carcinoma include $p16^{Ink4a}$, $p15^{Ink4b}$, the retinoblastoma (*RB*) tumor suppressor gene, and *cyclin D1*.

Histologic Subtypes

If not otherwise specified (NOS), vulvar squamous cell carcinomas are of the well to moderately differentiated, keratinizing type. Basaloid carcinoma is composed of relatively small cells with scant cytoplasm. It occurs in the younger patient population with a mean age of 54 years and is often associated with basaloid VIN. The majority of basaloid carcinomas are positive for HPV, mostly type 16. Basaloid carcinoma must be distinguished from basal cell carcinoma, which typically displays a palisading array of the outermost cells.

Similarly, warty (condylomatous) carcinoma presents at a mean age of 55 years, frequently shows associated warty VIN and is also associated with HPV, usually type 16. It is characterized by pronounced cytologic pleomorphism and koilocytotic changes. Of note, both basaloid and warty vulvar carcinomas may be associated with a synchronous cervical or vaginal squamous neoplasm.

Verrucous carcinoma is a well differentiated squamous cell carcinoma with a broad, "pushing" front of invasion that grows in a locally destructive fashion, but almost never metastasizes. Formerly known as "giant condyloma" of Buschke-Löwenstein, that designation is confusing and therefore no longer recommended. It has been found in association with lichen simplex chronicus and with vulvar acanthosis with "altered differentiation", characterized by loss of the granular cell layer and multilayered parakeratosis,[25] which may represent a precursor lesion. It is not clear whether verrucous carcinoma is causally related to HPV infection, but at least a subset of cases has been reported positive for various types, including the "low-risk" HPV type 6.[8] Basal cell carcinoma, although generally very common elsewhere on the skin, occurs only rarely on the vulva. Its histopathologic hallmarks are the parallel alignment of the peripheral cells of the tumor nests ("palisading"), and the surrounding stromal retraction artifact. Basal cell carcinoma is locally aggressive, does not usually metastasize and has a good prognosis if completely excised.

Additional rare types of vulvar carcinoma include spindle cell, giant cell, adenoid squamous, adenoid basal, lymphoepithelioma-like, basosquamous and sebaceous cell carcinoma.

Staging

As is true for many other tumors, the single most important prognostic factor of vulvar carcinoma is its extent at the time of presentation, recorded as the tumor stage. Gynecologic oncologists tend to use the Fédération Internationale de Gynécologie et d'Obstétrique (FIGO) staging system,[26] while the College of American Pathologists' (CAP) guidelines for pathology reports on cancer cases require indication of the tumor stage in the Tumor-Node-Metastasis (TNM) format as published by the American Joint Committee on Cancer (AJCC).[27] The TNM categories have been defined to correspond to the FIGO stages, but due to the different approaches some cases may fall into different stage groups depending on the system applied. Notably, the presence of any unilateral or bilateral regional lymph node metastasis will result in FIGO stage III or IVA, respectively, regardless of the size or depth of invasion of the primary tumor. FIGO stage IVB is defined by the presence of distant metastasis (Table 1).

Carcinomas with a depth of invasion of 1 mm or less (T1a, FIGO stage IA) are referred to as "superficially invasive" tumors. While the risk of metastatic disease in these cases is less than 5%, it sharply increases once the 1 mm threshold is passed. At 3 mm depth of invasion, regional lymph node metastases are seen in approximately 10% of cases. Depth of invasion is measured from the dermo-epidermal junction of the most superficial adjacent dermal papilla to the point of deepest invasion (Fig. 7). It is most accurately obtained by using a calibrated ocular under consideration of the magnification used. For practical purposes, if the diameter of the microscopic field at a specific magnification is known (e.g. at a magnification of 40× using a 4× objective and a 10× ocular, the diameter of the observed microscopic field is typically 5.0 mm), the depth of invasion can often be estimated with

Table 1. Staging of Vulvar Carcinoma[27]

TNM category	FIGO stage	Definition
		Primary Tumor (T)
TX	—	Primary tumor cannot be assessed
T0	—	No evidence of primary tumor
Tis	0	Carcinoma *in situ*, high grade VIN
T1	I	Greatest tumor diameter 2 cm or less; confined to vulva or vulva and perineum
T1a	IA	Stromal invasion 1 mm or less in depth, as measured from the dermoepidermal junction of the adjacent most superficial dermal papilla to the deepest point of invasion
T1b	IB	Stromal invasion greater than 1 mm in depth
T2	II	Greatest tumor diameter more than 2 cm; confined to vulva or vulva and perineum
T3	III	Tumor of any size with contiguous spread to the lower urethra and/or vagina or anus
T4	IVA	Tumor invades any of the following: upper urethra, bladder mucosa, rectal mucosa, or pelvic bone
		Regional Lymph Nodes (N)
NX	—	Regional lymph nodes cannot be assessed
N0	—	No regional lymph node metastasis
N1	III	Unilateral regional lymph node metastasis
N2	IVA	Bilateral regional lymph node metastases
		Distant Metastasis (M)
MX	—	Distant metastasis cannot be assessed
M0	—	No distant metastasis
M1	IVB	Distant metastasis (including pelvic lymph node metastasis) present

Legend: Regional lymph nodes are the femoral and inguinal lymph nodes. The involvement of pelvic lymph nodes, including internal, external, common iliac and obturator lymph nodes, is considered distant metastasis. Vascular invasion has no impact on staging. The stage cannot be changed on the basis of disease progression, recurrence or response to radiation or chemotherapy prior to surgery. This classification applies to all subtypes of squamous cell carcinoma, Paget disease of the vulva, basal cell carcinoma and vulvar adenocarcinoma including Bartholin gland carcinoma. It does not apply to mucosal malignant melanoma.

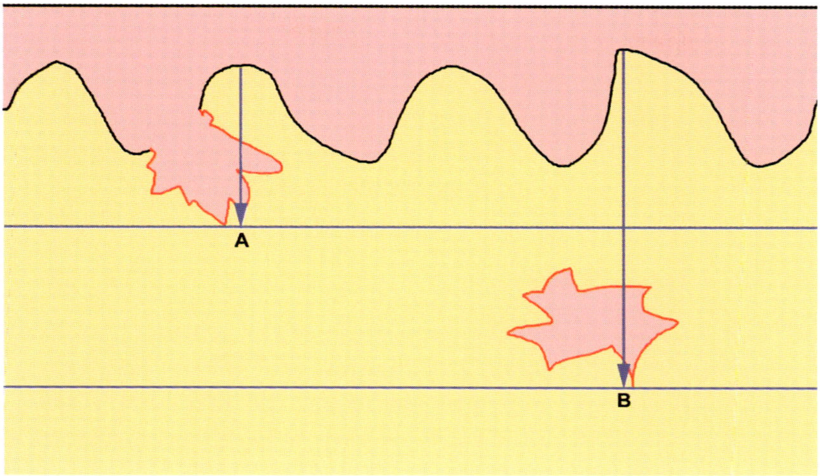

Fig. 7 Measurement of depth of invasion. Pink = epidermis; tan = dermis; black line = intact basement membrane; red line = front of invasive carcinoma. The depth of invasion is measured from the dermoepidermal junction of the most superficial adjacent dermal papilla to the point of deepest invasion. (a) Tumor is extending directly from the epidemis. (b) An isolated invasive tumor cell nest underneath an intact basement membrane.

sufficient accuracy, at least with respect to the 1 mm threshold. As opposed to carcinoma of the uterine cervix, the term "microinvasive carcinoma" is not clearly defined and should not be used to report on vulvar carcinoma. Instead, the pathology report should contain accurate measurements of the horizontal and deep tumor dimensions. The finding of vascular space involvement does not affect the staging, however, the pathology report should always contain a statement as to whether or not vascular space involvement was identified.

According to the FIGO report on the results of treatment, the five-year survival rates for vulvar carcinoma are 78.5%, 58.8%, 43.2% and 13.0% for FIGO stages I, II, III and IV, respectively. If inguinal lymph nodes are negative, the five-year survival rate is 80.7% as opposed to 62.9% with one positive lymph node, 30.4% with two and under 20% with more positive lymph nodes.[28]

Since the pathologist depends on accurate clinical information with respect to laterality and location of lymph nodes or the presence of distant metastases that may not have resulted in a surgical specimen, it is prudent to report the tumor stage as pathologic ("pTNM") stage with a disclaimer that this classification was determined based on the material and/or clinical information provided.

Sentinel Lymph Nodes

The clinical utility of selective extirpation of the sentinel lymph node in vulvar cancer is still under investigation. The idea is that the status of the sentinel lymph node, by definition the first lymph node to receive lymph fluid from the tumor region, is highly predictive for the presence of lymphatic metastases. Therefore, if the sentinel lymph node is negative, a complete inguinal lymph node dissection would not be necessary. However, it still remains to be determined whether the selective removal of the sentinel lymph node leads to a significant reduction of complications that are otherwise associated with a complete lymph node dissection (e.g. lymphedema), and how frequently groin recurrences will occur despite a negative sentinel lymph node, a scenario that carries a rather poor prognosis.

Grading

The AJCC suggests the following grading system: GX — grade cannot be assessed, G1 — well differentiated, G2 — moderately differentiated, G3 — poorly differentiated, and G4 — undifferentiated. However, the criteria to determine the grade if differentiation of vulvar squamous cell carcinoma are not defined. In fact, there is presently no generally agreed upon grading system that correlates well with clinical outcome and is applicable to the different histologic subtypes of vulvar carcinoma.

Adenocarcinoma

Primary vulvar adenocarcinomas are rare; the majority of cases fall under either Paget disease or Bartholin gland carcinomas.

Paget Disease

Vulvar Paget disease tends to occur in postmenopausal Caucasian women at a median age of 70 years. It usually presents as an erythematous, pruritic lesion that may have been present for years and even treated under various working hypotheses until finally the correct diagnosis is made based on a biopsy.

Histopathologically, Paget disease is characterized by relatively large malignant cells, occurring single or in clusters, located within the epidermis (Fig. 8) or extending into the dermis if it has become invasive. Depending upon the presumed cell of origin, a classification into three subtypes has been proposed:

Type 1: Primary vulvar Paget disease

(a) Intraepithelial, including surface epithelium and skin appendages.
(b) Invasive.

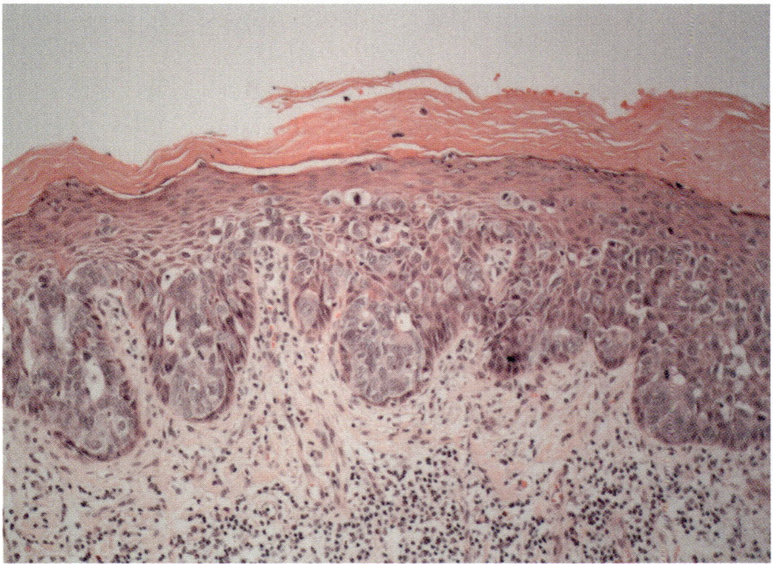

Fig. 8 Paget disease of the vulva. Large atypical cells are present within the epidermis, in clusters and individually. Hematoxylin/eosin, original magnification 100×.

(c) Presenting as a manifestation of an underlying primary vulvar invasive adenocarcinoma (e.g. of the Bartholin gland).

Type 2: Secondary Paget disease as a manifestation of an associated primary anal, colorectal or other non-cutaneous adenocarcinoma.

Type 3: Secondary Paget disease as a manifestation of an associated urothelial neoplasia, also known as pagetoid urothelial intraepithelial neoplasia (PUIN), or "pseudopaget disease".

The histogenesis of vulvar Paget disease type 1a and 1b has long been a subject of debate. Among others, eccrine and apocrine glands, ectopic mammary glands, or pluripotential basal cells have been implicated. The recent discovery of Toker cells as a normal constituent of mammary-like glands in the vulvar region has added another potential cell of origin. Toker cells were first described in the breast as intraepithelial cells with clear cytoplasm that are found in approximately 10% of normal nipples. They are thought to be the cell of origin in rare cases of mammary Paget disease that are not associated with intraductal carcinoma. An analogous process has been proposed to occur in the vulva.[29,30]

While it is not usually possible to distinguish cells of the various Paget types on routine hematoxylin/eosin stained slides, the following adjunct studies may be helpful. Paget type 1a–c cells are positive for cytokeratin (CK) 7 and negative for CK20, much like epithelia of Müllerian origin. In addition, they tend to be positive for gross cystic disease fluid protein-15 (GCDFP-15) and carcinoembryonic antigen (CEA). Conversely, type 2 Paget cells are positive for CK20, negative for CK7, and negative for GCDFP-15. The caudal-related homeobox gene nuclear transcription factor (CDX-2) is expressed in intestinal cells of both the small and large bowel; limited reports on the expression of CDX-2 in the various subtypes of Paget disease suggest that it may be a specific and sensitive marker for type 2 Paget disease.[31,32] Cells of Paget types 1 and 2 contain mucin and are positive on mucicarmine, Alcian blue and PAS (diastase-resistant) stains, whereas type 3 Paget cells (PUIN) are negative for mucin and negative for GCDFP-15. Similar to urothelial neoplasias, PUIN cells are positive for CK7 and uroplakin III, and may be positive for CK20.

Paget cells are HPV negative, unless they are a manifestation of an associated endocervical adenocarcinoma.

Immunohistochemical positivity for p53 and fatty acid synthase has been reported to be associated with invasive primary vulvar Paget disease (type 1(b)).[33,34] Positivity was seen in Paget cells of both the intra-epithelial and the invasive component. To distinguish Paget disease from malignant melanoma, which is its closest look alike, a marker for melanocytes (S-100 protein, HMB-45 or Melan-A) should be included in the panel of special stains (Table 2). Furthermore, the differential diagnosis includes pagetoid VIN (usually negative for CK7 and GCDFP-15) and mycosis fungoides (positive for lymphoid markers).

Table 2. Adjunct Studies in the Work-Up of Paget Disease and Its Differential Diagnosis

	Paget disease			Pagetoid VIN	Malignant melanoma	Mycosis fungoides
	Type 1	Type 2	Type 3			
Mucin markers						
Mucicarmine	+	+	–	–	–	–
PAS	+	+	–	–	–	–
Alcian blue	+	+	–	–	–	–
CK7	+	–*	+	–*	–	–
CK8	+	–	–	–	–	–
CK20	–*	+	+/–	–	–	–
Pan-CK	+	+	+	+	–*	–
GCDFP-15	+/–	–	–	–	–	–
CDX-2	–	+	–	–	–	–
Uroplakin III	–	–	+/–	–	–	–
CEA	+	+	+/–	–	–	–
Melanocytic markers						
S-100	–	–	–	–	+	–
HMB-45	–	–	–	–	+	–
Melan-A	–	–	–	–	+	–
LCA	–	–	–	–	–	+

Legend: + positive; – negative; +/– most cases positive; – * usually negative, rarely positive; CK = cytokeratin; GCDFP = gross cystic disease fluid protein-15; CDX-2 = caudal-related homeobox-2; HMB-45 = human melanoma black-45; CEA = carcinoembryonal antigen; LCA = leukocyte common antigen.

Obviously, the correct diagnosis not only of vulvar Paget disease, but preferably of the subtype is of great clinical importance. Based on the results of histopathologic and adjunct studies, a thorough clinical work-up should be performed to rule out an associated carcinoma elsewhere. Of note, many patients with extramammary Paget disease also develop synchronous or metachronous breast carcinoma. Whether this is a true association, and whether there is a correlation with one of the subtypes of vulvar Paget disease, is unclear. Be that as it may, it is certainly warranted to include a breast examination in the work-up of patients with vulvar Paget disease. Similar to squamous cell carcinoma, the risk of lymph node metastases in invasive primary vulvar Paget disease (types 1b and 1c) increases sharply once the depth of invasion exceeds 1 mm.[35]

Bartholin Gland Carcinoma

Primary Bartholin gland carcinomas are rare. They occur at an average age of 50 years typically as a solid mass, deeply located in the soft tissue, while the overlying skin may be intact and unremarkable. Some cases are associated with vulvar Paget disease (type 1c). A variety of different histologic subtypes of Bartholin gland carcinomas have been described, including adenocarcinoma (40%); squamous cell carcinoma (40%); adenoid cystic carcinoma (15%); transitional cell carcinoma; and adenosquamous carcinoma. To establish the diagnosis of a Bartholin gland carcinoma, three criteria must be fulfilled: the tumor must arise at the site of a Bartholin gland, it must be histologically consistent with Bartholin gland origin, and metastasis from a distant primary tumor must be ruled out.

Squamous cell and adenocarcinomas of the Bartholin gland are usually positive for CEA, which may be helpful to support the diagnosis. A subset of primary Bartholin gland carcinomas, especially of squamous differentiation, is positive for high risk HPV types, which may contribute to its pathogenesis.

Skene Gland Carcinoma

Adenocarcinoma of the Skene glands is extremely rare. Its diagnosis can be supported by immunohistochemical positivity for PSA and prostate acid phosphatase, due to its phylogenetic analogy with the male prostate gland.

Malignant Melanoma

Malignant melanoma of the vulva occurs predominantly in white women and in the postmenopausal population. It is the second most frequent vulvar malignancy after squamous cell carcinoma and accounts for 6%–9% of all vulvar malignancies. Three histopathologic subtypes are distinguished: superficial spreading melanoma, nodular melanoma and mucosal/acral lentiginous melanoma. Tumor cells may display a wide morphologic spectrum, including epithelioid, dendritic and spindle cells (Fig. 9). Malignant melanoma may or may not produce melanin. Whenever a poorly differentiated malignant neoplasm is encountered on the vulva that is difficult to classify, melanoma needs to be ruled out.

The main differential diagnosis of superficial spreading melanoma is Paget disease. Cells of Paget disease tend to be larger and form clusters with occasional gland formation. VIN and squamous cell carcinoma may clinically mimic melanoma, especially if they are darkly pigmented.

Immunohistochemically, melanoma cells are positive for S-100 protein, HMB45 and Melan A, whereas Paget cells and squamous epithelial cells are negative for these markers. Conversely, Paget cells are positive for mucicarmine, PAS, CEA and/or cytokeratins, which are negative in melanoma.

For staging of vulvar melanoma, a modified Clark classification is applied, as proposed by the American College of Obstetricians and Gynecologists (ACOG) (Fig. 10):

Level I — Melanoma *in situ*.
Level II — Melanoma extends into superficial papillary dermis.

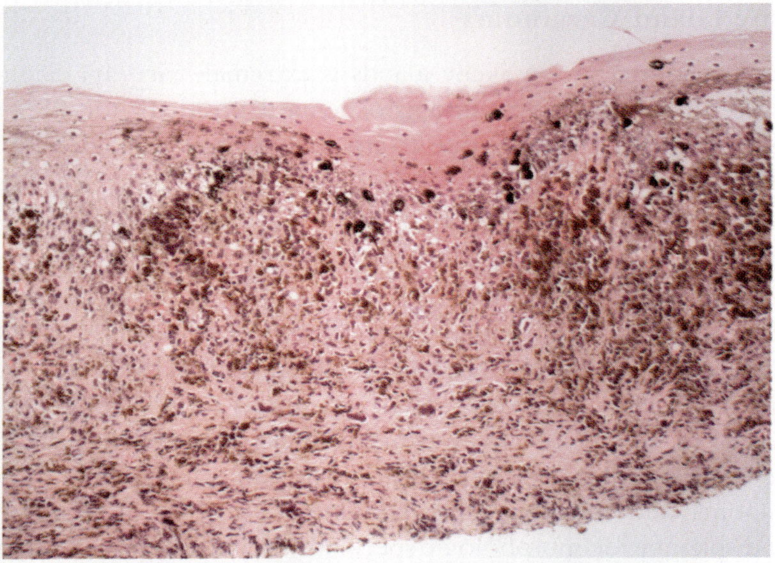

Fig. 9 Malignant melanoma. Tumor cells are present within the epidermis and dermis. There is abundant melanin production. Hematoxylin/eosin, original magnification 100×.

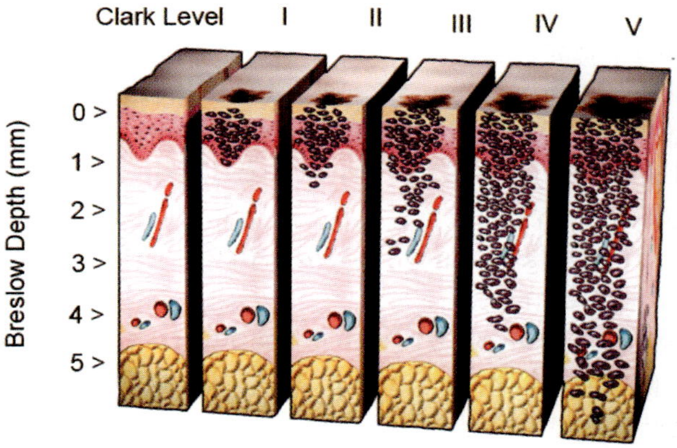

Fig. 10 Staging of malignant melanoma. In the Clark classification, levels are defined by the tissue layers involved. The Breslow system measures tumor thickness in mm from the lower border of the granular cell layer. Modified from http://www.med-ars.it. Illustration by Davide Brunelli, MD, with kind permission.

Level III — Melanoma fills and expands the papillary dermis.
Level IV — Melanoma extends into the reticular dermis.
Level V — Melanoma invades into fat or other subjacent tissues.

In addition, tumor thickness is correlated with prognosis. The Breslow system proposes measurement from the deep border of the granular layer to the deepest point of invasion. Lesions with a thickness of 0.75 mm or less have an excellent prognosis in that they virtually never metastasize or recur if completely excised.

Mesenchymal Tumors

Mesenchymal tumors of the vulva are generally rare, the most frequent entity being the benign leiomyoma. Not much is known about the pathogenesis and early stages of mesenchymal malignancies, and clinical management will be determined on a case by case basis. When faced with a spindle cell lesion of the vulva, the spindle cell variant of a squamous cell carcinoma should always be borne in mind, which can easily be confirmed due to its immunohistochemical positivity for cytokeratins. The following entities are somewhat specific to the vulva, or are frequently within the differential diagnosis of vulvar lesions.

Embryonal rhabdomyosarcoma typically is a tumor of infancy, although rare cases have been reported in young adults. It occurs more frequently in the vagina, and when both vulva and vagina are involved, it should be diagnosed as a primary vaginal tumor. The tumor presents as a fleshy, dark colored grape like mass that may ulcerate and bleed. Histologically, it is characterized by a proliferation of immature round to spindle shaped malignant cells. Cross striation may not be seen in all cases and is not required for the diagnosis. Cells are separated by a loose myxoid intercellular matrix. The most frequent subtype, sarcoma botryoides, is distinguished by the presence of a condensed layer of rhabdomyoblasts (cambium layer) underneath an epithelial surface.

Immunohistochemical markers for muscle differentiation (myoglobin, desmin, actin) as well as electron microscopy may be helpful to support the diagnosis. Surgery or radiotherapy, in combination with chemotherapy, is very efficient, and disease-free survival rates exceed 70% at five years.[36]

Dermatofibrosarcoma protuberans (DFSP) is a locally aggressive tumor, usually occurring in adults at a median age of 54 years. The tumor arises in the dermis and is thought to be of fibrohistiocytic origin. Microscopically, it is composed of spindle cells arranged in a "storiform" pattern of radial whorls. The lesion is highly cellular, and entrapped adipocytes indicate infiltration of the underlying adipose tissue. Cytologically, cells are monomorphic and exhibit a moderate mitotic activity. The tumor tends to recur if not completely excised, but distant metastases are very rare. Tumor cells are positive for CD34, which is useful for confirmation of the diagnosis.

Aggressive angiomyxoma is typically seen in adult women younger than 40 years of age. It may arise in the vulva or in the pelvis, extending to the vulva. It presents as a subcutaneous mass, and if present in the posterior part of the labia majora, it may be clinically mistaken for a Bartholin gland cyst. Histologically, the tumor is composed of bland appearing spindle cells with low mitotic activity and abundant intercellular myxoid material, which gives the lesion a rather hypocellular appearance. A characteristic feature is the presence of clustered thick-walled muscular vessels (Fig. 11). Entrapped adipocytes or nerves reflect the locally invasive nature of the tumor. The spindle cells are positive for desmin, smooth muscle actin and muscle specific actin, but negative for S-100. CD34 is expressed in approximately 50% of cases. Aggressive angiomyxoma may recur locally, but distant metastases are extremely rare.[37]

Rearrangements of the high mobility group gene *HMGA2*, which encodes a non-histone chromatin associated protein that is thought to play a role during transcription, have been reported in about one-third of aggressive angiomyxomas.[38] Similar alterations of the same gene are found in a variety of other benign mesenchymal tumors, including uterine leiomyomas, but not in angiomyofibroblastomas.

In the differential diagnosis, the most important entity is angiomyofibroblastoma. This is a well circumscribed benign tumor, composed of more epithelioid appearing cells with perivascular hypercellularity

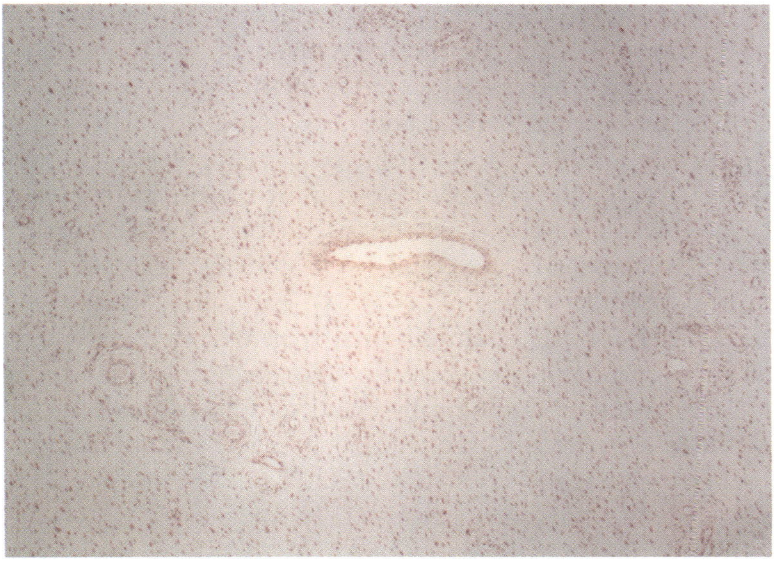

Fig. 11 Aggressive angiomyxoma. The lesion is composed of bland appearing spindle shaped cells with abundant myxoid intercellular substance. Numerous vessels are present, some of them are thick walled. Hematoxylin/eosin, original magnification 40×.

and occasional multinucleation. It may have myxoid areas, but lacks thick walled vessels. Angiomyofibroblastoma tends to be positive for vimentin and desmin, but negative for actin. Myxoid malignant fibrous histiocytoma (myxofibrosarcoma) usually shows areas of higher cellularity displaying the typical "storiform" architecture. Marked cytologic atypia and mitotic activity including atypical mitotic figures are present at least focally. It may be immunoreactive for α1-antitrypsin and α1-antichymotrypsin. Myxoid neurofibroma diffusely expresses S-100. Myxoid leiomyoma lacks a prominent vascular pattern and is composed of myocytes with cigar-shaped nuclei that tend to be arranged in fascicles.

Also to be considered in the differential diagnosis of aggressive angiomyxoma is a peculiar tumor that may present as a unilateral labial swelling in prepubertal girls and has been variably termed "prepubertal vulval fibroma", "childhood asymmetrical labium majus enlargement (CALME)" or "prepubertal fibrous hyperplasia of the labium majus."[39–41] Although a benign tumor, it is discussed here within the differential diagnosis of malignant entities, with which it shares certain clinical and histologic features. It is rare in absolute case numbers and has only been recognized recently as a distinctive entity. However, it may comprise more than 20% of all pediatric vulvar soft tissue masses. It can be associated with *peau d'orange* changes of the overlying skin and may extend to pelvic structures on radiologic images. It is both macroscopically and microscopically poorly circumscribed, such that it may be difficult or impossible to completely resect it. Histologically, it is hypocellular and composed of cytologically bland spindle-shaped cells, growing without a particular architectural pattern, and surrounded by collagenous or edematous stroma (Fig. 12). The mitotic index is less than one mitotic figure per 10 HPF. Fat, nerves, vessels or skin adnexal structures may be entrapped in the lesion. Spindle cells are positive for CD34 in the majority of cases, but negative for muscle and neural markers. Despite its infiltrative growth pattern, the tumor appears to behave in a benign fashion, although recurrences have been observed after incomplete resection. Conservative surgery with an emphasis on cosmetically acceptable results is recommended. No metastatic disease has been reported. Clinically, the differential diagnosis includes lipoma, hemangioma and lymphangioma, furthermore embryonal rhabdomyosarcoma due to its similar age and site specificity. Histologically, the prepubertal fibrous lesion shares similarities with aggressive angiomyxoma and angiomyofibroblastoma. However, the latter two entities usually occur in adult women and are positive for desmin. In addition, angiomyofibroblastoma is well demarcated.

Although not specific to the vulva, a wide variety of other soft tissue tumors have been reported to occur there, including leiomyosarcoma; malignant fibrous histiocytoma; epithelioid sarcoma; malignant rhabdoid tumor; angiosarcoma; lymphangiosarcoma; angiomyofibrosarcoma; hemangiopericytoma; Kaposi sarcoma; alveolar soft part sarcoma; malignant schwannoma; malignant granular cell tumor; liposarcoma; and eosinophilic granuloma. For more detailed information

(a)

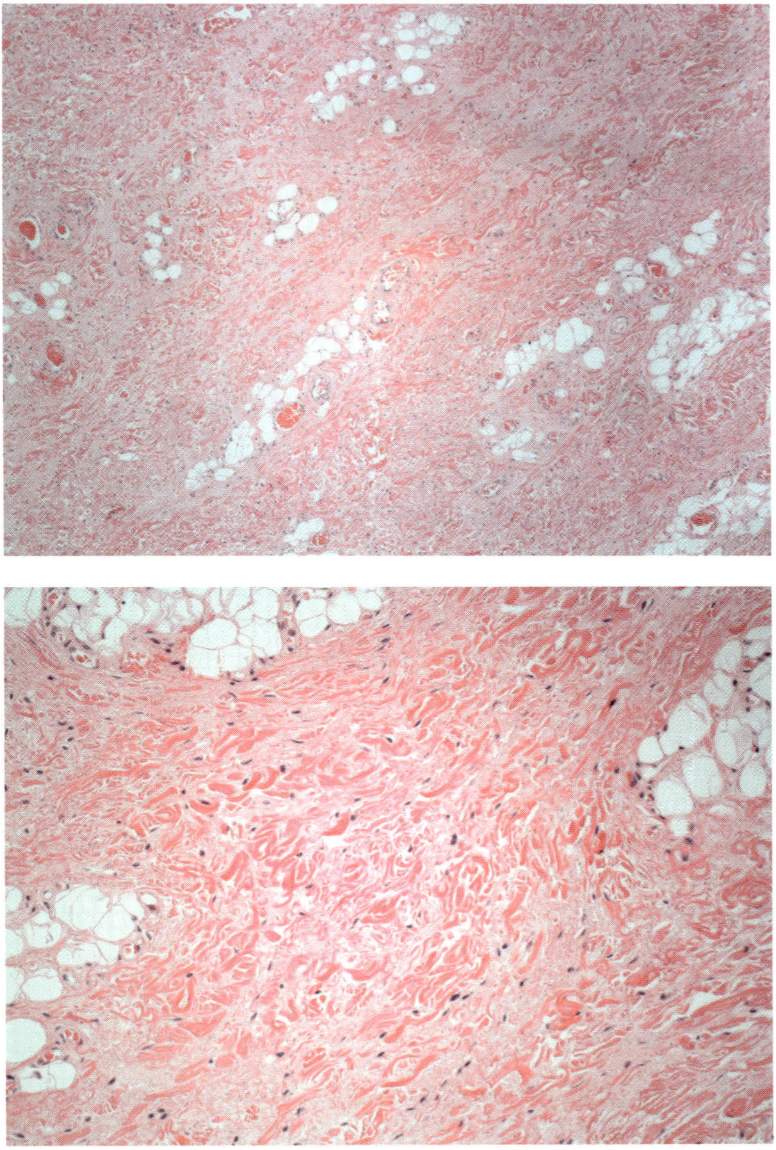

(b)

Fig. 12 Prepubertal vulval fibrous hyperplasia. (a) The lesion is composed of fibroblasts and collagen bundles. Entrapped adipocytes reflect the invasive nature of the lesion. Hematoxylin/eosin, original magnification 40×. (b) Higher magnification shows thick collagen bundles. Hematoxylin/eosin, original magnification 100×.

on these entities the reader is referred to textbooks of soft tissue pathology or review articles.

Other Malignant Tumors of the Vulva

Urethral carcinoma is rare and occurs mostly in elderly women. It tends to arise in the distal urethra or within diverticula and may present with bleeding and dysuria. Squamous cell carcinoma is the most frequent histologic type, followed by transitional cell carcinoma. The latter may be associated with pagetoid urothelial intraepithelial neoplasia (PUIN, type 3 Paget disease). Urethral adenocarcinomas have been subclassified into mucinous, clear cell or colloid types. For staging of urethral carcinoma, see Table 3.

Other malignancies that have been reported as primary vulvar tumors include yolk sac tumor (endodermal sinus tumor), malignant lymphoma, and Merkel cell tumor. Since these entities are extremely rare on the vulva, no experience has been accumulated as to their early detection. They display the same morphologic and immunophenotypic characteristics as in other sites. Once thought of in the differential diagnosis, they can be correctly identified by appropriate ancillary studies.

Accounting for about 8% of all vulvar neoplasms, metastatic tumors to the vulva are not infrequent. In the majority of cases, there is a primary malignancy of the genitourinary tract, squamous cell carcinoma of the uterine cervix being the most frequent. A metastatic tumor to the vulva always implies late stage disease, portends a poor prognosis and is generally treated palliatively.

Ancillary Studies

In the context of diagnosing early stage malignancies of the vulva and their precursor lesions, ancillary studies will be most useful in one of three scenarios: (1) Identification of HPV related lesions and differentiation from benign mimickers; (2) identification of very early and superficial stromal invasion; (3) the work-up of Paget disease, its subtypes and differential diagnosis. Additional applications are rather

Table 3. Staging of Urethral Carcinoma as Suggested by the AJCC[27]

TNM category	Definition
	Primary Tumor (T)
TX	Primary tumor cannot be assessed
T0	No evidence of primary tumor
Ta	Non-invasive papillary, polypoid or verrucous carcinoma
Tis	Carcinoma *in situ*
T1	Tumor invades subepithelial connective tissue
T2	Tumor invades corpus spongiosum or prostate periurethral muscle
T3	Tumor invades anterior vagina or bladder neck
T4	Tumor invades other adjacent organs
	Regional Lymph Nodes (N)
NX	Regional lymph nodes cannot be assessed
N0	No regional lymph node metastasis
N1	Metastasis in a single lymph node, 2 cm or less in diameter
N2	Metastasis in a single lymph node more than 2 cm in greatest dimension, or in multiple nodes
	Distant Metastasis (M)
MX	Distant metastasis cannot be assessed
M0	No distant metastasis
M1	Distant metastasis present

Legend: Regional lymph nodes are the inguinal (superficial or deep), iliac (common, internal [hypogastric], obturator, external), presacral, sacral, and pelvic lymph nodes.

rare, except for the occasional metastatic tumor with an unknown primary.

Identification of HPV associated lesions

The most useful immunohistochemical markers to support the diagnosis of an HPV associated lesion are Ki-67 and p16^{Ink4a}. The Ki-67 antigen (recognized by the MIB-1 antibody) is expressed in the nuclei of proliferating cells during all phases of the cell cycle except G0. It is physiologically present in parabasal cells (while basal cells are usually negative!) of the vulvar squamous epithelium, which serve as a convenient internal control. Positivity for Ki-67 in the upper two thirds of the epithelium has been shown to correlate with HPV-infection.[42] Note that although Ki-67 expression will be stronger and more diffuse in high grade lesions, positivity can be seen in the upper layers of the epithelium even in low grade lesions. Therefore, the Ki-67 reactivity can be used to differentiate HPV-associated lesions from non-HPV related changes, but is less helpful for the grading of VIN. Lymphocytes are frequently positive for Ki-67 and may lead to false positive interpretation, especially in heavily inflamed epithelia. Similarly, parabasal cells that appear to be located in higher epithelial layers due to tangential sectioning in suboptimally oriented biopsy specimens, or in the vicinity of stromal papillae extending towards the surface, should not be overinterpreted. Since koilocytotic changes on the vulva tend to be more subtle than on the uterine cervix, a Ki-67 stain can be very helpful to correctly identify a condyloma acuminatum and differentiate it from non-HPV related mimickers, e.g. fibroepithelial polyp, squamous papilloma or micropapillomatosis labialis. Dysplastic lesions of the vulva are usually characterized by mitotic activity beyond the parabasal cell layer, in which case a Ki-67 stain does not add much information. It is, however, very valuable when VIN is suspected in the absence of mitotic figures.

P16, also known as *inhibitor of cyclin dependent kinase 4a* (INK4a), is a tumor suppressor protein that inhibits cell cycle progression at the G1-S interphase. It is regulated by the expression status of the retinoblastoma tumor suppressor protein. Because the E7 protein of high risk HPV types inactivates the retinoblastoma protein, p16 expression is upregulated and seen in nuclei and cytoplasm of infected cells. Thus, although p16 positivity is not specifically associated with an HPV infection, in the correct clinical setting, it is interpreted as a surrogate marker for the presence of high risk HPV types. P16 is strongly and diffusely positive in the basaloid and warty types of VIN (Fig. 13), but not in the HPV-unrelated differentiated (simplex) form of VIN, and not in verrucous carcinoma.[43] On the other hand, p16 is expressed in the subset of vulvar low-grade lesions, which is caused by high-risk HPV type infection. For unknown reasons, p16 positivity is also

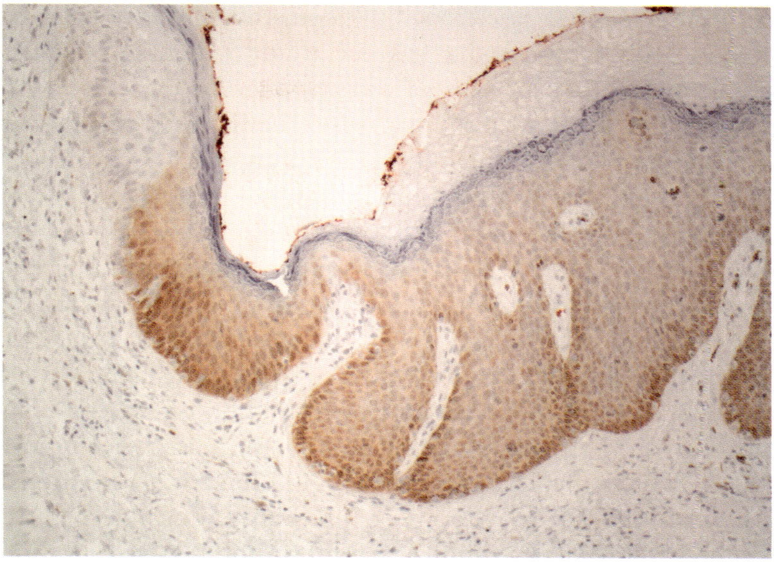

Fig. 13 p16 expression in basaloid VIN. Diffuse cytoplasmic and nuclear positivity in the dysplastic epithelium. Note the small portion of non-dysplastic epithelium in the upper left corner which is negative for p16. Original magnification 100×.

seen in 60% of basal cell carcinomas, and in the malignant cells of Paget disease.[43]

Direct identification of HPV particles within the tissue is possible but less practical. The gold standard would be to extract DNA from the tissue and PCR-amplify HPV type-specific sequences. This, however, is too costly and labor intensive for routine purposes. *In situ* hybridization for specific HPV types or groups of HPV types can be done on tissue sections, but this method is fraught with low sensitivity.

Identification of superficial stromal invasion

The correct identification of early stromal invasion obviously has significant impact on patient prognosis and clinical management. While on most other sites of the skin it may be practical, in case of doubt, to simply excise widely a questionable lesion, the vulva poses particular challenges: vulvar carcinoma has metastatic potential even if not deeply invasive; wide margins of excision may be difficult to obtain because of important adjacent structures, i.e. urethra or clitoris; and surgical treatment may include inguinal lymph node dissection. Therefore, the distinction between *in situ* and invasive disease is particularly critical on the vulva. In cases of questionable very superficial stromal invasion, the visualization of the basement membrane using antibodies against collagen type IV or laminin can be useful. While the basement membrane is interrupted in areas of recent or active invasion, some foci of clearly invasive or even metastatic tumor may be secondarily surrounded by basement membrane material. This is consistent with the theory that invasion happens in cycles of growth surges, in which the basement membrane is actively destroyed by tumor cells, followed by periods of quiescence, during which reformation of basement membrane material may occur, especially in well differentiated tumors. Hence, the finding of an interrupted basement membrane supports the diagnosis of an invasive process, whereas the presence of basement membrane material surrounding tumor cell nests does not rule out invasive disease. To highlight epithelial cells breaking through the basement membrane, double immunostaining for cytokeratin and basement membrane components has been proposed (Fig. 14). This may further enhance diagnostic accuracy, especially in cases where the dermoepidermal interface at the site of questionable invasion is obscured by a heavy inflammatory infiltrate.[44]

Paget disease and its differential diagnosis

The mucin containing cells of Paget disease types 1 and 2 can be demonstrated on mucicarmine, PAS (diastase resistant) and Alcian blue stains. In the majority of cases, one of these will be the single most important special stain to support the diagnosis of Paget disease. To rule out the possibility of a superficially spreading malignant melanoma, a melanocytic marker (S-100, HMB-45 or Melan-A) should be included in the panel. A lymphocytic marker (LCA) will help to identify mycosis fungoides.

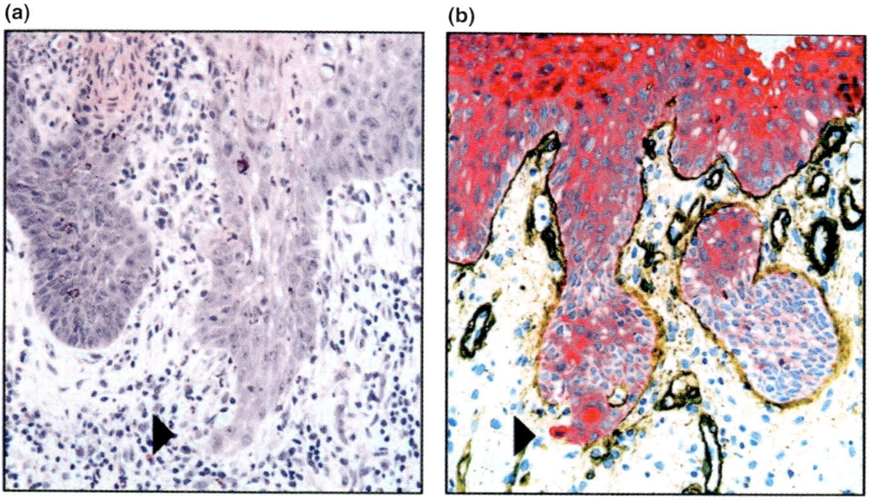

Fig. 14 VIN with focus of early invasion. (a) Hematoxylin/eosin, orginal magnification 200×. (b) Double immunostain for cytokeratin (red) and collagen IV (dark brown), orignal magnification 200×. Arrowheads indicate areas of early invasion. Note defect in the continuity of the basement membrane. Reprinted with permission from *Archives of Pathology & Laboratory Medicine*. Copyright 2005. College of American Pathologists.

To further classify the subtype of Paget disease, CK7 and CK20 are most useful: type 1 is typically positive for CK7 and in 85% of cases, negative for CK20, while the reverse is true for type 2. Positivity for CDX-2 appears to be specific for type 2 Paget disease, although experience with this intestinal marker is still limited. PUIN is positive for CK7, and frequently coexpresses CK20 and/or uroplakin III.

GCDFP-15 tends to be positive in type 1 Paget disease. This protein is also expressed in up to 50% of metastatic breast carcinomas, as well as in sweat gland and salivary gland carcinomas. Positivity is meaningful even if very focal and weak, which is often the case. CK8 (CAM5.2) is expressed in type 1 Paget cells, and similar to CK7, the surrounding squamous epithelium is negative for these markers. Along with mucin stains, CK7 and/or CK8 are useful tools not only to diagnose the disease but also to assess surgical resection margins or potential stromal invasion. Pagetoid VIN is positive for pan-cytokeratins

(AE1/AE3), but usually negative for CK7 and CK8, although rare CK7 positive cases have been reported. CEA positivity can be seen in all three types of Paget disease, including the majority of PUIN cases.

Immunohistochemical positivity for p53 or fatty acid synthase in intraepithelial Paget cells suggests that there may be an invasive component and should prompt careful examination of the specimen to rule out invasion.[33,34] A summary of markers and their expression patterns that may be useful in the work-up of Paget disease and lesions in the differential diagnosis is provided in Table 2.

Metastatic tumors

Extensive discussion of metastatic tumors to the vulva is beyond the scope of this chapter. Most frequently, the primary tumor is located in the genitourinary tract. If ancillary studies are needed to determine the likely site of a primary tumor, it may be more cost effective to perform selected special stains in two or more successive rounds rather than a large battery of immunostains at once. For example, the first round may include few markers to determine the cell lineage (e.g. pan-CK for epithelial cells, vimentin for mesenchymal cells, S-100 as a melanocytic marker, and LCA as a lymphocytic marker), followed by a panel of markers for more specific differentiation analysis, depending on the results from the first round. Note that vimentin is not specific for mesenchymal cells, but is frequently coexpressed in endometrial endometrioid carcinoma, serous ovarian tumors, renal cell carcinoma (but not clear cell carcinoma of Müllerian origin!), and papillary thyroid carcinoma. Likewise, occasional melanocytic, mesenchymal (endometrial stroma) and lymphoid cells may be reactive for pan-CK.

Additional special stains that may be helpful in the diagnosis of early vulvar neoplasms include the following: the D2-40 antibody is directed against podoplanin, a membrane protein of lymphatic endothelium. It can be used to identify lymphvascular space invasion by various tumors and rule out tissue retraction artifact.

Overexpression of p53 has been reported in the basal and parabasal keratinocytes of differentiated (simplex) VIN, and may be helpful to support that diagnosis. Of note, p53 positivity can also be seen in lichen sclerosus, in which case this is thought to be a reactive change rather than a marker of premalignancy.[12,45]

REFERENCES

1. Prowse DM, Ktori EN, Chandrasekaran D, Prapa A, *et al.*, Human papillomavirus-associated increase in p16(INK4A) expression in penile lichen sclerosus and squamous cell carcinoma, *Br J Dermatol* **158**: 261–265, 2008.
2. Tapp RA, Feng J, Jones JW, *et al.*, Single base instability is promoted in vulvar lichen sclerosus, *J Invest Dermatol* **127**:2563–2576, 2007.
3. Carlson JA, Ambros R, Malfetano J, *et al.*, Vulvar lichen sclerosus and squamous cell carcinoma: a cohort, case control and investigational study with historical perspective; implications for chronic inflammation and sclerosis in the development of neoplasia, *Hum Pathol* **29**:932–948, 1998.
4. Carlson JA, Lamb P, Malfetano J, *et al.*, Clinicopathologic comparison of vulvar and extragenital lichen sclerosus: histologic variants, evolving lesions, and etiology of 141 cases, *Mod Pathol* **11**:844–854, 1998.
5. Raspollini MR, Asirelli G, Moncini D, *et al.*, A comparative analysis of lichen sclerosus of the vulva and lichen sclerosus that evolves to vulvar squamous cell carcinoma, *Am J Obstet Gynecol* **197**: 592.e1–592.e5, 2007.
6. Nordenvall C, Chang ET, Adami HO, *et al.*, Cancer risk among patients with condylomata acuminate, *Int J Cancer* **119**:888–893, 2006.
7. Traiman P, Bacchi CE, De Luca LA, *et al.*, Vulvar carcinoma in young patients and its relationship with genital warts, *Eur J Gynaecol Oncol* **20**:191–194, 1999.
8. Downey GO, Okagaki T, Ostrow RS, *et al.*, Condylomatous carcinoma of the vulva with special reference to human papillomavirus DNA, *Obstet Gynecol* **72**:68–73, 1988.
9. Judson PL, Habermann EB, Baxter NN, *et al.*, Trends in the incidence of invasive and *in situ* vulvar carcinoma, *Obstet Gynecol* **107**:1018–1022, 2006.
10. van Seters M, ten Kate FJ, van Beurden M, *et al.*, In the absence of (early) invasive carcinoma, vulvar intraepithelial neoplasia associated with lichen sclerosus is mainly of undifferentiated type: new insights in histology and aetiology, *J Clin Pathol* **60**:504–509, 2007.

11. Chiesa-Vottero A, Dvoretsky PM, *et al.*, Histopathologic study of thin vulvar squamous cell carcinomas and associated cutaneous lesions: a correlative study of 48 tumors in 44 patients with analysis of adjacent vulvar intraepithelial neoplasia types and lichen sclerosus, *Am J Surg Pathol* **30**:310–318, 2006.
12. Yang B, Hart WR, Vulvar intraepithelial neoplasia of the simplex (differentiated) type: a clinicopathologic study including analysis of HPV and p53 expression, *Am J Surg Pathol* **24**:429–441, 2000.
13. van der Avoort IA, van der Laak JA, Paffen A, *et al.*, MIB1 expression in basal cell layer: a diagnostic tool to identify premalignancies of the vulva, *Mod Pathol* **20**:770–778, 2007.
14. Rolfe KJ, Eva LJ, MacLean AB, *et al.*, Cell cycle proteins as molecular markers of malignant change in vulvar lichen sclerosus, *Int J Gynecol Cancer* **11**:113–118, 2001.
15. Sideri M, Jones RW, Wilkinson EJ, *et al.*, Squamous vulvar intraepithelial neoplasia: 2004 modified terminology, ISSVD vulvar oncology subcommittee, *J Reprod Med* **50**:807–810, 2005.
16. Srodon M, Stoler MH, Baber GB, *et al.*, The distribution of low and high-risk HPV types in vulvar and vaginal intraepithelial neoplasia (VIN and VaIN), *Am J Surg Pathol* **30**:1513–1518, 2006.
17. Skapa P, Zamecnik J, Hamsikova E, *et al.*, Human papillomavirus (HPV) profiles of vulvar lesion: possible implications for the classification of vulvar squamous cell carcinoma precursors and for the efficacy of prophylactic HPV vaccination, *Am J Surg Pathol* **31**:1834–1843, 2007.
18. Jones RW, Rowan DM, Stewart AW, Vulvar intraepithelial neoplasia: aspects of the natural history and outcome in 405 women, *Obstet Gynecol* **106**:1319–1326, 2005.
19. Bae-Jump VL, Bauer M, Van Le L, Cytological evaluation correlates poorly with histological diagnosis of vulvar neoplasias, *J Low Genit Tract Dis* **11**:8–11, 2007.
20. Hillemanns P, Wang X, Integration of HPV-16 and HPV-18 DNA in vulvar intraepithelial neoplasia, *Gynecol Oncol* **100**:276–282, 2006.
21. Brustmann H, Galectin-3 and CD1a-positive dendritic cells are involved in the development of an invasive phenotype in vulvar squamous lesions, *Int J Gynecol Pathol* **25**:30–37, 2006.
22. Taube JM, Nichols AD, Bornman LS, *et al.*, Langerhans cell density and high-grade vulvar intraepithelial neoplasia in women with human immunodeficiency virus infection, *J Cutan Pathol* **34**:565–570, 2007.

23. Hantschmann P, Sterzer S, Jeschke U, *et al.*, P53 expression in vulvar carcinoma, vulvar intraepithelial neoplasia, squamous cell hyperplasia and lichen sclerosus, *Anticancer Res* **25**:1739–1745, 2005.
24. Holway AH, Rieger-Christ KM, Miner WR, *et al.*, Somatic mutation of PTEN in vulvar cancer, *Clin Cancer Res* **6**:3228–3235, 2000.
25. Nascimento AF, Granter SR, Cviko A, *et al.*, Vulvar acanthosis with altered differentiation: a precursor to verrucous carcinoma? *Am J Surg Pathol* **28**:638–643, 2004.
26. Benedet JL, Bender H, Jones H, *et al.*, FIGO staging classifications and clinical practice guidelines in the management of gynecologic cancers. FIGO committee on gynecologic oncology, *Int J Gynaecol Obstet* **70**:209–262, 2000.
27. Greene FL, Page DL, Fleming ID, *et al.*, *AJCC Cancer Staging Manual*, 6th edn., Springer Verlag, New York, 2002.
28. Beller U, Quinn MA, Benedet JL, *et al.*, Carcinoma of the vulva. FIGO 6th annual report on the results of treatment in gynecological cancer, *Int J Gynaecol Obstet* **95** (Suppl 1):S7–S27, 2006.
29. Willman JH, Golitz LE, Fitzpatrick JE, Vulvar clear cells of toker: precursors of extramammary Pagets' disease, *Am J Dermatopathol* **27**: 185–188, 2005.
30. Belousova IE, Kazakov DV, Michal M, *et al.*, Vulvar toker cells: the long-awaited missing link: a proposal for an origin-based histogenetic classification of extramammary Paget disease, *Am J Dermatopathol* **28**: 84–86, 2006.
31. De Nisi MC, D' Amuri A, Toscano M, *et al.*, Usefulness of CDX2 in the diagnosis of extramammary Paget disease associated with malignancies of intestinal type, *Br J Dermatol* **153**:677–679, 2005.
32. Zeng HA, Cartun R, Ricci A, Potential diagnostic utility of CDX-2 immunophenotyping in extramammary Pagets' disease, *Appl Immunohistochem Mol Morphol* **13**:342–346, 2005.
33. Zhang C, Zhang P, Sung CJ, *et al.*, Overexpression of p53 is correlated with stromal invasion in extramammary Pagets' disease of the vulva, *Hum Pathol* **34**:880–885, 2003.
34. Alo PL, Galati GM, Sebastiani V, *et al.*, Fatty acid synthase expression in Paget's disease of the vulva, *Int J Gynecol Pathol* **24**:404–408, 2005.
35. Crawford D, Nimmo M, Clement PB, *et al.*, Prognostic factors in Pagets' disease of the vulva: a study of 21 cases, *Int J Gynecol Pathol* **18**:351–359, 1999.

36. Martelli H, Oberlin O, Rey A, *et al.*, Conservative treatment for girls with nonmetastatic rhabdomyosarcoma of the genital tract: a report from the study committee of the international society of pediatric oncology, *J Clin Oncol* **17**:2117–2122, 1999.
37. Blandamura S, Cruz J, Faure VL, *et al.*, Aggressive angiomyxoma: a second case of metastasis with patient's death, *Hum Pathol* **34**:1072–1074, 2003.
38. Medeiros F, Erickson-Johnson MR, Keeney GL, *et al.*, Frequency and characterization of HMGA2 and HMGA1 rearrangements in mesenchymal tumors of the lower genital tract, *Genes Chromosomes Cancer* **46**:981–990, 2007.
39. Iwasa Y, Fletcher CD, Distinctive prepubertal vulval fibroma: a hitherto unrecognized mesenchymal tumor of prepubertal girls: analysis of 11 cases, *Am J Surg Pathol* **28**:1601–1608, 2004.
40. Vargas SO, Kozakewich HP, Boyd TK, *et al.*, Childhood asymmetric labium majus enlargement: mimicking a neoplasm, *Am J Surg Pathol* **29**:1007–1016, 2005.
41. Altchek A, Deligdisch L, Norton K, *et al.*, Prepubertal unilateral fibrous hyperplasia of the labium majus: report of eight cases and review of the literature, *Obstet Gynecol* **110**:103–108, 2007.
42. Pirog EC, Chen YT, Isacson C, MIB-1 immunostaining is a beneficial adjunct test for accurate diagnosis of vulvar condyloma acuminatum, *Am J Surg Pathol* **24**:1393–1399, 2000.
43. Santos M, Montagut C, Mellado B, *et al.*, Immunohistochemical staining for p16 and p53 in premalignant and malignant epithelial lesions of the vulva, *Int J Gynecol Pathol* **23**:206–214, 2004.
44. Rush D, Hyjek E, Baergen RN, *et al.*, Detection of microinvasion in vulvar and cervical intraepithelial neoplasia using double immunostaining for cytokeratin and basement membrane components, *Arch Pathol Lab Med* **129**:747–753, 2005.
45. Liegl B, Regauer S, p53 immunostaining in lichen sclerosus is related to ischaemic stress and is not a marker of differentiated vulvar intraepithelial neoplasia (d-VIN), *Histopathology* **48**:268–274, 2006.

CHAPTER 2

EARLY DIAGNOSIS OF CERVICAL AND VAGINAL CANCER

Peter Schlosshauer

INTRODUCTION

Cervical cancer continues to be a major health problem and a leading cause of cancer mortality in females worldwide. In developed countries, where efficient cancer screening programs are in effect, we have witnessed a dramatic decrease in the incidence of invasive cervical squamous cell carcinoma over the past decades. Consequently, the clinical focus has shifted to the diagnosis and treatment of precursor lesions and early stage invasive carcinomas. For unknown reasons, during the same time the incidence of cervical adenocarcinoma has increased in both absolute and relative numbers. This chapter reviews our current approach to the diagnosis of cervical cancer with an emphasis on precursor lesions and early stage invasive disease. In this context, numerous clinical and morphologic "look-alikes" will be discussed, along with ancillary studies that are used to resolve diagnostic problems. Also included is a summary of the etiology and pathogenesis, the role of human papilloma virus (HPV), and an update on the recently introduced HPV vaccines.

The single most effective tool to identify malignant and premalignant cervical lesions continues to be the cytologic evaluation of exfoliated cells ("Pap smear"), which will be discussed in chapter 7.

Malignant tumors of the vagina are rare, and most of them share epidemiologic, etiopathogenetic and pathologic features with their respective cervical counterparts. Therefore, this chapter covers tumors of both cervix and vagina; entities specific to the vagina are discussed in a designated paragraph.

NORMAL ANATOMY, HISTOLOGY AND PHYSIOLOGIC CHANGES

The vagina extends from the hymenal ring at the introitus to the uterine cervix. It is lined by a non-keratinizing stratified squamous epithelium. The collapsed lumen has a roughly H-shaped cross section. Transversely oriented mucosal folds (rugae) allow for considerable distension of the lumen, as necessary during parturition. At its superior end, the uterine cervix protrudes into the vagina, separating the vaginal vault into the anterior and posterior fornix. The normally developed vaginal wall does not contain glandular structures. Lubrification is achieved through transudation. Rarely encountered foci of endocervical-type glandular epithelium, either on the vaginal surface or as intramucosal inclusions, are referred to as *vaginal adenosis* and result from a defect during the epithelialization of the vaginal lumen. Occasionally, the lateral vaginal wall contains remnants of the mesonephric duct, which can give rise to Gartner duct cysts. The vaginal lamina propria is composed of connective tissue that frequently contains fibroblasts with multiple and/or bizarre-shaped nuclei, known as "floret cells". These can also occur in the cervical stroma and are entirely benign. The muscular cuff of the vagina consists of portions of the pelvic floor musculature, i.e. the levator ani muscle, deep transverse perineal and bulbocavernous muscles. The urinary bladder is attached to the anterior wall of the vagina and the uterine cervix through a layer of loose connective tissue. The urethra runs parallel and anterior to the lower third of the vagina. Posteriorly, the fibroconnective plate of the rectovaginal septum separates the vagina from the rectum. This rectovaginal septum ends just below the posterior fornix, the rear surface of which forms part of the recto-uterine pouch (pouch of Douglas, cul-de-sac). The blood supply of the vagina is provided by branches of the internal iliac vessels. The lymph vessels of the superior anterior portion of the vagina and the vaginal vault join those of the cervix and drain to the external iliac nodes, while lymph fluid from the inferior anterior vaginal wall is drained to the femoral lymph nodes. Lymph from the posterior vaginal wall is directed to the inferior gluteal, sacral and anorectal lymph nodes.

The uterine cervix is the lower portion of the uterus, inferior to the uterine isthmus. Its dense fibromuscular stroma surrounds the centrally located endocervical canal, which connects the vaginal lumen with the endometrial cavity. The *portio* (*vaginalis*) is that part of the cervix that protrudes into the vaginal vault. Its surface, the ecto (or exo-) cervix, is covered by non-keratinizing stratified squamous epithelium, which is histologically indistinguishable from that of the vagina. Within this epithelium, four cell layers can be distinguished. The cuboidal basal cells form a single cell layer adjacent to the basement membrane. Overlying the basal cells are one to three layers of parabasal cells. These are mitotically active and provide the cells necessary for the constant regeneration of the epithelium. Consequently, parabasal cells are physiologically positive for proliferation markers like MIB-1 (Ki-67). The intermediate cell layer contains maturing squamous cells with polygonal cytoplasm, round to oval nuclei and numerous intercellular “bridges”, corresponding to desmosomes. Normal intermediate cells are not mitotically active. They assume a more horizontal orientation as they move closer to the surface. During reproductive life and under the influence of estrogen they accumulate cytoplasmic glycogen. The superficial cell layer is composed of very flat, horizontally oriented squamous cells with pyknotic nuclei. At the end of their life cycle, the superficial cells are shed into the vaginal lumen. The turnaround time for cells that enter the maturation process is four to five days.

The endocervical canal extends from its external os in the center of the ectocervix to the internal os at the junction with the endometrial cavity. In nulliparous women, the external os is round, while in parous women it forms a horizontally oriented slit, which divides the ectocervix into an anterior and a posterior lip. On gross inspection the surface of the endocervical canal often shows obliquely oriented folds ("herringbone" pattern). Between these folds there are clefts and infoldings that may extend 5 mm–7 mm into the cervical stroma. The surface of the endocervical canal is lined by a single cell layer of tall columnar mucinous glandular epithelium. Nuclei are located close to the basement membrane. Mitotic figures are rare in normal mature endocervical epithelium. The so-called "endocervical glands" visible on tissue sections are not true glands, because there are no encapsulated glandular structures, no lobules and no ducts. Instead, the "endocervical glands" are the result of the complex infoldings of the endocervcial surface.

The endocervical glandular epithelium meets the ectocervical squamous epithelium at the squamocolumnar junction (SCJ). This is where the vast majority of HPV-associated cervical lesions arise. In the newborn baby girl, the *original* SCJ is located at the external os of the endocervical canal. Growth of the cervix during puberty leads to an eversion of endocervical epithelium onto the ectocervical surface. Induced by the increasingly acidic vaginal milieu, the everted glandular epithelium is then replaced by squamous epithelium — a process known as squamous metaplasia. After successful completion of this process, the new *functional* SCJ is ideally located again at the ectocervical os. The area between the original and the functional SCJ is called the transformation zone. During reproductive life, the SCJ may move to a variable extent on the surface of the endo- and ectocervix. As a result, glandular epithelium may cover parts of the ectocervix, which is visible on inspection and known as "ectopy" or "ectropion". The term "erosion" is a misnomer for this condition, because the epithelial lining is actually intact. After menopause, the squamocolumnar junction moves back into the endocervical canal; it is then no longer amenable to colposcopic inspection. If metaplastic squamous epithelium achieves full maturation, it becomes histologically indistinguishable from the non-metaplastic squamous epithelium of the vagina and ectocervix. However, all degrees of immaturity can be encountered in metaplastic squamous epithelium within the transformation zone. Histologically, this is manifested by a lack of glycogen formation, failure to align the cytoplasm horizontally and a relatively high nuclear/cytoplasmic ratio.

Cystically dilated endocervical "glands", also known as Nabothian cysts, result from an obstruction of the orifice by ingrown metaplastic squamous epithelium. *Tunnel clusters*, a variant of Nabothian cysts, are tightly packed groups of cystic spaces lined by a flattened mucinous epithelium. Metaplastic squamous epithelium can partially or entirely replace previously existing endocervical epithelium and fill the glandular spaces. In this context, a condition named *microglandular hyperplasia* is often observed. It is characterized by an intimate admixture of glandular structures and metaplastic squamous epithelium, often displaying a cribriform architecture. It is usually accompanied by a prominent acute inflammatory infiltrate and exudate. Cytologic features are bland, and mitotic figures are virtually absent (Fig. 1). Microglandular hyperplasia is an entirely benign condition.

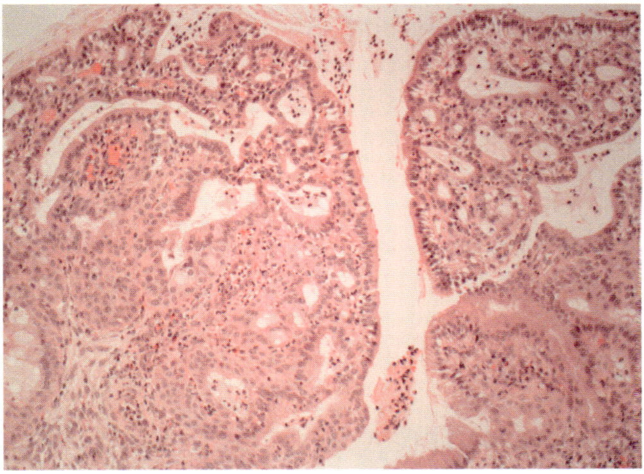

Fig. 1 Endocervical microglandular hyperplasia. Cribriform architecture in the upper and right part of the image, foci of squamous metaplasia on the left. Prominent acute inflammatory infiltrate and exudate. Hematoxylin/eosin, original magnification 100×.

Traditionally it has been linked to elevated progesterone levels, during pregnancy or under oral contraceptives, but this association has been recently questioned.[1] Practical experience has shown that the term "microglandular hyperplasia" may be misunderstood; if used in a pathology report, it is prudent to add the word "benign" in order to prevent unnecessary surgery.

Since the cervix is frequently exposed to infectious agents and other irritants, it usually exhibits acute and chronic inflammation to variable degrees. The inflammatory infiltrate is composed of neutrophils, T- and B-lymphocytes and numerous plasma cells. Formation of lymphoid follicles however is rare, and if present, leads to the diagnosis of *follicular cervicitis.* Dendritic (Langerhans) cells are present in the intermediate cell layer of the squamous epithelium. Antibodies of the IgG and IgA classes are present in the endocervical mucus and the vaginal transudate.

Remnants of the mesonephric (Wolffian) duct are occasionally found deep in the stroma of the lateral cervical walls. They are lined by a single cell cuboidal epithelium that is devoid of mucin or glycogen. The lumen typically contains eosinophilic PAS-positive amorphous material. In most cases, the duct-like architecture can be appreciated on the tissue section. However, sometimes there are exuberant collateral glandular structures that give rise to the designation *mesonephric hyperplasia.* This is again an entirely benign condition, and cytologic features are accordingly bland.

The cervix is connected to the pelvic side wall through the parametrial tissue, which contains the uterine blood vessels. Blood supply to the cervix is provided by the inferior branch of the uterine artery. Lymphatic drainage is directed to the exterior and common iliac, obturator, hypogastric and sacral lymph nodes. Occasional lymph nodes can be present within the parametria.

CLINICAL IDENTIFICATION OF EARLY VAGINAL AND CERVICAL NEOPLASMS

As opposed to the vulva, small cervical or vaginal lesions are not usually apparent to the patient, and self-examination has virtually no role in early detection of this disease. Most patients with early disease are completely asymptomatic. If symptoms exist, they are non-specific: patients may complain about discharge, vaginal bleeding (especially post-coital), discomfort or pain. However, once the patient finds the way into the gynecologist's office, cervix and vagina are readily amenable to examination. Before the actual exam, anamnestic information may reveal risk factors that increase the clinician's index of suspicion. Since the vast majority of all cervical and vaginal carcinomas are causally related to human papillomaviruses (HPV), they are basically considered sexually transmitted diseases (STD). Hence, risk factors for cervical/vaginal neoplasia are the same as for other STDs and include promiscuity and sexual activity at an early age. The risk of development and/or progression of neoplastic lesions is significantly increased in patients with immunodeficiencies, including HIV/AIDS, chemotherapy and post-transplantation immunosuppression. If the patient has a known vulvar HPV-related lesion, there is an up to 50% chance of a concomitant cervicovaginal lesion. Cigarette smoking appears to be an additional independent risk factor for cervical carcinoma, the biologic mechanism of which is not fully understood.

If during the gynecologic examination a cytologic smear is to be taken, it should be done first in order to minimize alterations or artifacts caused by other manipulations. A routine gynecologic examination includes inspection of the vaginal and cervical mucosae with the help of a speculum, and bimanual palpation. Grossly visible big polypoid tumors or mucosal ulcers represent either advanced neoplasms, benign polyps or infectious diseases. Early neoplastic lesions tend to be rather subtle on inspection. During colposcopy the cervical/vaginal mucosa is inspected through an optical apparatus (the colposcope) under up to 25-fold magnification. Foci of neoplastic epithelium are often recognized because of abnormal vascular patterns known as *punctation* or *mosaicism*. Application of 5% acetic acid results in a whitish discoloration of dysplastic epithelium. This "acetowhite" test is quite sensitive, but not very specific: it also highlights immature squamous metaplasia. Iodine containing Lugol's solution turns the color of glycogenated normal mature cervical and vaginal squamous epithelium into a dark brown, while dysplastic epithelium remains pink or pale. Once visualized, the lesion can be biopsied and histopathologically evaluated. The endocervical canal cannot be adequately inspected. Therefore an endocervical curettage is frequently performed, especially if in the presence of an abnormal cytologic finding there is no colposcopically visible lesion on the ectocervix.

When taking multiple biopsies, it is advised not to use Monsel's solution (20% ferric subsulfate) as a hemostatic agent until the very end of the procedure. Monsel's solution causes severe pigmentation artifacts on the hematoxylin/eosin stained tissue section that may make interpretation of the biopsy impossible. Although there are methods to remove Monsel's artifact from the slide, it is preferable to avoid this problem.[2]

PROCESSING OF A SURGICAL SPECIMEN FOR PATHOLOGIC EVALUATION

The following types of specimens are frequently received by the pathologist: cervical biopsies, endocervical curettings, tissue resulting from a Loop Electrosurgical Excision Procedure ("LEEP") or Large Loop Excision of Transformation Zone ("LLETZ"), traditional "cold knife" cone biopsies, simple and radical hysterectomy specimens. A trachelectomy (amputation of the cervix) is performed, when preservation of fertility is desired. In addition, there are ablative procedures like LASER vaporization or cryotherapy, which do not result in a tissue specimen that can be histologically examined.

Tissue pieces taken for biopsy should be at least 2 mm–3 mm in diameter to improve chances that an accurate diagnosis can be rendered. If the epithelial surface is recognizable, the tissue must be oriented such that a perpendicular section through the epithelium will be obtained. Tiny tissue fragments and oblique or tangential sectioning compromise diagnostic accuracy, especially when grading squamous lesions or assessing the presence of stromal invasion is required. Blood, mucus and inflammatory exudate, which often constitute the bulk of the biopsy volume, have virtually no diagnostic value. When there is a discrepancy between the amount of tissue seen on the histologic slide and the size of material documented in the gross description, the pathologist should not hesitate to request deeper levels or even melt down the paraffin block to make sure that the limited tissue available is adequately analyzed. The same is true for endocervical curettings, which notoriously contain large amounts of mucus and very small tissue pieces.

LEEP, LLETZ or cold knife cone biopsies can be performed with a diagnostic and/or therapeutic intention. LEEP specimens are most frequent in today's practice. This technique reduces blood loss during the procedure and allows resection of very shallow tissue pieces in order to minimize potential future obstetric complications. Cold knife cone biopsies are preferred when a lesion is located deep in the endocervical canal, i.e. an endocervical adenocarcinoma, adenocarcinoma *in situ* or lesions in postmenopausal women. For two reasons, it is preferred that the specimen be resected as a single piece: first to minimize cautery artifact; second it is impossible to determine whether a positive margin is the margin against another resected tissue fragment or against the remaining uterus. In such cases, a phrasing like "the lesion extends to an undesignated tissue edge" may be appropriate in the report. For optimal assessment of margin involvement, the stromal surfaces of LEEP/cone specimens are routinely inked before sectioning. In addition, it is useful to place a dot of a different color ink onto the apex (proximal end) of the cone. This will help to orient the tissue section in case the endo- and ectocervical margins cannot be differentiated on the slide (e.g. the section shows squamous mucosa on both ends). The cautery artifact seen in LEEP specimens is an unequivocal indicator for the true resection margin. Unfortunately, cautery artifact also obscures morphologic details, which may make it impossible to distinguish dysplastic from normal epithelium. Best tissue sections are obtained if the LEEP/cone specimen is received fresh, opened along the endocervical canal, rolled out and fixed in a linear position (e.g. by pinning down onto a cardboard), thus unfolding the epithelial lining of the endocervical canal. The tissue can then be serially sectioned, maximizing the chance that the epithelial surface will be represented on the slide. LEEP/cone specimens are always submitted entirely for histopathologic evaluation.

Specimens are often oriented by the surgeon with a stitch designating a certain "o'clock" position. This orientation should be maintained, and sections should be labeled according to their position. Traditional cone biopsies used to be quite large and were submitted in 12 cassettes, each representing one "hour" of the clock face. LEEPs tend to be much smaller and can usually be submitted in four cassettes, each representing one quadrant. When evaluating the tissue sections, it is important to examine not only the mucosal surfaces, but also the entire thickness of the stroma: an invasive tumor may be present despite an unremarkable surface epithelium; a squamous intraepithelial lesion may extend to the deep stromal margin if it involves endocervical glandular spaces. In most cases, endocervical curettings are obtained subsequently to the LEEP/cone procedure in order to rule out residual disease in the endocervical canal. Alternatively, an additional segment of endocervix ("top hat") may be resected.

If a hysterectomy (simple or radical) is performed for a cervical lesion that is not grossly recognizable, the cervix should be amputated at the level of the internal endocervical os and submitted entirely like a cone biopsy. Radical hysterectomy specimens usually come with attached vaginal cuff and parametria, which will have to be removed and submitted for histologic examination before opening and examining the cervix. If the tumor is grossly visible, representative sections including the area of deepest stromal invasion and the relation to resection margins are sufficient. Similar considerations apply for trachelectomy specimens.

BENIGN DISORDERS

Hyperkeratosis and Parakeratosis

Hyperkeratosis and/or parakeratosis is the most frequently encountered non-specific change of the vaginal and ectocervical squamous epithelium. Since hyper- and parakeratosis can give rise to abnormal cytology results and may be colposcopically visible, these alterations are frequently biopsied. Often this is the only pathologic change identifiable in the biopsy. Probably the most common cause of hyperkeratosis is uterine descensus or prolapse. However, hyper- and parakeratosis are often associated with HPV-related lesions ranging from condylomata to invasive carcinoma.

Polyps

Endocervical polyps are the most frequent abnormal growths of the cervix. The term "endocervical polyp" is routinely used for a benign pedunculated neoplasm that has a fibrovascular core and an endocervical-type lining epithelium. The stroma contains variable amounts of inflammatory cells, while the epithelium may exhibit squamous metaplasia and/or microglandular hyperplasia. It should be kept in mind, however, that the word "polyp" merely denotes a circumscribed growth projecting from a mucosal surface. It specifies neither the constituent type of tissue, nor its biologic behavior. Thus, a huge variety of benign and malignant conditions may clinically appear as "polyps", including granulation tissue, leiomyomata, decidual casts, squamous papillomas, condylomata acuminata, carcinomas and sarcomas. Certain malignancies, like adenosarcomas, embryonal rhabdomyosarcomas or malignant mixed Müllerian tumors, are known for their propensity to grow in a polypoid fashion.

So-called "fibroepithelial" or "mesodermal stromal" polyps are benign neoplasms arising from the vaginal mucosa. They have a fibrovascular core, often containing multinucleated floret cells, and are covered by normal maturing squamous epithelium. Some of these lesions show a worrisome combination of high cellularity, cytologic atypia, high mitotic count (more than ten mitotic figures per ten high power fields), including atypical mitoses, and have been referred to as cellular pseudosarcomatous fibroepithelial stromal polyps. Although some of these cases suffered recurrences, none developed metastatic disease.[3] Squamous papilloma is a benign lesion with morphologic features between a fibroepithelial polyp and a condyloma acuminatum. It has a thickened (acanthotic) epithelium covering a relatively thin fibrovascular core. No koilocytes are present. Some may be associated with viral infections, but no correlation with specific viral species has been established.

Not infrequently, the pathologist receives biopsies from the vaginal vault. This usually implies that the patient had a (recent) hysterectomy, and on follow-up a polypoid lesion is seen in the scar area of the vaginal apex. In most cases this is granulation tissue, histologically characterized by heavily inflamed, richly vascularized loose connective tissue, which may or may not be covered by stratified squamous epithelium. The differential diagnosis includes a malignant tumor, especially (recurrent) endometrial or cervical carcinoma. Therefore it is important that the clinical information be provided if, when and why a hysterectomy was performed. Occasionally the tissue will turn out to be a prolapsed fallopian tube. The typical scenario for this is when a vaginal hysterectomy was performed, in which case the adnexa are often left behind. If a wound dehiscence at the vaginal apex occurs, the fimbriated end of the fallopian tube can prolapse into the vagina. This can lead to vaginal discharge and/or ascending infections. Unlike granulation tissue or tumor, biopsy of the fallopian tube is painful, which may be the first clue to the nature of the lesion. Histologically, the tubal tissue can be very inflamed and vascularized, similar to granulation tissue. The finding of a tubal-type ciliated epithelium is diagnostic and should be searched for in any granulation tissue-like biopsy from the vaginal vault. Another entity seen in the vaginal vault is the rare *postoperative spindle cell nodule.* As the name implies, it develops within weeks to months after a surgical procedure. Histologically it is composed of fascicles of plump spindle cells with interspersed chronic inflammatory cells. Although mitotic figures may be numerous, cytologic features of this benign lesion are otherwise bland.

Endometriosis

Endometriosis can occur in the cervix and vagina. In the rectovaginal septum it may cause pain and dyspareunia. Even if asymptomatic, endometriosis may be visible as pigmented mucosal lesions and thus targeted for biopsies. For the definite diagnosis of endometriosis, three histologic features should be present: endometrial-type glands, endometrial-type stroma, and hemosiderin deposits as evidence of hemorrhage. The glandular epithelium may show tubal metaplasia or mild reactive atypia. The amount of stromal tissue is variable. If the patient is pregnant or treated with progesterone, the stromal element can undergo decidual changes and may appear much less cellular than usual endometrial stroma. *Stromal endometriosis* is characterized by the presence of endometrial-type stroma with hemorrhage, but absence of endometrial-type glands. Being a dark-bluish, richly vascularized spindle cell lesion that contains extravasated red blood cells, it shares clinical and histological features with Kaposi sarcoma, for which it should not be mistaken. Rarely, malignancies can arise in foci of endometriosis, including carcinomas of endometrioid or clear cell type, endometrial stromal sarcomas and malignant mixed Müllerian tumors (MMMT). Although endometriosis is not generally considered a premalignant lesion, patients with this condition in any location should be followed closely to rule out associated neoplasia.

Cysts

The most frequent type of vaginal wall cysts are epidermoid inclusion cysts. Usually being the result of birth trauma or episiotomy, they are encountered in the distal portion of the vagina near the introitus. Cystically dilated remnants of the mesonephric duct (Gartner duct cyst) are located in the lateral vaginal wall. Occasionally, a solid tumor (leiomyoma, angiomyofibroblastoma) may clinically appear as a cystic lesion. Nabothian cysts of the cervix are an extremely common finding. They can be numerous, can form polypoid structures or deeply penetrate the cervical wall and thus simulate neoplasms.

Condylomata

Human papilloma virus (HPV) plays an important role in both infectious and neoplastic lesions of the cervicovaginal mucosa. While the molecular pathogenetic mechanisms of HPV-associated tumorigenesis are discussed in the following section, wart-like conditions represent a "connecting link" between infectious and neoplastic diseases. Condylomas are the most frequent manifestation of cervicovaginal HPV infection. As opposed to the typically exophytic vulvar condylomata acuminata, cervical lesions tend to be flat ("condylomata plana"; not to be confused with "condylomata lata", which are a manifestation of secondary syphilis!). They are most frequently located in the cervical transformation zone, often appear as multiple raised and/or acetowhite lesions on colposcopy and are among the most common findings on cervical biopsies. Histologically a condyloma is defined by the presence of koilocytes, which are abnormal cells exhibiting an atypical (hyperchromatic, enlarged, irregularly shaped) nucleus and a cytoplasmic perinuclear halo. Mitotic figures are rare and confined to the basal or parabasal layer, and no atypical mitoses are present. The squamous epithelium may or may not be thickened (acanthotic). The mere finding of perinuclear clearing is not diagnostic for koilocytes, because it is also seen in normal maturing squamous cells due to cytoplasmic glycogen accumulation. Nuclear atypia tends to be more striking in cervical condylomas than in their vulvar counterparts and can reach extreme degrees, especially in adolescents (Fig. 2).[4] Multinucleated cells and parakeratosis are frequent findings associated with, but not specific for condylomata. Although condylomata display cytologic atypia throughout the full thickness of the epithelium, this must not be construed as evidence for a dysplastic change. If there is no increase in mitotic activity or expansion of immature basaloid cells, koilocytotic changes are considered a purely infectious phenomenon. On the other hand, koilocytes are often seen in association with dysplastic lesions as well as with invasive carcinomas, in which case they are usually located towards the surface of the epithelium. While vulvar condylomata are usually caused by HPV types 6 and 11, cervical condylomata can be associated with a wide range of HPV types. Morphology of the cervical condyloma does not allow determining whether it is caused by high risk or low risk HPV types. Of note, most "low grade" cervical lesions are associated with "high risk" HPV types![5,6] The vast majority of condylomata are self-limited and regress spontaneously, although the natural course may take several years.

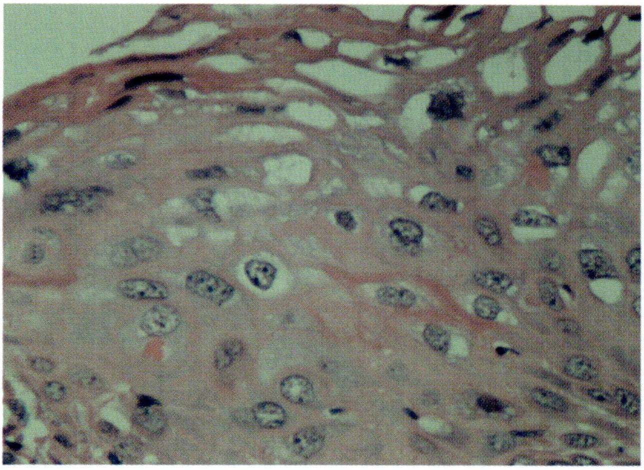

Fig. 2 Condyloma planum of the cervix. Marked nuclear atypia, including enlargement, hyperchromasia, irregular shape and multinucleation. Many cells have perinuclear halos. Hematoxylin/eosin, original magnification 400×.

Clearance of the lesions results in humoral immunity, which is specific for the causative HPV type.

Diethylstilbestrol

Intrauterine exposure to Diethylstilbestrol (DES) is another condition associated with mostly benign disease but occasional malignancies. DES was in clinical use from 1938 to 1971 for the treatment of threatened abortion. Individuals that were exposed to DES *in utero* often develop certain otherwise rare abnormalities of the female genital tract: the finding of vaginal adenosis and cervical ectropion in over one-third of affected patients suggests that DES interferes with the normal epithelialization of the vagina and ectocervix. Other structural abnormalities include cervical "hoods", vaginal ridges or pseudopolyps, seen in approximately 20% of patients. Both epithelial and structural abnormalities often regress spontaneously and do not require treatment. Also, DES-exposed women have an 80% increased risk of endometriosis.[7] A very small proportion of exposed women (less than 1%) presented with vaginal or cervical clear cell carcinoma at a median age of 20 years which led to withdrawal of the drug from the market.

HUMAN PAPILLOMA VIRUS (HPV): LIFE CYCLE AND ROLE IN TUMORIGENESIS

An infectious HPV particle consists of a non-enveloped capsid that contains a double stranded circular DNA. The capsid is composed of 72 identical capsomeres that are assembled into an icosahedral particle measuring 55 nm in diameter. The viral genome contains approximately 8000 basepairs and encodes a number of genes designated E1-E7 and L1-L2, which are expressed early and late during the viral life cycle, respectively (Fig. 3). Important functions of the viral proteins include the following: E1 is a DNA helicase involved in episomal replication. E2 is a transcription factor that controls the expression of viral proteins E6 and E7. E5 stimulates cell growth through activation of EGFR and PDGFR, and inhibits apoptosis. E6 and E7 promote host cell cycle progression, retard terminal differentiation and suppress

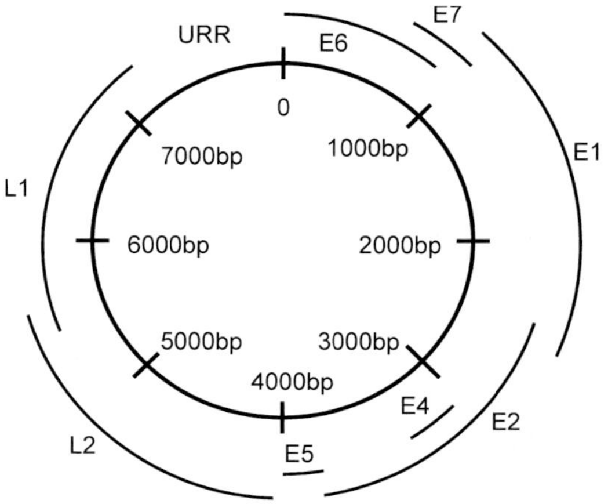

Fig. 3 Organization of the Human Papillomavirus Genome. URR: Upstream Regulatory Region; E1-E7 early proteins; L1-L2 late proteins (major and minor capsid proteins).

apoptosis, allowing for further viral replication. Specifically, E6 induces degradation of the tumor suppressor protein p53 and of the pro-apoptotic BAK, activates telomerase, and interferes with PDZ proteins that have a variety of functions in signal transduction and cell development. E7 alters the retinoblastoma tumor suppressor protein (RB), leading to its degradation and release of transcription factor E2F, which induces expression of cyclins A and E and drives the cell cycle from the G1 into the S-phase. It also blocks the cyclin dependent kinase inhibitors $p21^{CIP1}$, and indirectly reduces $p27^{KIP1}$.[8–11] Through association with γ-tubulin, E7 can induce aberrant centrosome duplication, which facilitates the emergence of aneuploidy.[12] The L1 gene encodes the major capsid protein, which forms the entire exterior surface of the virion. The L2 minor capsid protein is a constituent element of the interior surface of the capsid and may have a function in DNA packaging.

In a latent infection, viral DNA is present as an episome that does not replicate independently and does not induce functional or morphologic changes of the host cell. For a productive infection, the HPV virion must enter a host cell in the basal layer that then undergoes maturation and thereby provides the necessary environment for the virus to complete its life cycle. Access to the basal cell layer is easiest at the squamocolumnar junction (Fig. 4), which explains the fact that this is by far the most frequent site for HPV-associated lesions. Alternatively, HPV can reach the basal cell layer after (micro-)trauma to the epithelium. In basal and parabasal cells, viral DNA replicates episomally within the nucleus, independently from the host cell DNA synthesis. When the host cell matures to become an intermediate or superficial cell, capsid proteins L1 and L2 are expressed and the viral particles are assembled. New virions are not released until superficial cells exfoliate and degrade.

HPV exists and replicates in an "immunologic niche" where it is relatively protected from the host's immune system. During the entire course of the infection there is neither a blood borne phase nor lysis of infected cells with a subsequent inflammatory reaction, which would expose the virus to the host's immune system. No intraepithelial antigen presenting (Langerhans) cells are infected. Viral proteins E5, E6 and E7 interfere with the processing of antigenic peptides, interferon

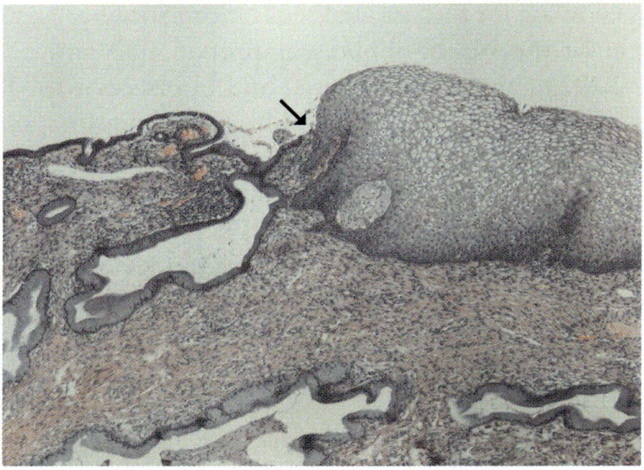

Fig. 4 Squamocolumnar junction. The stratified squamous ectocervical epithelium (right) meets the single cell layered mucinous endocervical epithelium (left and lower part of the image). At the squamocolumnar junction (arrow) the basal cell layer is easily accessible. Hematoxylin/eosin, original magnification 40×.

signaling and intraepithelial dendritic cell function.[13,14] The L1 major capsid protein, which is the most immunogenic of the viral proteins, is not synthesized until late in the viral life cycle in the intermediate and superficial layer of the squamous epithelium. These immune-evasive mechanisms make the virus practically invisible to the host's defense system and are the reason why it takes a relatively long time — months to years — for an HPV infection to be naturally cleared.

The morphologic correlate of a productive HPV-infection is the koilocytotic change of the infected cells. It is important to keep in mind that koilocytes are terminally differentiated cells; they will not turn into cancer cells. The emergence of dysplastic host cells, i.e. cells that display a lack of maturation and uncontrolled proliferation, requires a number of events that happen "accidentally" to the viral and host cell genomes. The malignant transformation of the host cell does not provide any advantage for viral replication, which is reflected by the fact that high grade dysplastic epithelium and carcinoma cells contain far less viral copies than koilocytes. The statistical likelihood of all necessary events to happen in the same cell is very small, which is part of the reason that carcinoma develops in only a minute proportion of all HPV-infected individuals. Initially the circular HPV DNA breaks and becomes a linear strand. This linearized DNA fragment can then integrate into the host cell genome, i.e. it does not exist as an episome any more. If the breakpoint is located within the E2 gene, the resulting loss of a functional E2 protein leads to uncontrolled overexpression of viral proteins E6 and E7. While their limited expression is beneficial for viral replication, they now massively interfere with the host cell cycle control mechanisms, especially through alterations of p53 and RB. Consequently, this leads to acceleration of the cell cycle, inhibition of apoptosis and accumulation of additional mutations, opening the way to become a cancer cell.[8,11]

Papillomaviruses are highly species- and site-specific, and there are more than 100 different identified human types. Separate types are defined as having a greater than 10% divergence in the DNA sequence of the L1, E6 and E7 genes. If the difference is less than 10% compared to an already known type, it is referred to as a variant or subtype. About 40 HPV types target the skin and mucosae of the human anogenital region. Based on the frequency of their association with invasive carcinoma, they are classified into low risk (including HPV 6, 11, 40, 42, 43, 44, 54) and high risk (including 16, 18, 31, 33, 35, 39, 45, 51, 52, 58) types. Some of the abovementioned HPV E6/E7 functions are specific to high risk types, and/or the high risk type viral proteins have a higher affinity to their cellular target proteins than the low risk type proteins. This explains why HPV 16 is the most frequent type associated with invasive carcinoma, accounting for 54% of squamous cell carcinomas and over 40% of adenocarcinomas.[15–17]

PREMALIGNANT EPITHELIAL LESIONS

Squamous Lesions

Terminology

Precursor lesions of invasive cervical carcinoma have been described since the late 19th century. Terminology and classification have changed several times since. At present, the three-tiered Cervical Intraepithelial Neoplasia (CIN) system and the two-tiered Squamous Intraepithelial Lesion (SIL) system are most frequently used. In the CIN classification lesions are graded as mild, moderate and severe dysplasia (CIN 1, 2, and 3, respectively), based on the proportion of the full thickness of the squamous epithelium that is occupied by immature dysplastic cells: in CIN 1, dysplastic cells are confined to the lower third, in CIN 2, they extend into the middle third, and in CIN 3, they extend into the upper third of the epithelium. The term *carcinoma in situ* refers to those lesions within the CIN 3 category that show virtually no maturation at all. The analogous classification for Vaginal Intraepithelial Neoplasia is VAIN 1–3, respectively. The CIN nomenclature was introduced under the assumption that the different grades of CIN represent a continuum on a spectrum of the same disease process, invasive carcinoma being the end point. With improved understanding of the molecular pathogenesis, including the facts outlined above, it is now thought that intraepithelial lesions can be divided into purely infectious lesions and those in which integration of the viral DNA into the host cell genome has led to transformation into a neoplastic lesion. Based on this biologic dichotomy, and in analogy with the Bethesda system used for cervical cytology reports, histopathologic findings have recently been classified as low grade (LG) versus high grade (HG) Squamous Intraepithelial Lesions (SIL). LG-SIL encompasses condylomas and CIN 1, whereas HG-SIL comprises CIN 2, CIN 3 and *carcinoma in situ.* (This is the classification commonly used in the USA; note that in many European countries, CIN 2 is classified as a low-grade lesion!). This two-tiered system is felt to better reflect the different biologic behavior of the lesions, and parallels clinical management: the vast majority of low grade lesions regresses spontaneously and does not need active treatment, while high grade lesions have a greater risk of progressing to invasive carcinoma and therefore are surgically removed.

Epidemiology

The identification of HPV as a causative agent has explained the well known observation that cervical cancer and its precursor lesions exhibit the epidemiologic features of a sexually transmitted disease (STD). Early age at first vaginal intercourse, number of sexual partners, oral contraceptive use and a history of other STDs (herpes, chlamydia, syphilis) are risk factors for cervical carcinoma. HPV infection is a necessary, but not sufficient, condition for developing almost all cervical carcinomas. Other, much less well understood factors must also play a role in carcinogenesis. Probably the most important of those is the immune system. It is known that precursor lesions have a much higher risk of progression, and can progress more rapidly under immunocompromised conditions, including HIV/AIDS, post-transplantation immunosuppression or chemotherapy. In addition, tobacco smoking is another independent risk factor for cervical squamous cell carcinoma (but not adenocarcinoma) and is associated with an increased prevalence of HPV infections.[18,19]

Worldwide, 660 million people (20 million in the USA) are infected with HPV, with an incidence of 30 million (6.2 million in the USA) new cases annually. By the age of 50 years, 80% of all women have been exposed to HPV. The vast majority of infections is cleared spontaneously by the host's immune system. As a result of the "immune-evasive" mechanisms discussed above, this takes a relatively long time, compared to other common viral infections: the median duration of an HPV infection, as defined by the time when HPV DNA can no longer be detected on the cervix and specific serum antibodies appear, is eight months. After three years approximately 90% of infections will be spontaneously cleared. While a "persistent" HPV infection is postulated to be a prerequisite for progression to neoplastic disease, the long duration of the uncomplicated infection makes it difficult to precisely define what a "persistent" infection is. According to the WHO, a "persistent" infection is characterized by identification of the same HPV type in two analyses 6–12 months apart, but this definition is not universally accepted.

The mean ages for CIN 1–2, CIN 3 and invasive carcinoma are 25 years, 35–42 years and 54 years, respectively. This supports the concept of a slowly progressive process, with an average progression time of more than 10 years from a high grade SIL to invasive carcinoma. However, not every dysplastic lesion will progress. In fact, a significant proportion of high grade lesions will regress spontaneously, although it may take many months to years.[20,21] It is estimated that approximately 12% of CIN 3 lesions and less than 2% of CIN 1 lesions will ultimately progress to invasive carcinoma. Unfortunately we are presently unable to predict by morphologic, molecular or other criteria, which lesions will progress. To be on the safe side, HG-SIL is therefore usually surgically removed, knowing that many of these cases will be overtreated.

The above-mentioned numbers are true for immunocompetent individuals. Incidence and progression rates are significantly higher in immunocompromised (e.g. HIV positive) patients.[22,23] In view of the greatly increased risk of disease progression, invasive cervical carcinoma in HIV positive women under the age of 35 years is an AIDS defining illness.

Histomorphology

Morphologic criteria to grade SIL are well defined. As stated above, classification is based on the proportion of the epithelial thickness that is occupied by immature dysplastic cells. While this definition sounds straightforward, in practical terms it is not always easily applicable. There is a good inter- and intraobserver reproducibility at the extremes of the spectrum, but intermediate lesions are notoriously difficult to classify. There is no straight line separating immature from maturing cells, and this is where the inherent subjectivity of morphologic evaluation comes into play. In addition, the epithelium may be sectioned obliquely or tangentially, or its full thickness may not be visible, which further confounds the picture. The diagnosis of CIN 2 is particularly prone to intra- and interobserver variability.[24] Use of the two-tiered SIL system somewhat alleviates this problem when consolidation of CIN 2 and CIN 3 into one group eliminates the potential source of disagreement towards the high grade end of the spectrum.[25] However, the dilemma persists towards the low grade end, since the distinction of LG-SIL from HG-SIL is based on the same criteria as the distinction of CIN 1 from CIN 2; and clinically this means the difference between no treatment and surgery.

The following adjunct morphologic criteria may be helpful to grade a lesion:

1. Mitotic figures above the parabasal cell layer are abnormal, indicating a proliferation disorder and lack of cellular maturation. Mitoses are frequent findings in cervical dysplasia and a useful diagnostic criterion. In typical cases, mitotic figures are seen within the layer of immature dysplastic cells. Hence, the presence of mitotic figures in the middle or upper third of the epithelium strongly supports the diagnosis of a high grade lesion. A mitotic figure with visible individual chromosomes is definitely better recognizable and leaves less room for interpretation than an imaginary line separating immature from mature cells. One must be sure, though, that the epithelium is perpendicularly sectioned and the full thickness of the epithelium is visible. If a fibrovascular core is present close by, the mitosis may not be as far away from the basement membrane as its position within the epithelium may suggest (Fig. 5(a)). Apoptotic bodies should not be mistaken for mitotic figures.
2. Atypical mitotic figures (AMFs; especially two- or three group metaphases, V-shaped metaphases and ring mitoses) have been linked to aneuploidy, which in turn is associated with high grade SIL.[26] The absence of AMFs, however, does not exclude a high grade lesion. Some authors recommend that any lesion containing AMFs should be considered high grade, but this is not universally accepted. If AMFs are seen in a lesion that otherwise appears to be low grade, the finding should be included in the pathology report such that it may be incorporated into clinical decision making.
3. Dysplastic cells of a high grade lesion tend to have indistinct cell borders and lack intercellular bridges.
4. High grade lesions are composed of cells with higher nuclear/cytoplasmic ratio, resulting in apparent nuclear crowding and nuclear overlapping.
5. Involvement of endocervical glands by dysplastic squamous epithelium (Fig. 5(b)) is seen approximately four times more frequently

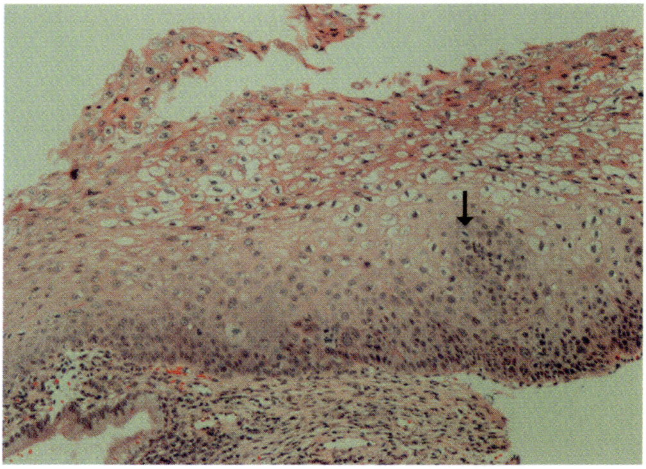

(a)

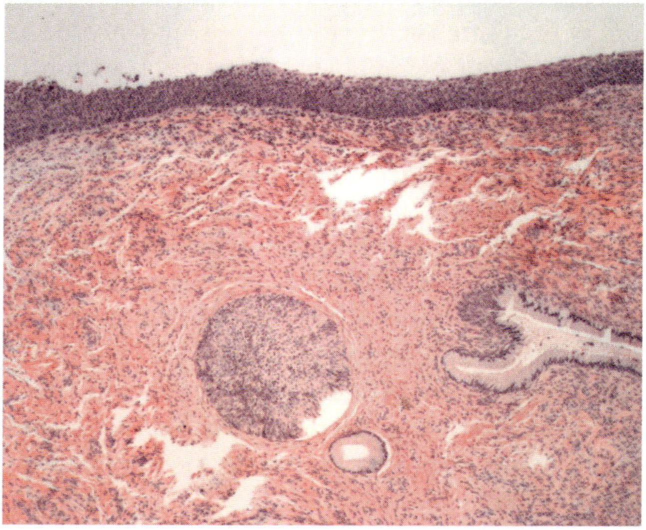

(b)

Fig. 5 (a) Low grade SIL (CIN 1). Increased mitotic activity within the mildly expanded parabasal cell layer. One mitotic figure (arrow) appears to be located within the middle third of the epithelium, however it is close to a basement membrane of a fibrovascular core. Hematoxylin/eosin, original magnification 100×. (b) High grade SIL (CIN 3), with endocervical glandular involvement. Hematoxylin/eosin, original magnification 100×.

in high grade lesions than in low grade lesions.[27] It has also been associated with a higher recurrence rate after LEEP/cone biopsy.[28] This condition needs to be distinguished from lesions of the endocervical glandular epithelium, see below.

Many but not all of the above features may be present to support a diagnosis of a high grade lesion. It is important to remember that there are koilocytotic changes and full thickness cytologic atypia in virtually all HPV associated lesions, including condylomas, low grade, high grade and invasive disease. In fact, koilocytes often exhibit greater pleomorphism and nuclear atypia than high grade dysplastic cells, while some high grade lesions have quite uniform nuclei.

The absence of koilocytes should raise the suspicion that one is dealing with a benign mimicker. These include immature squamous metaplasia, reactive atypia and atrophy. Immature metaplastic squamous epithelium may display cells with a high nuclear/cytoplasmic ratio, occasional mitotic figures, lack of glycogen and failure to align the cellular axis horizontally. Reactive (inflammatory) atypia is characterized by an expansion of immature appearing cells that tend to have well demarcated cell borders and nuclei with finely dispersed chromatin and one or two nucleoli. Since even the HPV-free cervix is almost always inflamed to some degree, inflammatory atypia is an extremely common finding and may be difficult to distinguish from dysplasia. Epithelial atrophy occurs due to lack of estrogen, i.e. in prepubertal girls and in postmenopausal women. Atrophic epithelium is thin and composed of only basal and parabasal cells, which lack glycogen. All these mimickers do not reach the degree of nuclear atypia usually seen in high grade dysplasia, and have only rare if any mitoses, which are never atypical.

Follicular cervicitis can sometimes mimic a high grade lesion involving an endocervical gland, especially when the lymphoid follicle has a large germinal center and is sharply demarcated. Cells of the germinal center can display significant pleomorphism and high mitotic activity. Tingible body macrophages are an important diagnostic clue and must not be mistaken for apoptotic cells (Fig. 6). A debatable entity called "atypical immature metaplasia" (AIM) may be described

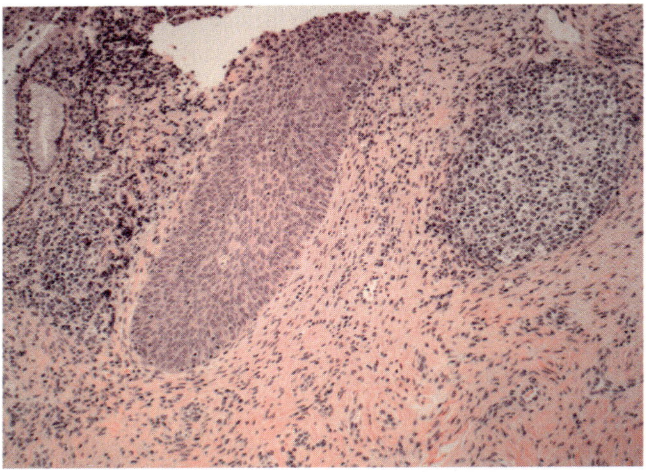

Fig. 6 Follicular cervicitis. A lymphoid follicle (right) containing numerous tingible body macrophages. A focus of dysplastic squamous epithelium occupying an endocervical glandular space is present in the center, a normal endocervical gland is visible on the left. Hematoxylin/eosin, original magnification 100×.

as a lesion that has all the features of a high grade dysplasia, except for the mitotic activity. The use of this term is not recommended, because neither the pathologist nor the clinician knows what it actually means and what to do about it. If morphology is inconclusive, immunohistochemical stains for p16 and MIB-1 (Ki-67) are very helpful for identification of HPV-related lesions (see section on ancillary studies).

Preinvasive Glandular Lesions

Terminology, Epidemiology and Clinical Aspects

Neoplastic appearing atypical endocervical epithelium lining architecturally normal endocervical glands was first observed adjacent to invasive endocervical adenocarcinoma. The existence of such lesions in the absence of invasive disease is now well established. It is thought to be the direct precursor lesion of invasive endocervical adenocarcinoma, and the currently used designation is endocervical *adenocarcinoma in situ* (AIS). For unknown reasons, a significant increase in incidence of AIS has been reported over the past decades, in both absolute and relative numbers.[29] Like invasive adenocarcinoma, the vast majority of AIS is HPV associated. Hence, the same risk factors as for squamous lesions are operative and it is not unusual to find both squamous and glandular lesions side by side in the same patient: 50% of patients with AIS also have a SIL.[30] Often the AIS is only identified because the patient is worked up for a known or suspected squamous lesion.

Most AIS patients are asymptomatic; some complain about vaginal discharge. Unfortunately, AIS is much less amenable to early detection than squamous lesions. On colposcopy AIS is difficult to identify because it extends into the endocervical canal, is not morphologically distinctive and cannot be highlighted with acetic acid or Lugol's solution. Cervical cytology is not an efficient screening tool for glandular lesions, although the diagnosis can be made on cytology if specific findings are present. AIS is one of the entities that may lead to a cytologic diagnosis of "atypical glandular cells" (AGC). However, when evaluating biopsies taken subsequently to a cytologic "AGC" diagnosis, one must also be aware of the possibility of a squamous lesion, present in a significant proportion of cases.

Histomorphology

AIS is characterized by malignant glandular epithelium lining normally shaped endocervical glands. On low magnification, the neoplastic glandular epithelium may appear hyperchromatic, with a typically very abrupt transition to residual normal endocervical epithelium (Fig. 7). Epithelial proliferation into the glandular lumen may result in papillary or cribriform formations. Cytologic features include high nuclear/cytoplasmic ratio, mucus depletion, nuclear enlargement, hyperchromasia, elongation ("pencil-shaped") and pseudostratification, and numerous mitotic figures, which are often located in the apical portion of the cells. Of note, mitoses are quite rare in normal endocervical epithelium. Although the isolated finding of occasional mitoses in otherwise normal appearing endocervical epithelium does not warrant a specific diagnosis, it should prompt a careful search

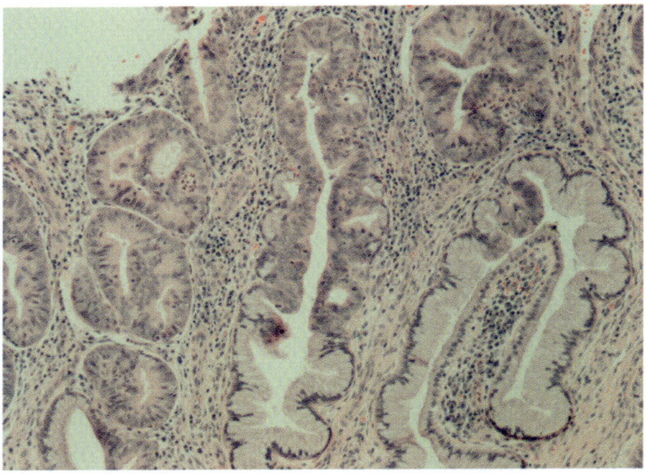

Fig. 7 Endocervical adenocarcinoma *in situ*. The abnormal epithelium shows increased nuclear/cytoplasmic ratio, numerous mitotic figures and mucus depletion. Note the abrupt transition between normal and malignant epithelium. Hematoxylin/eosin, original magnification 100×.

to rule out a glandular lesion. Findings on endocervical curettings (ECC) from a patient with AIS can be extremely subtle and may be reduced to cytologic dimensions. On the other hand, the possibility of an AIS must be kept in mind in every patient who is being worked up for HPV-related disease. Identification of a squamous lesion does not rule out the simultaneous presence of a glandular lesion, and *vice-versa*!

Endometrioid, mucinous, intestinal-type and adenosquamous differentiation of AIS is distinguished based on the resemblance of the neoplastic epithelium to related normal epithelium. The endometrioid variant shows the highest degree of mucus depletion and highest nuclear/cytoplasmic ratio. "Mucinous" refers to endocervical-type epithelium, while intestinal-type AIS contains goblet cells. This latter variant may be difficult to appreciate on low magnification, because it has ample cytoplasm and does not appear hyperchromatic. High magnification will show significant nuclear atypia and mitotic activity. A tubal type AIS has been described but appears to be extremely rare.[31]

Reports about the multifocality and frequency of "skip lesions" in AIS are conflicting. Be that as it may, residual disease (including invasive adenocarcinoma) is found in up to 44% of follow-up hysterectomy specimens, even when the resection margins of the preceding cone biopsy were histologically negative.[30,32] Therefore it has been recommended to achieve an at least 10 mm margin around the endocervical glandular lesion, and to state the closest distance between AIS and resection margin in the pathology report.[33]

The discussion about putative precursor lesions to AIS is ongoing. Theoretically it may be assumed that AIS does not occur *de novo*, but as the result of a gradually progressing process, similar to squamous lesions. There is at present no general agreement about identification and terminology of such antecedent lesions. Proposed entities include superficial AIS (SAIS),[34] glandular dysplasia, atypical hyperplasia and cervical intraepithelial glandular neoplasia.[35] The term "endocervical glandular dysplasia", although listed in the WHO classification of diseases, is neither uniformly defined nor universally accepted, and the biological significance of such lesions is unclear.[30,36] When all features of AIS as described above are present, there is little doubt about the diagnosis and its clinical significance. Cases with findings suspicious but not diagnostic of AIS are probably best designated descriptively as "endocervical glandular atypia" and clinically managed on an individual basis.

The long list of benign conditions that can mimic AIS includes the following:

1. Tubo-endometrioid metaplasia is the most notorious look-alike of AIS and always needs to be excluded before making the latter diagnosis. This condition can usually be recognized by the presence of ciliated cells, reflecting a state of high differentiation (Fig. 8). The epithelium can display different cell types, similar to fallopian tube epithelium, which results in a somewhat pleomorphic appearance. Mitoses may be present, but no AMFs.
2. Cervical endometriosis may also display a mitotically active epithelium closely resembling benign endometrium. An endometrial-type stromal cuff around these glands provides the diagnostic clue.

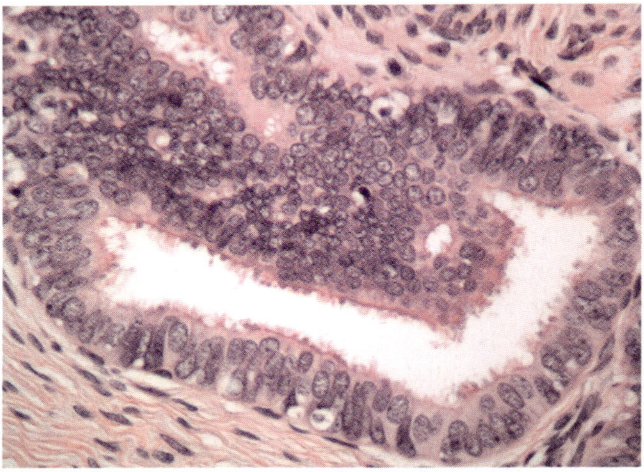

Fig. 8 Tubo-endometrioid metaplasia. Different cell types mimic cellular pleomorphism; tangential sectioning suggests epithelial stratification. Note the well-formed ciliae at the apical cell border. Hematoxylin/eosin, original magnification 400×.

3. Endocervical microglandular hyperplasia is a benign condition, which however displays a cribriform architecture. It is usually intimately associated with squamous metaplasia. Cytologic features are bland and mitotic figures virtually absent. Typically there is a prominent neutrophilic inflammatory infiltrate and exudate (Fig. 1).
4. Viral infection of endocervical epithelial cells can lead to significant atypia. HPV and herpes simplex are the two viruses encountered most frequently on histopathologic examination of cervical material. Herpes simplex (usually type 2) affects the genital skin and mucosae and typically manifests with painful blisters and ulcers. When seen on biopsy, there is destruction of the mucosa accompanied by severe acute and chronic inflammation. The pathognomonic finding are multinucleated epithelial cells that display nuclear molding and a transparent ("ground glass") appearance of the nuclei. Although herpetic lesions tend to affect the squamous mucosa, the degree of ulceration may obscure whether a biopsy was taken from the ecto- or endocervix.

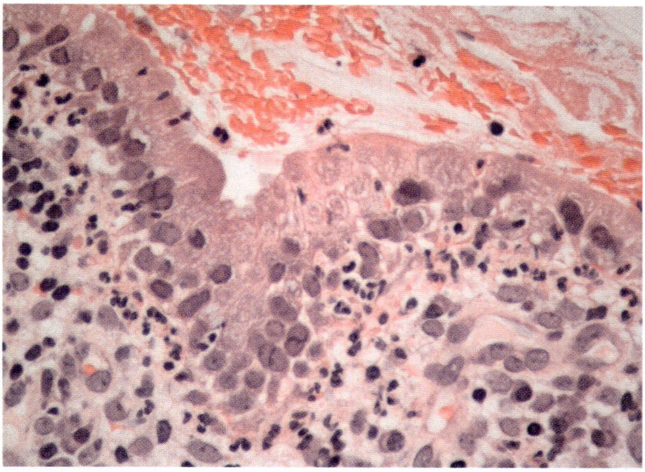

Fig. 9 Viral cytopathic changes of endocervical epithelium. Numerous multinucleated epitheial cells with smudged nuclear chromatin texture are present. Note the severe acute and chronic inflammatory infiltrate. Hematoxylin/eosin, original magnification 400×.

Multinucleation is a well-known effect of HPV infection and is almost always present in squamous lesions. Sometimes HPV also causes multinucleation of endocervical glandular cells (Fig. 9). If pronounced and accompanied by severe inflammation, it may be difficult to distinguish between HPV and herpes (in which case immunohistochemistry will be helpful). As long as multinucleated cells show not more than mild nuclear atypia and lack mitotic activity, it is thought to have no clinical significance. If on the other hand, in addition to multinucleation, cytologic features become atypical and occasional mitotic figures are present, AIS comes into the differential diagnosis. As described above, this is a scenario where currently there is no agreement on terminology and very limited clinical experience regarding the biologic significance of such (fortunately rare) "atypical" lesions.

5. Arias-Stella changes can affect the endometrial and endocervical epithelium. They are seen during or shortly after pregnancy. The typical cytologic features consist of an atypical (hyperchromatic,

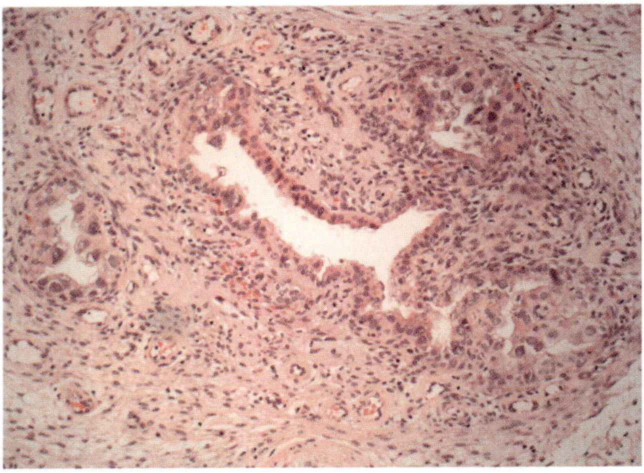

Fig. 10 Arias-Stella change. Numerous epithelial cells show nuclear enlargement and hyperchromasia. Some exhibit nuclear hobnailing. Some cells have clear cytoplasm. These findings were present in an endocervical polyp of a patient who recently had a spontaneous abortion. Hematoxylin/eosin, original magnification 100×.

enlarged, irregularly shaped) nucleus and ample clear or eosinophilic cytoplasm. Nuclear enlargement and hyperchromasia are due to polyploidy, although no aneuploidy has been reported. "Hobnailing" (protrusion of the nucleus into the lumen) is often present (Fig. 10). Mitotic activity, including AMFs, may be seen, albeit rarely.[37] Hence, Arias-Stella changes are a close mimicker of clear cell carcinoma. Unless there is a history of DES esposure, primary endocervical clear cell carcinoma is extremely rare. No clear cell-AIS has been described. Therefore the diagnosis of cervical clear cell carcinoma has to be made with extreme caution and only after exclusion of a current or recent pregnancy.

6. Post-radiation atypia affects not only the epithelium but also the stroma and vascular endothelial cells. It can persist for decades after radiation. Cytologic features include large cells with enlarged nuclei that have a smudged texture, nuclear and cytoplasmic vacuoles, and lack of mitotic activity. Note that the nuclear/cytoplasmic ratio is not necessarily altered. A history of radiation

often implies the history of a malignancy, therefore recurrent tumor must be carefully searched for. Also, radiation itself can induce neoplasia, generally after a latent period of at least ten years. Viable tumor cells can usually be distinguished by their higher nuclear/cytoplasmic ratio, coarse chromatin pattern and mitotic activity.

INVASIVE CARCINOMA OF THE CERVIX

The WHO classification distinguishes three groups of primary cervical carcinomas: squamous cell carcinoma, adenocarcinoma and "other" epithelial tumors. The incidence of invasive cervical cancer worldwide is approximately 470,000 per year, making it the second most frequent cancer in women after breast carcinoma. The mortality rate is 233,000 cases per year worldwide, of which over 80% occur in developing countries. In the USA, 11,070 new cases and 3,870 deaths due to cervical carcinoma are expected in 2008.

Although the objective of the screening programs is to detect and treat precursor lesions before they become invasive, early stage invasive cervical carcinoma still has an excellent prognosis. This section will address specific diagnostic considerations of early invasive carcinoma. Risk factors for invasive carcinoma are the same as for the precursor lesions as discussed above. More than 99% of squamous cell carcinomas and almost as many adenocarcinomas are associated with HPV infection. Some infectious diseases like genital herpes or granuloma inguinale can clinically mimic an invasive carcinoma. Therefore the latter diagnosis should always be based on the histologic evaluation of a biopsy.

Squamous Cell Carcinoma

Microinvasive Carcinoma

Although the term *microinvasive carcinoma* is generally accepted and widely used, it is not universally defined. Most authors refer to the

Fédération Internationale de Gynécologie et d'Obstétrique (FIGO) stage IA1, which is defined as invasive carcinoma with a measured stromal invasion 3.0 mm or less in depth and 7.0 mm or less in horizontal spread, provided the tumor is not macroscopically visible. All macroscopically visible tumors are automatically classified as at least FIGO stage IB. This does not mean that the cervical surface has to appear entirely normal. Colposcopic findings consistent with an intraepithelial lesion (abnormal vessels, puckered surface, acetowhite area) do not preclude the diagnosis of microinvasive disease. The FIGO classification does not take into account the presence or absence of vascular involvement. The Society of Gynecologic Oncologists (SGO) defines microinvasion as 3.0 mm or less in depth below the basement membrane in the absence of lymphvascular involvement, but does not specify a limit to the horizontal extension.

Tumor dimensions can be best measured using a calibrated ocular under consideration of the magnification factor. For practical purposes, comparison of the tumor dimension to the diameter of the microscopic field allows in most cases to determine whether the lesion falls below or above the "microinvasion" threshold. On most microscopes, a magnification of 40× (10× ocular and 4× objective) visualizes a field of 5.0 mm in diameter. For measurements of depth of invasion, one must assure that the section was taken perpendicularly to the surface. Oblique sections will result in falsely increased measurements. Examination of several levels is recommended, since the difference in tumor extension from level to level can be astounding in these small dimensions. Depth of invasion is measured as the distance between two (imaginary) parallel lines through the deepest point of the invasive focus and the closest adjacent basement membrane. The invasive focus may appear in continuation with HG-SIL covering the surface, emerging from SIL involving an endocervical gland, or discontinuous from the point where it broke through the basement membrane (Fig. 11). When multiple foci of invasion are present, their horizontal dimensions are added. Care must be taken not to count the same focus twice, which may happen if it has been bisected and the two halves appear on different tissue pieces. The third dimension of tumor extension is difficult to assess accurately. Tissue sections should

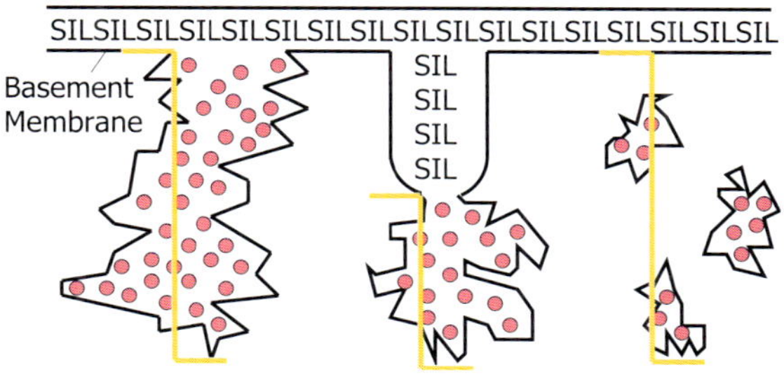

Fig. 11 Measurement of depth of stromal invasion. Left: Invasive carcinoma emerges directly from HG-SIL. Center: Invasive carcinoma emerges from HG-SIL involving an endocervical gland. Right: Nests of invasive carcinoma are present within the stroma, the site of emergence is not visible.

ideally be about 2.0 mm thick. Hence, if tumor is present on more than three different pieces of a sequentially sectioned specimen, it is likely that the lesion exceeds 7.0 mm in the third (i.e. second horizontal) dimension.

A diagnosis of "microinvasive" carcinoma can only be made if the lesion is completely excised. Hence, it cannot normally be rendered on a biopsy. LEEP/cone specimens must be entirely submitted and margins must be free of disease. Microinvasion is usually an unsuspected finding, since by (FIGO) definition it is not grossly recognizable.

Clinical features of patients with microinvasive carcinoma do not differ from those with non-invasive lesions. The peak age is 35–45 years, which overlaps with the mean age for HG-SIL and is about 10 years younger than the mean age for overall invasive cervical carcinoma.

Histopathologically, invasion is defined as tumor cells moving across the level of the basement membrane that underlies the basal cells of normal squamous epithelium. Normal squamous cells as well as cells of an intraepithelial lesion never trespass the boundary of the basement membrane. Invasion requires a breach in the integrity of the basement membrane, which is presumably achieved by newly acquired capabilities of the neoplastic cells. On light microscopy, the basement membrane corresponds to the distinct line separating epithelial basal cells from the underlying stroma. Several morphologic features are indicative of early stromal invasion: the interface between epithelial and stromal cells, which in the presence of an intact basement membrane is smooth, becomes irregular and rugged. Paradoxically, invasive cells appear to display a higher degree of maturation (accumulation of eosinophilic cytoplasm) than HG-SIL cells. They do exhibit, however, the characteristic features of malignancy including nuclear atypia, nucleoli, mitotic activity and AMFs. A desmoplastic stromal reaction is often present around the foci of invasion, consisting of loose stromal cells with a prominent inflammatory infiltrate (Fig. 12). Discontinuation of the basement membrane can be visualized on immunohistochemistry using antibodies against collagen IV or laminin (see chapter 1, pp. 40–41). Gaps in the basement membrane may occur in areas of heavy inflammation. This by itself does not qualify for invasive disease unless tumor cells are seen migrating through that gap. Conversely, nests of obviously invasive

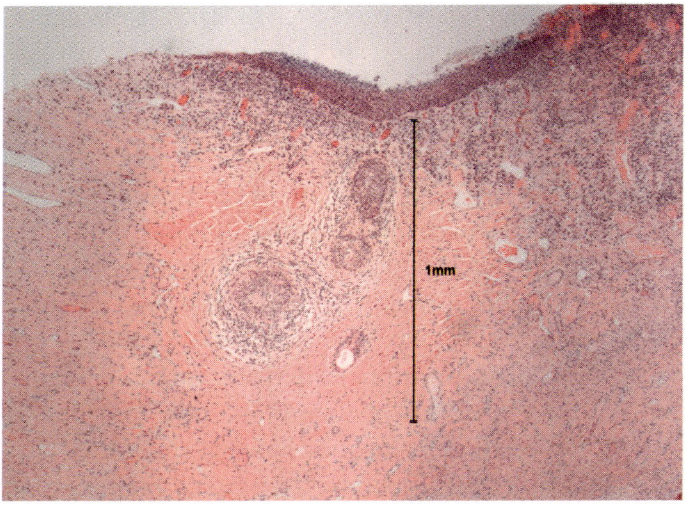

Fig. 12 Microinvasive squamous cell carcinoma. Several nests of invasive squamous cell carcinoma are present, surrounded by a desmoplastic stromal reaction. The deepest point of invasion is less than 1 mm below the basement membrane. The surface epithelium shows high grade SIL. Hematoxylin/eosin, original magnification 40×.

tumor cells can form a basement membrane around them when they are not actively invading.

Lymphvascular involvement must be carefully searched for. It is recognized as tumor cell emboli occupying endothelium-lined lymphatic or venous spaces. To exclude overinterpretation of tissue retraction artifact, immunohistochemical stains specific for vascular or lymphatic endothelium (Factor VIII, podoplanin [D2-40]) can be performed. Microinvasive cervical cancer without lymphvascular involvement can be treated with cone biopsy, trachelectomy or simple hysterectomy. It has a good prognosis with a recurrence rate of less than 3%.[38] Tumors beyond FIGO stage IA1 have a significantly higher risk of lymph node involvement or distant metastasis and require more aggressive treatment.

FIGO Stage IA2 and Up

Although higher stage cervical carcinomas can continue to remain asymptomatic, the appearance of clinical symptoms (vaginal, especially postcoital bleeding, malodorous discharge) usually means that the tumor is past the microinvasive stage. Pain, fistulas, edema of legs, hematuria and weight loss are signs of advanced disease.

On gross examination, early stage cervical carcinoma is located in and close to the transformation zone. In later stages the entire cervix may be involved, exhibiting either an exophytic or an endophytic tumor growth, the latter resulting in a "barrel-shaped" cervix.

Microscopically, irregular clusters, nests and cords of polygonal squamoid cells pervade the stroma, exceeding the limits defined for microinvasive disease. Areas of necrosis may be present. Keratinizing squamous cell carcinomas by definition form keratin "pearls" (a single pearl is sufficient), while non-keratinizing carcinomas may have individual cell keratinization, but no pearls.

The HPV type identified in the tumor has implications on the prognosis, type 18 being associated with more aggressive behavior.[39,40] Most recurrences occur within two years of the initial therapy. If a carcinoma "recurs" after more than five years, it may actually represent a second primary tumor, caused by persisting risk factors

(HPV infection) or even induced by radiation/chemotherapy for the previous tumor.

Carcinoma During Pregnancy

Cervical carcinoma occurring during pregnancy deserves special consideration: pregnancy care offers the chance of a gynecologic exam including cervical cytology to every pregnant woman, including those who otherwise might have never seen a gynecologist. This implies the opportunity of an early diagnosis of cervical neoplasia. Approximately 3% of all cervical cancers are diagnosed during pregnancy at a mean age of 32 years. Indeed, 84% of these cases are diagnosed in FIGO stage I. Despite reports to the contrary, most studies show that cervical carcinoma diagnosed during pregnancy has a similar prognosis as in the non-pregnant state when stratified stage by stage. Nevertheless, the diagnosis of invasive cervical carcinoma during pregnancy has always far more complex implications than in the non-pregnant patient. Management must be individualized and interdisciplinary, considering the patient's age, gestational age, obstetrical history, tumor size, etc.

Biopsies can be taken during pregnancy, and as long as the lesion is *in situ*, further treatment is generally deferred until after delivery. The only indication for a cone biopsy during pregnancy is to rule out or confirm invasive carcinoma, if this has immediate consequences for further management. Although a diagnosis of invasive carcinoma becomes a treatment priority, a delay of 6–12 weeks is considered acceptable if during that time fetal maturity can be achieved.[41]

Cervical biopsies obtained during pregnancy can show areas of stromal decidualization, sometimes very focally (Fig. 13). Because decidualized stromal cells assume a polygonal shape, this condition may simulate an invasive squamous cell carcinoma. Absence of cytologic atypia and lack of mitotic activity usually lead to the correct interpretation, but it is most important to provide the pertinent clinical information. In case of doubt, decidualized stromal cells are negative for cytokeratins on immunohistochemistry.

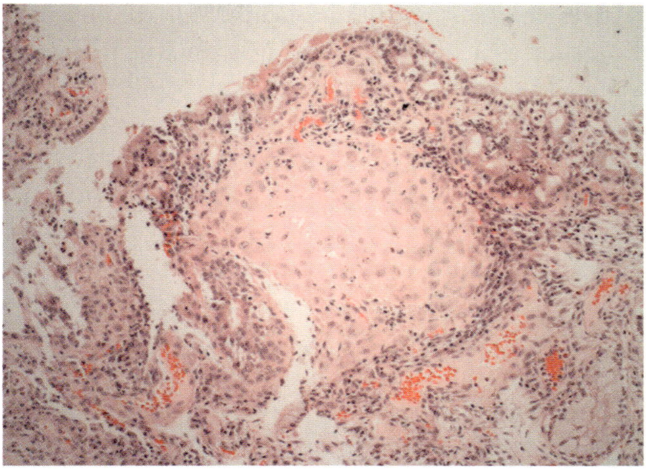

Fig. 13 Cervical biopsy from a patient who was 14 weeks pregnant. The image shows endocervical tissue with a focus of stromal decidualization (center). Also present is microglandular hyperplasia (upper right). Hematoxylin/eosin, original magnification 100×.

Histologic Subtypes

Most squamous cell carcinomas belong to the large cell type, either keratinizing or non-keratinizing. Occasionally, cells of a squamous cell carcinoma can accumulate abundant cytoplasmic glycogen and resemble clear cell carcinoma, but absence of nuclear hobnailing and lack of tubular or papillary structures favor a squamous cell differentiation.

Among the other histologic subtypes, the following are noteworthy:

Verrucous carcinoma (Buschke-Löwenstein "giant condyloma") can occur on the cervix and displays similar features as its vulvar counterpart. This includes a high degree of differentiation and a broad margin pushing against the underlying stroma. It virtually never metastasizes, unless it is radiated, which is therefore contraindicated. Complete surgical removal is usually curative.

Warty (condylomatous) carcinoma displays prominent cytologic atypia and koilocytotic changes. Papillary squamous cell carcinoma is rare and shares features with transitional cell carcinoma. The two forms often occur as a spectrum, and it is unclear if their distinction is of any value. Since this tumor forms large papillary structures with fibrovascular cores, it may be underdiagnosed on a cervical biopsy as intraepithelial disease when it is in fact part of an invasive tumor. Cone biopsy is required to rule out invasion. Lymphoepithelioma-like carcinoma is composed of undifferentiated cells growing in syncytium-like clusters with a heavy inflammatory infiltrate. It resembles nasopharyngeal carcinoma, however an association with Epstein Barr virus (EBV) has only been described in Asian women. In Caucasians, HPV has been detected in some cases. This entity is important to recognize because despite its undifferentiated phenotype it has a relatively good prognosis. In particular, it needs to be differentiated from glassy cell carcinoma, which is considered a poorly differentiated variant of cervical adenosquamous carcinoma and has a much worse prognosis. Glassy cell carcinoma also exhibits a poorly differentiated phenotype with pronounced inflammatory infiltrate, but has distinct cell borders. True lymphoproliferative disorders can be distinguished using immunohistochemical markers for lymphoid cells.

Grading

Tumor grading is based on the degree of differentiation as reflected by the amount of keratinization (grade 1 showing keratin pearls, grade 2 individual cell keratinization and grade 3 no keratinization at all) and the degree of cytologic atypia. However, the prognostic value of this grading system is questionable. In fact, keratinizing tumors tend to have a worse prognosis than non-keratinizing ones.

Adenocarcinoma

Epidemiology and Clinical Aspects

Similar to endocervical adenocarcinoma *in situ* (AIS), a significant increase in the incidence of invasive endocervical adenocarcinoma has been reported over the past decades in both relative and absolute numbers. The age-adjusted incidence rate of cervical adenocarcinoma increased from 1.34 in 1973 to 1.73 per 100,000 women in 1996 (a 29% increase in 24 years!).[29,42,43] At the same time, the proportion of adenocarcinomas relative to squamous cell carcinomas has doubled. Currently, 15%–20% of all cervical carcinomas are adenocarcinomas. The reasons for this increase are not entirely understood; one likely factor is that adenocarcinoma and its precursor lesions are less amenable to early detection by cytologic screening tests than squamous cell carcinoma. Given its association with HPV infections, cervical adenocarcinoma has basically the same risk factors as its squamous counterpart. HPV 16 is the most frequently found type (43% of cases), but the proportion of HPV 18 associated tumors is higher among adenocarcinomas (32% of cases) compared to squamous cell carcinomas.[17]

Early stage invasive endocervical adenocarcinoma may be asymptomatic or may present with non-specific symptoms like bleeding, discharge or pain. It has a good prognosis when excised completely. For lesions less than 3.0 mm in depth (FIGO stage IA1), the recurrence rate is less than 2%.[44] Adenocarcinoma appears to have a worse prognosis with a hazards ratio ranging from 1.39 to 1.94 depending on tumor stage at the time of diagnosis, compared to squamous cell carcinoma.[45] Therefore a more aggressive treatment is traditionally preferred for adenocarcinoma even in early stages. Recent evidence suggests that in the absence of lymphvascular involvement early invasive adenocarcinoma can be safely treated more conservatively, i.e. with simple hysterectomy or conization alone.[44,46]

Microinvasive Adenocarcinoma

The concept of "microinvasive" disease is accepted for endocervical adenocarcinoma, but its definition is even more problematic than for squamous cell carcinoma. Adenocarcinoma poses its own difficulties in recognizing when the process has progressed beyond the *in situ* stage. As opposed to the ectocervical epithelial-stromal interface, the endocervical subepithelial basement membrane does not form a straight line. Especially well differentiated endocervical adenocarcinoma can maintain an inconspicuous architecture and display a very dispersed

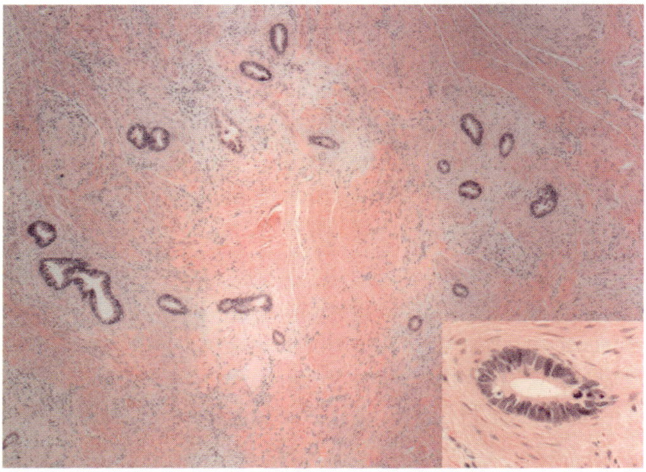

Fig. 14 Well differentiatied (G1) invasive endocervical adenocarcinoma. Note haphazard arrangement of well-formed glandular structures. Desmoplastic stromal reaction is often best appreciated on low magnification. On high magnification, the glands are lined by malignant epithelium showing high nuclear/cytoplasmic ratio, nuclear pleomorphism and mitotic activity. Hematoxylin/eosin, original magnification 40×, inset 400×.

pattern of invasion (Fig. 14). Features characteristic for early stromal invasion of a glandular lesion include the following:

1. Haphazard architecture with irregular borders that deviates from the usual lobular arrangement of normal endocervical glands.
2. A desmoplastic stromal response (loose edematous connective tissue that may show an inflammatory infiltrate) around the neoplastic glands (Fig. 14).
3. Individual cell or small cell group stromal invasion.
4. Buds of epithelial cells with more abundant eosinophilic cytoplasm emerging from neoplastic glandular structures (Fig. 15).
5. Presence of neoplastic glands deep in the cervical wall, beyond the level of adjacent residual normal endocervical glands.
6. Some authors also accept the finding of dilated glandular structures with architecturally complex intraglandular growth (cribriforming) as evidence of invasive disease.[30]

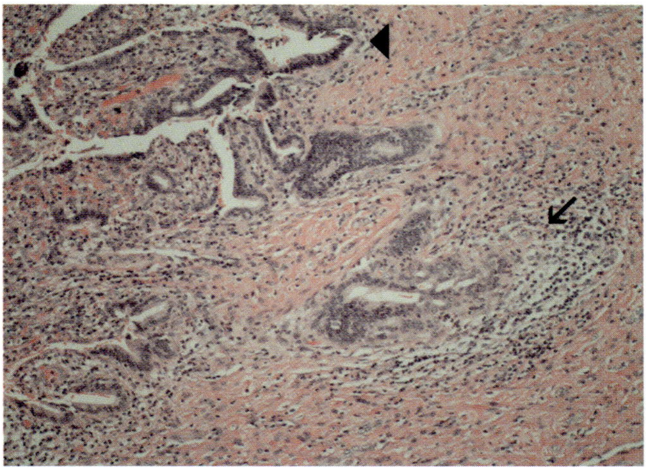

Fig. 15 Early invasive endocervical adenocarcinma. Invasive cells budding out from a glandular structure, surrounded by a desmoplastic stromal reaction (arrow). Also seen are foci of adenocarcinoma *in situ* (arrowhead).

For adenocarcinoma, the depth of stromal invasion is measured as the distance of the deepest point of invasion from the endocervical lumen.

Histologic Subtypes

Most endocervical adenocarcinomas are of mucinous differentiation. They can display endometrioid, endocervical, intestinal, signet ring cell or mixed phenotypes. Virtually all of these are HPV associated[16,47] and have a similar biologic behavior and prognosis. The rare villoglandular carcinoma is characterized by very slender papillary projections, lined by endocervical, endometrioid or intestinal-type epithelium. This is a well differentiated HPV (mostly type 16) — associated carcinoma, which has a relatively favorable prognosis.

The following tumors are rare and not associated with HPV infections: primary serous carcinomas of the endocervix are highly aggressive and morphologically resemble ovarian or endometrial serous carcinomas. This includes high grade cytologic features and nuclear hobnailing; psammoma bodies may be present. Clear cell carcinoma, when not DES-associated, tends to occur in postmenopausal women, and also has an aggressive behavior.

The so-called *minimal deviation* adenocarcinoma (MDA) is a very well differentiated invasive adenocarcinoma. Most display an endocervical-type mucinous phenotype (also known as *adenoma malignum)*, but endometrioid and clear cell variants have been described. It is characterized by glandular structures showing a great variability in size and shape (including "clover leaf"-like structures), which deeply penetrate the cervical wall. Normal endocervical glands are not usually seen beyond 7.0 mm into the cervical stroma. The neoplastic glands are lined by a bland appearing epithelium that shows occasional mitotic figures. Although mitoses are an important criterion, they are not diagnostic by themselves. The diagnosis of MDA should not be made unless at least rare foci of obvious stromal invasion (single cell invasion, desmoplastic reaction) are present. The clinical history of a slowly enlarging cervix is also important. Because of its bland morphology, the diagnosis of MDA is often challenging. The following adjunct studies may be helpful: like other mucinous endocervical adenocarcinomas, most MDAs show at least focal cytoplasmic CEA expression, and are negative for estrogen and progesterone receptors. Due to the production of abnormal mucins, MDA glands stain red on a combined Alcian Blue (pH 2.5)/PAS stain, whereas normal glands display a purple color;[48] MDA is also positive for the gastric mucin markers HIK1083 and/or MUC6.[49] When diagnosed correctly, the prognosis of MDA, stage by stage, is similar to that of other mucinous-type endocervical adenocarcinomas. The erroneous notion that (despite the well differentiated phenotype) this is a highly aggressive tumor is probably a result of diagnostic difficulties in early stage disease. MDA needs to be differentiated from benign look-alikes, including deep-seated Nabothian cysts, tunnel clusters and mesonephric hyperplasia. Lobular endocervical glandular hyperplasia (LEGH) is also in the differential diagnosis. Although generally considered a benign condition, LEGH has recently been suggested as a precursor to MDA, based on overlapping morphologic and immunohistochemical findings.[49] Patients with Peutz-Jeghers syndrome have an increased risk for developing cervical MDA as well as the peculiar ovarian sex cord stromal tumors with annular tubules; therefore these patients need close gynecologic surveillance. On the other hand, cervical MDA can be associated with ovarian mucinous tumors, which need to be carefully ruled out.

Adenocarcinoma arising from the mesonephric remnant is located deep in the lateral cervical wall and thus is not amenable to early diagnosis. It can be differentiated from its benign counterpart by the typical morphologic features of malignancy, including an infiltrative architectural pattern, cytologic atypia and mitotic activity.

Grading

Histologic grading of endocervical adenocarcinoma is based on the proportion of solid tumor versus glandular formations: a well differentiated tumor (G1) shows 10% or less of a solid component; a moderately differentiated (G2) tumor has 11%–50% solid elements; a poorly differentiated (G3) tumor is solid in more than 50% of its volume.

Other Epithelial Tumors

Depending upon the series reported, adenosquamous carcinoma constitutes up to 25% of all cervical carcinomas. It is defined by the presence of clearly identifiable malignant glandular and malignant squamoid areas. Adenosquamous carcinomas are HPV associated. They appear to have a somewhat worse prognosis compared to cervical squamous cell- and adenocarcinomas, which is reflected by the histopathologic findings of higher tumor grade and higher frequency of lymphvascular involvement.[50,51] Adenosquamous carcinoma is also less frequently associated with SIL or AIS, which makes it particularly difficult to detect at an early stage.[1] The rare but highly aggressive glassy cell carcinoma is considered a poorly differentiated variant of adenosquamous carcinoma. It is composed of undifferentiated polygonal cells with distinct cell borders, slightly granular ("ground glass" appearance) cytoplasm, prominent nucleoli and a high mitotic index. The stroma contains a chronic inflammatory infiltrate. Occasional glandular formations may be present. Glassy cell carcinoma must be differentiated from lymphoepithelioma-like carcinoma, which has indistinct cell borders.

Adenoid cystic carcinoma is composed of small basaloid cells with a cribriform architecture. The cystic spaces are filled with hyaline material. It needs to be distinguished from adenoid-basal carcinoma, which displays similar cytologic features. As opposed to adenoid-cystic carcinoma, tumor nests of adenoid-basal carcinoma tend to undergo central necrosis and contain cystic spaces filled with cellular debris. Adenoid-basal carcinoma has a relatively favorable prognosis, although at the time of diagnosis it is often found to have deeply invaded into the cervical stroma.

Neuroendocrine tumors of the cervix are rare and are classified as elsewhere in the body.[52] Except for small cell carcinomas, they are characterized by a typical growth pattern in nests, cords and acini, and a coarsely granulated ("salt and pepper") nuclear chromatin structure. Immunohistochemically, they are variably positive for chromogranin A, synaptophysin and/or neuron-specific enolase. Typical ("classical") carcinoid tumors have a low mitotic index (MI) of less than 5 mitoses per 10 high power fields (HPF) and no necrosis. Atypical carcinoids show a MI of 5–10 mitoses per 10 HPF and/or tumor necrosis. If the MI is even higher, the diagnosis of a large cell neuroendocrine carcinoma is made. Small cell carcinomas of the cervix may also display neuroendocrine features on electron microscopy and/or immunohistochemistry. They are composed of immature cells with high nuclear/cytoplasmic ratio, finely stippled chromatin, and high mitotic acitivity. Nuclear molding, crush artifact and extensive necrosis are characteristic morphologic features. While typical carcinoid tumors have a relatively favorable prognosis, large cell neuroendocrine carcinomas and small cell carcinomas are highly aggressive tumors. Most neuroendocrine tumors of the cervix are HPV-associated.

Staging

Tumor stage is the single most important prognostic factor for cervical carcinoma. The Fédération Internationale de Gynécologie et d'Obstétrique (FIGO) recommends determination of the tumor stage based on clinical (i.e. pretreatment) findings. The reason is that some patients will not come to operation if they are deemed inoperable or unfit to undergo surgery. Also, a clinical staging system will allow comparing treatment and prognostic data from developed countries to those from countries where advanced technology is not available. The following exams and procedures are accepted as contributions to the clinical staging: inspection, palpation, colposcopy, cervical biopsy including conization and amputation of the cervix, endocervical curettage, hysteroscopy, cystoscopy, proctoscopy, intravenous urography, X-ray exams of lungs and skeleton, and fine needle aspiration of lymph nodes. In contrast, results from optional examinations like laparoscopically or radiologically guided biopsy or aspiration, CT, MRI, PET, lymphangiography, arteriography and venography are not to be used for clinical staging, because these techniques are not universally available. Of course, any of these diagnostic procedures may be used to develop an optimized treatment plan. In case of doubt, the lesser stage should be utilized. If surgery is performed, the histopathologic information obtained from the specimen may be included for staging, but should be indicated as such. The clinical stage cannot be changed due to subsequent findings or treatment effects once the treatment has started.

For definition of tumor stages in the FIGO and AJCC classification systems, see Table 1. As for other carcinomas of the female genital tract, the definitions for primary tumor stages in the AJCC classification parallel that of the FIGO system; note however that any lymph node involvement results in a FIGO stage IIIB, regardless of the extent of the cervical tumor. Overall 5-year survival rates for all age groups as published in the FIGO report on the results of treatment for carcinoma of the cervix uteri are 97.5%, 94.8%, 89.1%, 75.7%, 73.4%, 65.8%, 39.7%, 41.5%, 22.0% and 9.3% for FIGO stages IA1, IA2, IB1, IB2, IIA, IIB, IIIA, IIIB, IVA and IVB, respectively.

Table 1. Staging of Cervical Carcinoma[62]

TNM category	FIGO stage	Definition
Primary Tumor (T)		
TX	—	Primary tumor cannot be assessed
T0	—	No evidence of primary tumor
Tis	0	Carcinoma *in situ*, high grade CIN
T1	I	Cervical carcinoma confined to uterus (extension to the corpus does not alter the stage)
T1a	IA	Invasive carcinoma diagnosed only by microscopy (not clinically visible)
$T1a_1$	IA1	Measured stromal invasion 3.0 mm or less in depth and 7.0 mm or less in horizontal spread
$T1a_2$	IA2	Measured stromal invasion more than 3.0 mm but not more than 5.0 mm in depth and 7.0 mm or less in horizontal spread
T1b	IB	Clinically visible lesion of any size confined to the cervix or microscopic lesion greater than $T1a_2$
$T1b_1$	IB1	Lesion 4.0 cm or less in greatest dimension
$T1b_2$	IB2	Lesion more than 4.0 cm in greatest dimension
T2	II	Cervical carcinoma invades beyond uterus but not to pelvic wall or to lower third of vagina
T2a	IIA	Tumor without parametrial invasion
T2b	IIB	Tumor with parametrial invasion
T3	III	Tumor extends to pelvic wall and/or involves lower third of vagina and/or causes hydronephrosis or non-functioning kidney
T3a	IIIA	Tumor involves lower third of vagina, no extension to pelvic wall
T3b	IIIB	Tumor extends to pelvic wall and/or causes hydronephrosis or non-functioning kidney
T4	IVA	Tumor invades mucosa of bladder or rectum (bullous edema is not sufficient to classify a tumor as T4) and/or extends beyond true pelvis
Regional Lymph Nodes (N)		
NX	—	Regional lymph nodes cannot be assessed
N0	—	No regional lymph node metastasis
N1	IIIB	Regional lymph node metastasis

(*Continued*)

Table 1. (*Continued*)

TNM category	FIGO stage	Definition
Distant Metastasis (M)		
MX	—	Distant metastasis cannot be assessed
M0	—	No distant metastasis
M1	IVB	Distant metastasis present

Legend: Vascular space involvement of primary tumor does not affect stage classification, but should be reported. Regional lymph nodes are the parametrial, paracervical, obturator, internal (hypogastric), external and common iliac, sacral and presacral lymph nodes. Para-aortic lymph node involvement is considered a distant metastasis (M1).

Stratified for the same stages, the frequency of lymph nodal involvement is 3.9%, 9.7%, 17.1%, 30.5%, 28.8%, 37.7%, 48.3%, 60.7%, 57.1% and 91.7%.[45]

Sentinel Lymph Nodes

As for other malignancies of the female genital tract, sentinel lymph node (SLN) analysis is not (yet) standard of care in the treatment of cervical cancer, and its clinical utility is still being investigated. The detection rate of SLNs, using a combination of a radiolabeled colloid and blue dye, varies from 80% to 100%. Most commonly the SLN is located in the external iliac area, followed by the common iliac and parametrial areas. The negative predictive value ranges from 87.5% to 100% in various recent studies.[53] Immunohistochemical analysis of nodal tissue sections for cytokeratins increases the sensitivity to detect micrometastases. Additional analysis for the presence of HPV DNA or mRNA in the nodal tissue may further enhance the negative predictive value of SLN examination. Unfortunately, these ancillary studies are not available at the time of intraoperative consultation when the decision has to be made whether or not a complete pelvic lymphadenectomy is necessary. It is hoped that by means of SLN examination the high frequency of lymphocele formation, lymphedema, bladder dysfunction and nerve damage associated with pelvic lymph node dissection can substantially be reduced in eligible patients. This is especially true for patients with early stage disease, who have a very low risk of lymph node metastases and frequently undergo unnecessary lymph node dissection. Conversely, only early stage patients are eligible for SLN analysis, because with increasing size of the primary tumor the detection rate of the SLN decreases substantially. SLN analysis has been successfully performed during minimally invasive (laparoscopic) radical hysterectomy.

Pathology Report

Early stage cervical or vaginal lesions are frequently treated with conservative surgical procedures, i.e. LEEP/cone biopsies, simple hysterectomy or excisional biopsies. The following issues should routinely be addressed in the pathology report of cervical or vaginal lesions:

1. Preinvasive disease: Presence of a lesion; type of lesion (squamous, glandular); grading (in the CIN/VAIN or SIL system); involvement of endocervical glands by SIL; status of resection margins (note that squamous lesions involving endocervical glands can extend to the deep stromal margin of a LEEP/cone specimen!); distance from closest resection margin in cases of adenocarcinoma *in situ*; for LEEP/cone biopsies, a statement whether the squamocolumnar junction and/or transformation zone is included in the specimen.
2. Invasive disease: Presence of invasive disease; histologic subtype; tumor grade; exact measurements of depth of stromal invasion and horizontal extent in mm; if a hysterectomy or trachelectomy specimen is available, percentage of full thickness of the cervical wall that is involved; presence of lymphvascular space involvement; status of resection margins. The College of American Pathologists (CAP) recommends including a statement on tumor stage in the American Joint Committee on Cancer (AJCC) classification (TNM system). It should be indicated that the report refers to the pathologic tumor stage (pTNM). The FIGO stage, which tends to be more popular among gynecologic oncologists,

may as well be provided. Detailed guidelines about the information to be included in a pathology report ("Cancer Protocols and Checklists") have been elaborated by the CAP and can be accessed under www.CAP.org.

CARCINOMA OF THE VAGINA

To qualify as vaginal primary carcinoma, there must be no involvement of either cervix or vulva. If there is a history of cervical carcinoma within the past five years, a vaginal tumor is classified as recurrence. This is of course an arbitrary definition and may result in under-estimation of the incidence of primary vaginal carcinoma. Uncertainty about the site of origin arises primarily in advanced stage cases when the tumor involves multiple adjacent organs at the time of diagnosis. In early stage disease it will generally be obvious where the primary site is located.

Primary vaginal carcinoma is rare; its incidence is only approximately 2% that of cervical carcinoma. 80% of vaginal carcinomas are squamous cell carcinomas, histologically similar to cervical squamous cell carcinomas. Most occur in the upper third of the vagina and on the posterior wall. Occasionally, vaginal adenocarcinomas, including non-DES associated clear cell carcinomas, arise from endometriosis of the rectovaginal septum. The diagnosis of "microinvasive" carcinoma is not defined for vaginal carcinoma. Regarding the morphologic identification of early stromal invasion, histologic subtypes, grading, HPV-association, and pathologic examination, similar principles apply as for cervical carcinoma. For staging of vaginal carcinoma, see Table 2. Reported 5-year survival rates for vaginal carcinoma are 90.3%, 77.6%, 52.2%, 42.5%, 20.5% and 12.9% for FIGO stages 0, I, II, III, IVA and IVB, respectively.[54]

DES-Associated Clear Cell Carcinoma

Clear cell adenocarcinoma of the vagina and/or cervix has been reported in approximately 0.1% of women who were exposed to DES *in utero*. The median age at diagnosis was 19 years, and the

Table 2. Staging of Vaginal Carcinoma[62]

TNM category	FIGO stage	Definition
Primary Tumor (T)		
TX	—	Primary tumor cannot be assessed
T0	—	No evidence of primary tumor
Tis	0	Carcinoma *in situ*, high grade VAIN
T1	I	Tumor confined to vaginal wall
T2	II	Tumor invades paravaginal tissue but does not extend to pelvic wall
T3	III	Tumor extends to pelvic wall
T4	IVA	Tumor invades mucosa of the bladder or rectum (bullous edema is not sufficient to classify a tumor as T4) and/or extends beyond the true pelvis
Regional Lymph Nodes (N)		
NX	—	Regional lymph nodes cannot be assessed
N0	—	No regional lymph node metastasis
N1	III	Pelvic or inguinal lymph node metastasis
Distant Metastasis (M)		
MX	—	Distant metastasis cannot be assessed
M0	—	No distant metastasis
M1	IVB	Distant metastasis present

Legend: Pelvic wall is defined as muscle, fascia, neurovascular structures or skeletal portions of the bony pelvis. Regional lymph nodes are the pelvic lymph nodes, including obturator, internal (hypogastric) and external iliac nodes for lesions of the upper two-thirds of the vagina; and inguinal and femoral lymph nodes for lesions of the lower third of the vagina.

risk appeared to be greater if the drug was administered early during pregnancy. Similar to vaginal adenosis, clear cell carcinoma most frequently involves the upper third of the anterior vaginal wall. The assumption that vaginal adenosis is a precursor lesion to clear cell carcinoma, however, has never been proven. Small tumors may be invisible if they are located submucosally, but they may be palpable. Histologically, the tumors are similar to other clear cell carcinomas of the Müllerian tract. They display various architectural patterns (solid, papillary, tubulo-glandular), glycogen containing cells with clear cytoplasm, distinct cell borders, nuclear "hobnailing" and variable nuclear pleomorphism. The differential diagnosis includes microglandular hyperplasia or Arias-Stella reaction occurring in vaginal adenosis, and metastatic clear cell carcinoma of either Müllerian or renal origin. The prognosis of DES-associated clear cell carcinoma appears to be somewhat better than if DES-unrelated, the 5-year survival rate being 84% versus 69%, respectively.[55] The youngest women that were still exposed to DES are by now beyond the peak age for DES-associated clear cell carcinoma, but it cannot be excluded that a second peak for this or another neoplasm will emerge in the future.

Embryonal Rhabdomyosarcoma

Vaginal embryonal rhabdomyosarcoma typically occurs in infants: the mean age at diagnosis is 2 years and 90% of all cases are diagnosed before the age of 5 years. However, it has been reported in women up into the fifth decade of life. The tumor presents as an exophytic, polypoid nodular mass, covered by an intact mucosa. Histologically it is composed of immature oval to spindle-shaped cells with occasional eosinophilic cytoplasm. Cross striation may be seen, but is not required for the diagnosis. The most frequent subtype, *sarcoma botryoides*, is characterized by subepithelial areas of cellular condensation (cambium layer). Immunohistochemical positivity for muscle specific actin, desmin and myoglobin as well as electron microscopy may be helpful to confirm the diagnosis. This tumor has a highly aggressive natural course, but with the advent of modern chemotherapy survival rates of up to 95% for *sarcoma botryoides* have been achieved. The differential diagnosis includes the benign entities of fibroepithelial polyp, Müllerian papilloma and rhabdomyoma. The rare vaginal yolk sac tumor shares a similar age distribution, natural course and responsiveness to chemotherapy with embryonal rhabdomyosarcoma. The Intergroup Rhabdomyosarcoma Study Group has elaborated a special clinical classification system for rhabdomyosarcomas (Table 3).

Table 3. Clinical Classification Groups for Rhabdomyosarcoma

Group	Clinical findings
I	Localized disease, completely resected, no regional nodes involved
Ia	Confined to organ or muscle of origin
Ib	Infiltration outside organ or muscle of origin
II	Regional disease
IIa	Microscopic residual disease, no regional nodes involved
IIb	Regional disease, completely resected, nodes may be involved and/or extension of tumor into adjacent organ
IIc	Regional disease with involved nodes, grossly resected, but with evidence of microscopic residues
III	Incomplete resection or biopsy with gross residual disease
IV	Distant metastases present at onset

Malignant Melanoma

Melanocytic lesions, including blue nevi and malignant melanomas, rarely occur as primary tumors in the cervix or vagina. Melanoma may or may not be pigmented. Early diagnosis is not impossible, but would be rather incidental because melanoma is not routinely screened for in this location. Although malignant melanoma may be noted as a pigmented mucosal lesion, and can be picked up on cervical cytologic smears,[56,57] this does not necessarily correspond to an early stage. Melanoma is known for its great histomorphologic variability. Therefore, whenever a malignant tumor with unusual histologic features is found in the vagina or cervix, malignant melanoma should be considered. Immunohistochemical positivity for S-100 protein, HMB-45 and/or Melan-A supports the diagnosis. As opposed to metastatic malignant melanoma, primary vaginal/cervical melanoma tends to have an extensive lateral junctional component. The further differential diagnosis includes blue nevus, poorly differentiated squamous cell carcinoma and sarcoma. Given the rarity of malignant melanoma in this location, a clinically identified "pigmented lesion" of the vagina/cervix more likely corresponds to foci of endometriosis, stromal endometriosis or a hemangioma.

The Chung classification for staging of mucosal melanoma of the female genital tract is defined as follows:

Level I — tumor confined to the surface epithelium.
Level II — invasion of 1 mm or less.
Level III — invasion 1 mm–2 mm.
Level IV — invasion greater than 2 mm.

Using this classification, most vaginal malignant melanomas are level IV at presentation. The prognosis is poor with an overall 5 year survival rate of 30%–40%.[54]

OTHER MALIGNANT TUMORS OF THE VAGINA AND CERVIX

Leiomyosarcoma of the vagina is histologically similar to that arising from other sites. In the vagina, any smooth muscle tumor larger than 3 cm in diameter, with a mitotic index of 5 or more MF per 10 HPF, moderate or marked cytologic atypia, and infiltrating borders should be considered a leiomyosarcoma.

Adenosarcoma may present as (recurrent) vaginal or endocervical "polyps". The presence of stromal mitoses in conjunction with perivascular hypercellularity (cuffing) is the clue for histopathologic identification.

For discussion of aggressive angiomyxoma see chapter 1, pp. 32–33.

Given the rarity of primary vaginal malignancies, the majority of malignant tumors involving the vagina are due to secondary extension, most frequently from cervix, endometrium, colorectum, bladder and vulva. Distant metastases to vagina or cervix are rare, and if encountered the likely primary sites are ovary, colon, stomach, breast, and choriocarcinoma.

ANCILLARY STUDIES

Markers specific for a certain entity are discussed in the respective section above. Ancillary studies helpful for the identification of early stromal invasion (collagen IV, laminin) and lymphvascular involvement (podoplanin/D2-40), and the work-up for metastatic tumors with unknown primaries are described in chapter 1, and can be similarly applied to lesions of the vagina or cervix. The same is true for p16 and MIB-1/Ki-67 as adjunct markers for diagnosing HPV-associated squamous lesions, although some considerations specific to the vagina and cervix are mentioned below. The following is a list of additional clinical scenarios in which special studies may help to establish the diagnosis of cervicovaginal malignant or premalignant lesions and differentiate them from benign mimickers.

Dysplastic Squamous Epithelium versus Atrophic Squamous Epithelium, Immature Squamous Metaplasia, Transitional Cell Metaplasia or Inflammatory Atypia

Due to its association with HPV infection, dysplastic squamous epithelium shows diffuse nuclear and cytoplasmic positivity for p16, whereas the mimickers are negative for p16. MIB-1 is expressed in nuclei of all layers in dysplastic epithelium, but only in the parabasal cell layer of benign squamous epithelium. Note that MIB-1 expression pattern is not helpful for grading of a squamous lesion, since even low-grade SIL can display MIB-1 positive nuclei in the upper layers. The combination of both p16 and MIB-1 can increase diagnostic accuracy. Atrophy is a notorious mimicker of high grade dysplasia on both cytology and histology and should always be considered in postmenopausal patients, especially when no mitotic activity is seen.

AIS versus Benign Mimickers

Since most endocervical glandular lesions are also HPV-related, they diffusely express p16, like squamous lesions. The utility of this expression pattern is however compromised because normal endocervical epithelium as well as areas of tubo-endometrioid metaplasia and cervical endometriosis may also exhibit focal p16-positivity. Similarly, a MIB-1 stain shows a proliferative index of more than 30% in AIS, but less than 10% in benign mimickers. CEA is frequently expressed in the cytoplasm of neoplastic glandular cells (cave: expression in the apical cell membrane or in extracellular mucus is non-specific!), whereas benign glandular cells are negative for CEA. Conversely, vimentin is expressed in normal and neoplastic endometrial epithelium, tubo-endometrioid metaplasia and endometriosis, but not in AIS. Bcl-2 has been reported positive in tubo-endometrioid metaplasia and endometriosis, but negative in AIS.

AIS versus Microinvasive Endocervical Adenocarcinoma

Desmoplastic stroma associated with an invasive process contains SMA-positive myofibroblasts and is negative for estrogen receptors, while normal cervical stroma is ER positive and does not contain myofibroblasts. These considerations may also be helpful to establish the diagnosis of a minimal deviation adenocarcinoma, see below.

Endocervical Microglandular Hyperplasia versus Endometrioid Adenocarcinoma

Fragments of well differentiated endometrial endometrioid adenocarcinomas can occasionally look strikingly similar to endocervical microglandular hyperplasia, which may give rise to a diagnostic dilemma on either endocervical or endometrial biopsies. This is especially true if the patient was placed on progesterone therapy, which results in suppression of mitotic activity and a very bland appearing cytology of cancer cells. In this scenario, stains for vimentin and MIB-1 may be helpful: cells of endocervical microglandular hyperplasia are negative for vimentin and have a proliferative index (MIB-1 nuclear positivity) of less than 1%. Conversely, endometrial endometrioid carcinoma tends to express cytoplasmic vimentin and has a proliferative index greater than 10%. In contrast to endocervical adenocarcinoma, microglandular hyperplasia is negative for CEA.

Endometrial versus Endocervical Adenocarcinoma

Not infrequently the pathologist is faced with the question whether an adenocarcinoma diagnosed on endocervical curettings is of endocervical or endometrial/lower uterine segment origin. Morphologic features that may be helpful in this setting include the following: the finding of AIS, which is thought to be the direct precursor lesion of endocervical adenocarcinoma, favors an endocervical origin. If tissue fragments resembling endometrial complex atypical hyperplasia are present, possibly with endometrial-type stroma and stromal foam cells (which can be seen in association with hyperestrogenism), an endometrial primary tumor is likely. Moreover, certain histologic subtypes (e.g. serous carcinoma) are extremely rare in the endocervix.

In addition, the following special stains may be useful: endometrial carcinoma tends to be positive for vimentin and negative for CEA, whereas the reverse is true for endocervical carcinoma. Note that only cytoplasmic positivity in glandular epithelium is diagnostic; membranous or extracellular CEA positivity, as well as staining of metaplastic squamous epithelium including squamous morules within an endometrioid carcinoma, is non-specific. Estrogen receptors are usually expressed in the nuclei of endometrial endometrioid carcinomas, but not in endocervical carcinomas. Evidence of HPV infection supports the diagnosis of an endocervical adenocarcinoma. p16 is frequently used as a surrogate (although by no means specific) marker for the presence of high risk HPV types. It can be useful in this scenario if the tumor has an endometrioid phenotype, in which case p16 positivity strongly favors an endocervical origin. However, endometrial serous carcinomas tend to be p16 positive for reasons unrelated to HPV.[58] In those histologic subtypes of adenocarcinoma that are not HPV-associated when arising from the endocervix (including serous, clear cell and minimal deviation adenocarcinoma), HPV analysis or p16 expression pattern cannot contribute to the determination of the primary site.

Müllerian Endometrioid Carcinoma versus Colon Carcinoma

Endometrioid carcinomas of Müllerian origin (i.e. arising from the endometrium, endocervix, ovaries, fallopian tubes or from foci of endometriosis) can display a remarkable morphologic variability and sometimes resemble primary colonic adenocarcinomas. The following stains are usually helpful: endometrioid carcinomas tend to be positive for cytokeratin 7, estrogen and progesterone receptors, but negative for cytokeratin 20 and CDX-2; the reverse is true for primary colonic carcinomas.

Müllerian Clear Cell Carcinoma versus Renal Clear Cell Carcinoma

In the absence of intrauterine DES exposure, primary cervical or vaginal clear cell carcinomas are extremely rare. Therefore a metastatic, especially renal origin should always be ruled out. Müllerian clear cell carcinomas are usually positive for cytokeratin 7, whereas renal carcinomas express CD10 and vimentin.

Pregnancy-related Changes

Arias-Stella reaction is a notorious mimicker of clear cell carcinoma. Stains for MIB-1 and p53 have been suggested to distinguish between these two entities. Cells of Arias-Stella reaction tend to show a proliferative index (nuclear MIB-1 positivity) of less than 5% and are negative for p53, while clear cell carcinomas display the reverse staining pattern. A minority of cases, however, exhibits an overlapping pattern.[59]

Intermediate trophoblast cells of a placental site nodule can be morphologically quite atypical and have irregular, hyperchromatic nuclei. They are positive for cytokeratins, including CK18, which is usually negative in carcinomas. In addition, they express human placental lactogen (hPL), placental alkaline phosphatase (PLAP) and inhibin. The proliferative index (MIB-1 nuclear positivity) is less than

5%. In contrast, squamous cell carcinomas are negative for the above markers, express p16 and have a proliferative index over 60%.

To differentiate various types of trophoblast cells and lesions derived from them, the following markers are useful: β-HCG is strongly expressed in syncytiotrophoblast and choriocarcinoma. HPL is positive in syncytial and intermediate trophoblast cells and strongly expressed in placental site trophoblastic tumor (PSTT). Mel-CAM (CD146) is a marker for implantation site-type intermediate trophoblast and is expressed in cells of exaggerated placental site and PSTT. PLAP is positive in syncytiotrophoblast and intermediate trophoblast, especially chorion-type. The Ki-67 proliferative index is low in placental site nodules (less than 5%), intermediate in epithelioid trophoblastic tumor (ETT) and PSTT (approximately 15%), and high in choriocarcinoma (greater than 50%). Care must be taken not to include interspersed lymphocytes into the analysis, which frequently express MIB-1. Double immunostains may be necessary to avoid this pitfall.

Small Round Blue Cell Tumors

Small cell carcinomas of the cervix or vagina may be positive for neuroendocrine markers (neuron specific enolase, synaptophysin or chromogranin). Positivity for one of these markers however is not required for the diagnosis, since one-third of the cases are negative on immunohistochemistry. Membranous expression of the CD99 antigen (Mic-2 gene product) is seen in peripheral primitive neuroectodermal tumors. Nuclear p63 expression is a marker for squamous differentiation and may help to distinguish between small cell neuroendocrine versus small cell non-keratinizing squamous cell carcinomas. The diagnosis of rhabdomyosarcoma can be supported by positivity for muscle specific actin, desmin or myoglobin. Positivity for lymphocyte common antigen (LCA) will identify lymphoproliferative disorders.

Ectopic Prostatic Tissue

As a curiosity, prostatic tissue can be encountered in the cervix and vagina, usually in the stroma. Immunohistochemical positivity for prostatic acid phosphatase and alpha-methylacyl-CoA racemase can confirm the diagnosis. PSA is expressed only in a subset of cases. The basal cell layer is positive for high molecular weight cytokeratin. No malignancies have been reported in association with this finding.[60]

HPV-VACCINE

Hailed by many as the greatest achievement in the battle against cervical cancer since the introduction of the "Pap smear", the first HPV vaccine became available in 2006. The two preparations currently on the world's markets (a bivalent vaccine covering HPV types 16 and 18, and a quadrivalent vaccine covering types 6, 11, 16 and 18) are based on virus-like particles (VLPs). In order to manufacture VLPs, the HPV type-specific L1 major capsid protein is recombinantly synthesized in eukaryotic cells. L1 proteins then self-assemble into an icosahedral particle that has a surface identical to the real virus, but does not contain a DNA core and therefore is non-infectious and non-oncogenic. The full immunization protocol calls for three injections over the course of six months and results in a strong humoral immune response with seroconversion rates of over 99%. Protection is conveyed by IgG antibodies that reach the vaginal lumen with the transudate and neutralize viral particles. The longest follow-up studies currently cover approximately six years, which is far too short to observe a decline in the incidence of cervical cancer. Substitute endpoints to assess the efficacy of the vaccine are squamous intraepithelial lesions (CIN 1–3) and endocervical adenocarcinoma *in situ* (AIS). Vaccine efficacy is measured as the reduction of endpoint events in the vaccine cohort as compared to the placebo cohort. In patients who received the full course of the vaccination and had no evidence of exposure to vaccine-type HPV until at least one month after administration of the last vaccine dose ("per protocol" population), vaccine efficacy approached 100% in several studies. If patients are included who had evidence of vaccine-type HPV infection prior to vaccination ("intention-to-treat" population), the efficacy drops to 40%–50%. When all patients (regardless of HPV status at the time of enrollment) and all lesions (regardless of associated HPV type, i.e. including HPV types not covered by the vaccine) are considered, the reduction of lesions is less than 20% in vaccinees compared to placebo recipients ("population impact"). These data demonstrate that the currently available vaccines have an excellent preventive efficacy against the vaccine HPV types; but no therapeutic effect can be expected, and cross protection against non-vaccine HPV types is at best very limited. The vaccines are considered safe, serious side-effects being extremely rare, and comparable to other vaccines that are generally accepted as beneficial.[61] The ideal target population for this vaccine are females before the onset of sexual activity, i.e. girls at the age of 11–12 years. After sexual debut, "catch-up" vaccination may still be beneficial or provide partial protection if the recipient has not been exposed to all HPV types covered by the vaccine. Males may benefit from the vaccine not so much in terms of protection against the rather rare penile carcinoma, but also against condylomata acuminata, which are a frequent cause of emotional embarrassment and reason for cumbersome medical interventions. Also, if herd immunity is desired, males need to be vaccinated in order to eliminate that viral reservoir. The usefulness of vaccinating other target groups (e.g. older adults, victims of sexual abuse, HIV positive individuals, infants born to HIV positive mothers) is still under investigation. In addition to cervical, vaginal and penile carcinomas, a significant subset of vulvar, anal, oropharyngeal and other carcinomas are associated with the same high risk HPV types, and it is expected that the vaccine will provide protection against those cancers, too. Since HPV types 16 and 18 together cause approximately "only" 70% of all cervical cancers, the vaccine does not provide protection against all cancers. Therefore it is most important to emphasize that vaccine recipients must not discontinue their screening programs!

Although it is hoped that the advent of the HPV vaccine marks the beginning of the end of cervical cancer, there is still a long way to go. Considering that it takes on average at least ten years for a high grade squamous intraepithelial lesion to progress to an invasive carcinoma, a significant reduction in the incidence of cervical cancer cannot be expected until about the year 2020. Developed countries have already experienced a dramatic reduction in cervical cancer numbers over the past decades due to efficient prevention programs. Here, the impact of the vaccine on a further reduction of morbidity and mortality will be relatively small. Most cases of invasive cervical carcinoma in industrialized countries occur in patients who did not participate in screening programs anyway, and this population is unlikely to volunteer for a vaccine. On the other hand, the greatest population impact of the HPV vaccine could be achieved in developing countries where no screening programs are in effect. There the major drawbacks of the currently available vaccines become evident: first of all, the high cost makes them practically unaffordable for the population in need. Furthermore, limited shelf life, the need to refrigerate the vaccine, and the protocol of three separate injections over the course of six months reduce the practicability in countries with compromised infrastructure. Current research efforts addressing these and other shortcomings of the first generation HPV vaccines include the following: VLP-based vaccines against more (e.g. a total of eight) HPV types; L2 (minor capsid protein)-based vaccines that evoke a broader cross protection covering numerous HPV types; single dose application vaccines; oral/nasal (inhalation) application vaccines; DNA vaccines (plasmid-based) that are stable at room temperature; therapeutic vaccines that elicit a cellular immunity against the viral E6 and E7 proteins; and chimeric vaccines that combine preventive and therapeutic properties.

REFERENCES

1. Wang SS, Sherman ME, Silverberg SG, *et al.*, Pathological characteristics of cervical adenocarcinoma in a multi-center US-based study, *Gynecol Oncol* **103**:541–546, 2006.
2. Schlosshauer PW, Chen W, Chanderdatt D, *et al.*, Monsel's artifact in gynecologic biopsies: a simple remedy, *J Histotechnol* **28**:161–162, 2005.
3. Nucci MR, Young RH, Fletcher CD, Cellular pseudcsarcomatous fibroepithelial stromal polyps of the lower female genital tract: an

underrecognized lesion often misdiagnosed as sarcoma, *Am J Surg Pathol* **24**:231–240, 2000.

4. Deligdisch L, de Resende Miranda CR, Wu HS, *et al.*, Human papillomavirus-related cervical lesions in adolescents: a histologic and morphometric study, *Gynecol Oncol* **89**:52–59, 2003.
5. Clifford GM, Rana RK, Franceschi S, *et al.*, Human papillomavirus genotype distribution in low-grade cervical lesions: comparison by geographic region and with cervical cancer, *Cancer Epidemiol Biomarkers Prev* **14**:1157–1164, 2005.
6. Evans MF, Adamson CS, Papillo JL, *et al.*, Distribution of human papillomavirus types in ThinPrep papanicolaou tests classified according to the Bethesda 2001 terminology and correlations with patient age and biopsy outcomes, *Cancer* **106**:1054–1064, 2006.
7. Missmer SA, Hankinson SE, Spiegelman D, *et al.*, *In utero* exposures and the incidence of endometriosis, *Fertil Steril* **82**:1501–1508, 2004.
8. Wise-Draper TM, Wells SI, Papillomavirus E6 and E7 proteins and their cellular targets, *Front Biosci* **13**:1003–1017, 2008.
9. Thomas M, Banks L, Human papillomavirus (HPV) E6 interactions with bak are conserved amongst E6 proteins from high and low risk HPV types, *J Gen Virol* **80**(Part 6):1513–1517, 1999.
10. Cho NH, Kim YT, Kim JW, Alteration of cell cycle in cervical tumor associated with human papillomavirus: cyclin-dependent kinase inhibitors, *Yonsei Med J* **43**:722–728, 2002.
11. Kim YT, Zhao M, Aberrant cell cycle regulation in cervical carcinoma, *Yonsei Med J* **46**:597–613, 2005.
12. Nguyen CL, Eichwald C, Nibert ML, *et al.*, Human papillomavirus type 16 E7 oncoprotein associates with the centrosomal component gamma-tubulin, *J Virol* **81**: 13533–13543, 2007.
13. Stanley MA, Pett MR, Coleman N, HPV: from infection to cancer, *Biochem Soc Trans* **35**:1456–1460, 2007.
14. Tindle RW, Immune evasion in human papillomavirus-associated cervical cancer, *Nat Rev Cancer* **2**:59–65, 2002.
15. Clifford GM, Smith JS, Aguado T, *et al.*, Comparison of HPV type distribution in high-grade cervical lesions and cervical cancer: a meta-analysis, *Br J Cancer* **89**:101–105, 2003.
16. Pirog EC, Kleter B, Olgac S, *et al.*, Prevalence of human papillomavirus DNA in different histological subtypes of cervical adenocarcinoma, *Am J Pathol* **157**:1055–1062, 2000.

17. Castellsague X, Diaz M, de Sanjose S, *et al.*, International Agency for Research on Cancer Multicenter Cervical Cancer Study Group. Worldwide human papillomavirus etiology of cervical adenocarcinoma and its cofactors: implications for screening and prevention, *J Natl Cancer Inst* **98**:303–315, 2006.
18. Appleby P, Beral V, Berrington de Gonzalez A, *et al.*, Carcinoma of the cervix and tobacco smoking: collaborative reanalysis of individual data on 13,541 women with carcinoma of the cervix and 23,017 women without carcinoma of the cervix from 23 epidemiological studies, *Int J Cancer* **118**:1481–1495, 2006.
19. Vaccarella S, Herrero R, Snijders PJ, *et al.*, Smoking and human papillomavirus infection: pooled analysis of the international agency for research on cancer HPV prevalence surveys, *Int J Epidemiol* **37**:536–546, 2008.
20. Chan JK, Monk BJ, Brewer C, *et al.*, HPV infection and number of lifetime sexual partners are strong predictors for 'natural' regression of CIN 2 and 3, *Br J Cancer* **89**:1062–1066, 2003.
21. Trimble CL, Piantadosi S, Gravitt P, *et al.*, Spontaneous regression of high-grade cervical dysplasia: effects of human papillomavirus type and HLA phenotype, *Clin Cancer Res* **11**:4717–4723, 2005.
22. Ellerbrock TV, Chiasson MA, Bush TJ, *et al.*, Incidence of cervical squamous intraepithelial lesions in HIV-infected women, *JAMA* **283**: 1031–1037, 2000.
23. Hawes SE, Critchlow CW, Sow PS, *et al.*, Incident high-grade squamous intraepithelial lesions in senegalese women with and without human immunodeficiency virus type 1 (HIV-1) and HIV-2, *J Natl Cancer Inst* **98**:100–109, 2006.
24. Carreon JD, Sherman ME, Guillen D, *et al.*, CIN2 is a much less reproducible and less valid diagnosis than CIN3: results from a histological review of population-based cervical samples, *Int J Gynecol Pathol* **26**:441–446, 2007.
25. Cai B, Ronnett BM, Stoler M, *et al.*, Longitudinal evaluation of interobserver and intraobserver agreement of cervical intraepithelial neoplasia diagnosis among an experienced panel of gynecologic pathologists, *Am J Surg Pathol* **31**:1854–1860, 2007.
26. Monsonego J, Valensi P, Zerat L, *et al.*, Simultaneous effects of aneuploidy and oncogenic human papillomavirus on histological grade of cervical intraepithelial neoplasia, *Br J Obstet Gynaecol* **104**:723–727, 1997.

27. Nagi CS, Schlosshauer PW, Endocervical glandular involvement is associated with high-grade SIL, *Gynecol Oncol* **102**: 240–243, 2006.
28. Livasy CA, Maygarden SJ, Rajaratnam CT, *et al.*, Predictors of recurrent dysplasia after a cervical loop electrocautery excision procedure for CIN3: a study of margin, endocervical gland, and quadrant involvement, *Mod Pathol* **12**:233–238, 1999.
29. Wang SS, Sherman ME, Hildesheim A, *et al.*, Cervical adenocarcinoma and squamous cell carcinoma incidence trends among white women and black women in the United States for 1976–2000, *Cancer* **100**: 1035–1044, 2004.
30. Zaino RJ, Symposium Part I: adenocarcinoma *in situ*, glandular dysplasia, and early invasive adenocarcinoma of the uterine cervix, *Int J Gynecol Pathol* **21**:314–326, 2002.
31. Schlesinger C, Silverberg SG, Endocervical adenocarcinoma *in situ* of tubal type and its relation to atypical tubal metaplasia, *Int J Gynecol Pathol* **18**:1–4, 1999.
32. Young JL, Jazaeri AA, Lachance JA, *et al.*, Cervical adenocarcinoma *in situ*: the predictive value of conization margin status, *Am J Obstet Gynecol* **197**:195.e1–7; discussion 195.e7–8, 2007.
33. Goldstein NS, Mani A, The status and distance of cone biopsy margins as a predictor of excision adequacy for endocervical adenocarcinoma *in situ*, *Am J Clin Pathol* **109**:727–732, 1998.
34. Witkiewicz A, Lee KR, Brodsky G, *et al.*, Superficial (early) endocervical adenocarcinoma *in situ*: a study of 12 cases and comparison to conventional AIS, *Am J Surg Pathol* **29**:1609–1614, 2005.
35. Lee KR, Symposium Part 4: should pathologists diagnose endocervical preneoplastic lesions "less than" adenocarcinoma *in situ*? Counterpoint, *Int J Gynecol Pathol* **22**:22–24, 2003.
36. Tavassoli FA, Devilee P, *Tumours of the Breast and Female Genital Organs*, IARC Press, Lyon, France 2003.
37. Arias-Stella J, The Arias-Stella reaction: facts and fancies four decades after, *Adv Anat Pathol* **9**:12–23, 2002.
38. Raspagliesi F, Ditto A, Solima E, *et al.*, Microinvasive squamous cell cervical carcinoma, *Crit Rev Oncol Hematol* **48**:251–261, 2003.
39. Lai CH, Chang CJ, Huang HJ, *et al.*, Role of human papillomavirus genotype in prognosis of early-stage cervical cancer undergoing primary surgery, *J Clin Oncol* **25**:3628–3634, 2007.

40. Schwartz SM, Daling JR, Shera KA, *et al.*, Human papillomavirus and prognosis of invasive cervical cancer: a population-based study, *J Clin Oncol* **19**:1906–1915, 2001.
41. Van Calsteren K, Vergote I, Amant F, Cervical neoplasia during pregnancy: diagnosis, management and prognosis, *Best Pract Res Clin Obstet Gynaecol* **19**:611–630, 2005.
42. Smith HO, Tiffany MF, Qualls CR, *et al.*, The rising incidence of adenocarcinoma relative to squamous cell carcinoma of the uterine cervix in the United States — a 24-year population–based study, *Gynecol Oncol* **78**:97–105, 2000.
43. Vinh-Hung V, Bourgain C, Vlastos G, *et al.*, Prognostic value of histopathology and trends in cervical cancer: a SEER population study, *BMC Cancer* 7:164, 2007.
44. Smith HO, Qualls CR, Romero AA, *et al.*, Is there a difference in survival for IA1 and IA2 adenocarcinoma of the uterine cervix? *Gynecol Oncol* **85**:229–241, 2002.
45. Quinn MA, Benedet JL, Odicino F, *et al.*, Carcinoma of the cervix uteri. FIGO 6th annual report on the results of treatment in gynecological cancer, *Int J Gynaecol Obstet* **95**(Suppl. 1):S43–S103, 2006.
46. Poynor EA, Marshall D, Sonoda Y, *et al.*, Clinicopathologic features of early adenocarcinoma of the cervix initially managed with cervical conization, *Gynecol Oncol* **103**:960–965, 2006.
47. An HJ, Kim KR, Kim IS, *et al.*, Prevalence of human papillomavirus DNA in various histological subtypes of cervical adenocarcinoma: a population-based study, *Mod Pathol* **18**:528–534, 2005.
48. Hayashi I, Tsuda H, Shimoda T, Reappraisal of orthodox histochemistry for the diagnosis of minimal deviation adenocarcinoma of the cervix, *Am J Surg Pathol* **24**:559–562, 2000.
49. Mikami Y, Kiyokawa T, Hata S, *et al.*, Gastrointestinal immunophenotype in adenocarcinomas of the uterine cervix and related glandular lesions: a possible link between lobular endocervical glandular hyperplasia/pyloric gland metaplasia and 'adenoma malignum', *Mod Pathol* **17**:962–972, 2004.
50. Farley JH, Hickey KW, Carlson JW, *et al.*, Adenosquamous histology predicts a poor outcome for patients with advanced-stage, but not early-stage, cervical carcinoma, *Cancer* **97**:2196–2202, 2003.
51. Yasuda S, Kojima A, Maeno Y, *et al.*, Poor prognosis of patients with stage Ib1 adenosquamous cell carcinoma of the uterine cervix with pelvic lymphnode metastasis, *Kobe J Med Sci* **52**:9–15, 2006.

52. Albores-Saavedra J, Gersell D, Gilks CB, *et al.*, Terminology of endocrine tumors of the uterine cervix: results of a workshop sponsored by the college of American pathologists and the national cancer institute, *Arch Pathol Lab Med* **121**:34–39, 1997.
53. Ayhan A, Celik H, Dursun P, Lymphatic mapping and sentinel node biopsy in gynecological cancers: a critical review of the literature, *World J Surg Oncol* **6**:53, 2008.
54. Beller U, Benedet JL, Creasman WT, *et al.*, Carcinoma of the vagina. FIGO 6th annual report on the results of treatment in gynecological cancer, *Int J Gynaecol Obstet* **95**(Suppl. 1):S29–S42, 2006.
55. Waggoner SE, Mittendorf R, Biney N, *et al.*, Influence of in utero diethylstilbestrol exposure on the prognosis and biologic behavior of vaginal clear-cell adenocarcinoma, *Gynecol Oncol* **55**:238–244, 1994.
56. Deshpande AH, Munshi MM, Primary malignant melanoma of the uterine cervix: report of a case diagnosed by cervical scrape cytology and review of the literature, *Diagn Cytopathol* **25**:108–111, 2001.
57. Schlosshauer PW, Heller DS, Koulos JP, Malignant melanoma of the uterine cervix diagnosed on a cervical cytologic smear, *Acta Cytol* **42**: 1043–1045, 1998.
58. Chiesa-Vottero AG, Malpica A, Deavers MT, *et al.*, Immunohistochemical overexpression of p16 and p53 in uterine serous carcinoma and ovarian high-grade serous carcinoma, *Int J Gynecol Pathol* **26**:328–333, 2007.
59. Vang R, Barner R, Wheeler DT, *et al.*, Immunohistochemical staining for Ki-67 and p53 helps distinguish endometrial Arias-Stella reaction from high-grade carcinoma, including clear cell carcinoma, *Int J Gynecol Pathol* **23**:223–233, 2004.
60. McCluggage WG, Ganesan R, Hirschowitz L, *et al.*, Ectopic prostatic tissue in the uterine cervix and vagina: report of a series with a detailed immunohistochemical analysis, *Am J Surg Pathol* **30**:209–215, 2006.
61. Villa LL, Overview of the clinical development and results of a quadrivalent HPV (types 6, 11, 16, 18) vaccine, *Int J Infect Dis* **11**(Suppl. 2): S17–S25, 2007.
62. Greene FL, Page DL, Fleming ID, *et al.*, *AJCC Cancer Staging Manual*, 6th edn., Springer Verlag, New York, 2002.

CHAPTER 3

EARLY DIAGNOSIS OF CERVICAL, VAGINAL AND VULVAR CANCER: A CLINICIAN'S VIEW

Albert Altchek

CERVICAL CANCER

General Considerations

The risk for cervical cancer in the US is 1 in 135 women with 11,070 new cases and 3870 deaths predicted for 2008. There has been a great decrease in the incidence of cervical cancer in the US because of Pap cytology and HPV testing. Worldwide there are about 500,000 new cases annually, mainly in the developing countries where it is the second leading cause of mortality due to cancer. The high-grade lesion biopsies or excisional procedures may be found to detect a small percentage of early cervical cancer, according to Creasman.[1] Other guidelines are more detailed with many exceptions and individualization depending on age (adolescent, postmenopausal), desire to preserve fertility, pregnancy and different life styles. Endocervical glandular (adenomatous) cytology is relatively unreliable and malignancy is readily overlooked. The American College of Obstetricians and Gynecologists, the American Cancer Society and the Bethesda System (2001) have slightly different guidelines. Of the 120 types of human papilloma virus (HPV), about 30 types affect the squamous epithelium of the lower genital and anal areas of females and males.[1] Types 6 and 11 (low-risk) cause condyloma acuminata. Types 16, 18, 31 and 45 (high-risk) may induce cancer if they persist over the years. Type 18 tends to be found in adenocarcinoma.[1]

Screening for Cervical Neoplasia Precursors

A simplified management of cervical cytology (with individual modifications) was outlined:[1]

1. For ASC-US: Atypical squamous cells of unknown significance. *Consider*: Repeat cytology, colposcopy or HPV DNA testing. Cone or loop excisional procedures should not be done if there is no proven cervical intraepithelial neoplasia (CIN) or in adolescents.
2. For ASC-H: Atypical squamous cells — cannot exclude HSIL (high-grade squamous intraepithelial lesion). *Recommend*: Should have colposcopy.
3. For low-grade squamous intraepithelial lesions (LSIL). *Consider*: Colposcopy; for adolescents repeat cytology.
4. For high-grade squamous intraepithelial lesions (HSIL). *Recommend*: Colposcopy and endocervical sampling; sometimes diagnostic excisional procedures; repeat cytology or HPV testing is unacceptable because there should be prompt investigation.[1]
5. For atypical glandular cells and adenocarcinoma *in situ* (AGC and AIS) (based on 2001 Bethesda system). *Recommend*: Colposcopy with endocervical sampling; consider endometrial sampling. If negative, consider cold knife conization. Repeat cytology is unacceptable.[1]

An excellent review of Cervical Cancer Screening (PDQ^{R}) Health Professional Version was prepared by the National Cancer Institute, last modified 4/10/2008.[2] The prevalence of CIN is highest among women in their 20s and 30s; however, mortality is rare under age 30. HSIL is rare in women older than age 65 who have been previously screened. About 70% of ASCUS and CIN 1 lesions regress within six years. About 6% of CIN 1 lesions progress to CIN 3 or worse. About 10% to 20% with CIN 3 progress to invasive cancer. Although mortality is higher in black women than white women, mortality in all is rare if there has been regular screening. In low resource, underdeveloped countries there is ongoing research of one-time "screen and treat" such as a one-time visual inspection of the cervix with acetic acid (VIA) and immediate colposcopy, directed biopsy and cryotherapy when indicated.

The accuracy of the Papanicolau (Pap) test is measured by sensitivity (percent of "true-positives") and specificity (percent of "true-negatives"). Such tests have rarely been done. For a single Pap test for high-grade lesions the sensitivity is 55% to 80%. With regular Pap testing it is higher. To determine the sensitivity and specificity of the Pap smear, both a test threshold (point at which it is "positive") and a reference-standard threshold (considered to be "positive") must be defined. Atypical squamous cells of undetermined significance is often used as the test threshold and cervical intraepithelial neoplasm (CIN) is used as the reference threshold. This gives a sensitivity of about 68% and a specificity of about 75%. A better test threshold may be low-grade squamous intraepithelial lesions with a reference threshold of CIN 2–3 which gives a sensitivity of 70% to 80%, with a specificity of about 95%.

An adequate specimen is critical. "Adequate training and using such techniques as the cytobrush may improve sensitivity"[2] (Fig. 1). Although the new liquid-based cytology (ThinPrep) gives mixed evidence for adequacy, it has the advantage of simultaneous HPV testing. (Comment: Advantages are simultaneous HPV testing and in the near future testing for other diseases, such as gonorrhea, chlamydia, herpes, trichomonads, candida, bacterial vaginosis. In addition, individual squamous cells are seen without overlapping other cells, therefore readings are faster). Women who have had a total hysterectomy with removal of the cervix for benign disease rarely have Pap smear

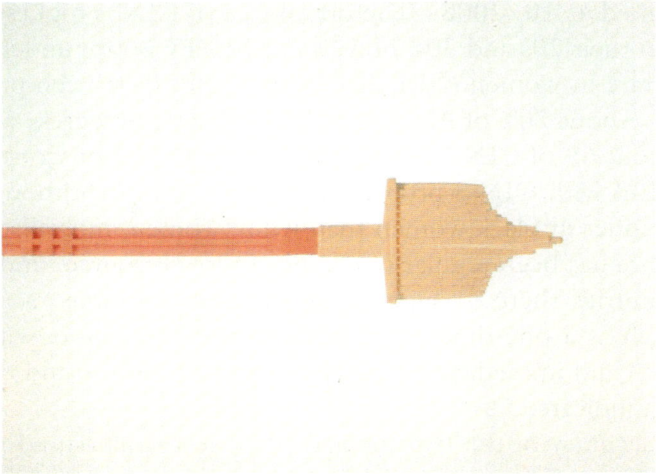

Fig. 1 Cytobrush for cervical cytology which might sample the distal endocervical canal of the cervix as well as the cervical portio. It cannot reach the upper endocervix.

abnormalities. There is uncertainty about the optimal screening interval. "The positive predictive value (PPV) of screening one year after a negative Pap test was 0%; after two years the PPV was 0.9%. The authors concluded that the Pap tests do not have to be repeated within two years of a prior negative test."[2]

(Comment: Professional medical societies recommend annual routine office visits with examination and Pap cytology. Pap cytology is not always ideal. The sample may not be adequate, and there may be a laboratory error. Women may not go for annual examination and might miss an opportunity to detect ovarian cancer, ectopic pregnancy, pelvic inflammatory disease, endometriosis, as well as general medical conditions. Women often use gynecologists as primary care doctors. There is another factor — patient selection such as in private practice or sexually transmitted infection clinics. In addition with evolving social mores, sexual activity is increasing with new sexual partners at a later age (now about 50%). Thus there is increased exposure to high risk (or new high risk) HPV of various types. Another reason for routine annual examination is to include doing and teaching breast examination which is often overlooked by primary care physicians.)

HPV Testing

Virtually all cervical cancers are associated with high-risk type human papillomavirus (HPV) infection. Not all patients infected with HPV develop cancer, fortunately. The Hybrid Capture 2 (HC 2) test is FDA approved and detects the presence of 13 types of HPV associated with cancer. The sensitivity for detecting cervical intraepithelial neoplasia (CIN 2–3) is from 84% to 95%. In women aged 30 to 69, the sensitivity of HPV (HC 2) was 95% and for Pap cytology it was 55%. HPV and Pap combined had 100% sensitivity with a referral rate of 7.9% for further testing. In women over 30, the Pap test had a 97% specificity compared with 94% for HPV DNA testing. Younger women may have frequent HPV infections. HPV testing of the large number of women with an ASCUS finding is more efficient than immediate colposcopy or repeat cytology.[2,3]

Screening Older Women (Age 60 and Over)

In women who have had negative cytologic screening mortality at all ages is low as is high-grade squamous intraepithelial lesions. (Comment: With changing social mores and increased longevity, there may be an increased exposure to sexually transmitted diseases in older women.) In the US, about 50 million women are screened annually. About 3.5 million or 7% will be referred for further evaluation. Of these, over 2 million were referred for ASCUS. Since about 11,000 cases of invasive cancer were expected in 2007, a large number of colposcopies were performed for benign conditions. Another review of screening[4] notes that despite the presumption that liquid based cytology is better than the traditional Papanicolaou (Pap) cytology, it is controversial. Liquid based cytology facilitates HPV DNA testing and in the future testing for chlamydia and gonorrhea. Liquid based cytology has a decrease in unsatisfactory specimens and can be read faster. Screening is less effective for the detection of endocervical adenocarcinoma and its precursors. Women diagnosed with low grade squamous intraepithelial lesions (LSIL) or high grade intraepithelial lesions (HSIL) may be treated with cryotherapy or loop electrosurgical excision, which have unknown effect on fertility and pregnancy.[2]

Cervical Neoplasms

Holschneider CH[3] wrote an excellent review on the subject of Cervical Intraepithelial Neoplasia (CIN), adenocarcinoma and squamous cell cervical cancer, which share many risk factors: early sexual activity, multiple sexual partners, high-risk sexual partner, partners with human papillomavirus infection, history of sexually transmitted disease, smoking, high parity, immunosuppresion, low socioeconomic status, prolonged use of oral contraceptives, and previous vulvar or vaginal squamous dysplasia. Although smoking is associated with squamous cell carcinoma, it is not with adenocarcinoma. Circumcised males have a lower risk of penile HPV infection and a reduced risk of cervical cancer in their current partners. Cervical adenocarcinoma has been increasing in incidence since 1970, especially in women younger than 35. It is probably due to increasing prevalence but also to improved screening and prevention of SIL. Adenocarcinoma has a stronger association with oral contraceptives than squamous cell cancer, especially with long use. The pathology of adenocarcinoma includes mucinous, endometrioid, clear cell and serous carcinomas.

Squamous cell carcinoma represents 70% of cervical cancer, adenocarcinoma 25% and adenosquamous carcinoma 3%–5% (see chapter on cervical pathology). The most common symptoms at presentation are abnormal vaginal bleeding, postcoital bleeding and vaginal discharge (may be watery, mucoid or purulent and malodorous). The cervical cytology may show severe inflammation. On clinical examination in most women with invasive cervical cancer there is variation from negative to gross tumor replacing the cervix. The symptoms of late disease include pelvic or low back pain radiating down the posterior legs; bowel or urinary symptoms (pressure, hematuria, hematochezia [passage of bloody stool] or vaginal passage of urine or stool). Squamous cell carcinoma usually begins at the squamocolumnar junction (transformation zone) and may present as a superficial ulcer, portio exophytic tumor or infiltration of the endocervix. Endophytic tumors may cause an enlarged, indurated smooth barrel-shaped cervix. About half of adenocarcinomas are exophytic, and others may diffusely enlarge or ulcerate the cervix. About 15% are not visible because they are in the endocervical canal. The differential diagnosis includes Nabothian cysts, glandular hyperplasia, mesonephric remnants or hyperplasia, reactive inflammatory glandular change and endometriosis.

Diagnosis and Management

For a grossly visible lesion a punch biopsy is done, including the edge of the tumor. Women with symptoms without a visible lesion but with abnormal cytology should have colposcopy with directed biopsy. An adequate colposcopy means that the entire squamocolumnar junction and all lesions are visualized and that biopsies explain the abnormal cytology. If colposcopy is not adequate and to diagnose microinvasion, a cold knife conization is done which might be adequate treatment for stage IA1. Loop electrosurgical excision may cause thermal artifact which may obscure the margins. (Comment: Many gynecologists do routine endocervical curettage when colposcopy is done.) That is my procedure but in addition, I do a 4 quadrant microendocervical punch biopsy to rule out an endocervical endophytic neoplasia (Fig. 2). If there is invasive cervical cancer, a clinical physical examination is done for gross staging. The vagina is inspected and palpated. Rectovaginal examination is done. The liver is palpated as well as inguinal and supraclavicular lymph nodes. Preoperative laboratory studies include chest X ray, intravenous pyelography, complete blood count, renal and hepatic function tests and cystoscopy and proctosigmoidoscopy. The patient is promptly referred to a gynecologic oncologist. Surgical staging with lymph nodes is more precise for early lesions.[3]

Most cases of invasive cervical cancer occur in women who have not been screened in the previous five years. That is why there are

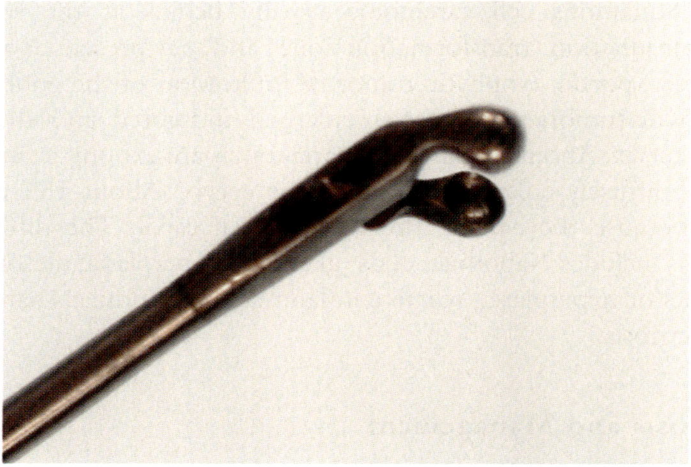

Fig. 2 Four quadrant microendocervical punch biopsy used by Altchek.

relatively few deaths in the US while it is one of the leading causes of cancer mortality in developing countries. HPV 16 accounts for 60% of cervical cancer, while HPV 18 accounts for 10%–20%. HPV 18 is found in 50% of adenocarcinomas. One screening approach is cytology and HPV testing for all women age 30, regardless of past testing. Presumably it would represent women who had been sexually active over three years and have a high risk HPV which persisted. HPV testing in mature women is helpful for triage of ASCUS.[4]

The 2006 Consensus Guidelines

The 2006 Consensus Guidelines for the management of women with abnormal cancer screening tests was reported in 2007.[5] Up to age 20, there is a high prevalence of HPV, atypical squamous cells (ASC) and low grade squamous intraepithelial lesions (LSIL). Most HPV positive cases become negative within two years. Invasive cervical cancer is very rare under age 20.[6,7] Atypical squamous cells are divided into two groups: ASC-US (undetermined significance) and ASC-H (cannot exclude high-grade intraepithelial neoplasia). The latter is more frequently associated with CIN 2 and 3. The recommended management of ASC-US in women over 20 includes testing for high-risk HPV or repeat cytology or colposcopy. If HPV DNA is negative in ASC-US, repeat cytology is done in one year. The patients HPV DNA positive with ASC-US should be colposcoped. If the colposcopy is negative or not adequate, then endocervical sampling is done. If there is no CIN it is recommended to repeat cytology in 6 and 12 months and HPV DNA in one year. Immunosuppressed women are treated as others. Women with ASC-H are colposcoped. If there is no CIN 2 or 3, repeat cytology at 6 and 12 months and HPV DNA in one year. The incidence of a biopsy report of CIN 2 and 3 is similar with cytology of LSIL and ASC-US with low-risk HPV DNA.

Women with LSIL should have colposcopy and possible endocervical sampling as well as HPV testing if colposcopy is negative or inadequate. For negative results, repeat the cytology and HPV at follow-up. For adolescents with LSIL, annual cytology is done. Colposcopy is done for HSIL, or after a two years follow-up for ASC-US. HPV DNA is not done for LSIL because the HPV infection usually disappears.[6,7] For postmenopausal women with LSIL, the patient might have HPV DNA testing or repeat cytology or colposcopy. Colposcopy is done for positive HPV or repeat ASC-US or high grade dysplastic lesions. One colposcopy for HSIL finds CIN 2 or 3 in 53%–66% cases, while using a loop excision 84%–97% is found. In 2% of cases diagnosed with HSIL there is invasive cancer. Colposcopy can "... miss a significant number of CIN 2 and 3 lesion ...."[5] For unsatisfactory colposcopy in HSIL a loop procedure or cone is recommended except in pregnancy or adolescents. Although atypical glandular cells (AGC) may be caused by harmless causes, it may be a sign of adenocarcinoma of the cervix, endometrium, ovary and tube. About 9%–38% of AGC have CIN 2 and 3 or/and *in situ* or invasive cancer. AGC requires colposcopy, endocervical and endometrial sampling and HPV DNA testing. All these methods have low sensitivity. In postmenopausal women, Pap cytology showing endometrial cells or histiocytes require investigation.

The sensitivity of colposcopy with biopsy is only 72.5%. Endocervical curettage adds 3%. In women over 40, endocervical curettage (ECC) sensitivity increases while colposcopic biopsy sensitivity decreases, therefore ECC is worthwhile even in CIN 1.[8] ECC is appropriate when colposcopy can not visualize the squamocolumnar junction, to detect CIN I, atypical squamous cells (ASC-US) or atypical glandular cells.[9] For adolescents with CIN 2 it is reasonable to do colposcopy and cytology at 4–6 months intervals, assuming satisfactory colposcopy and negative ECC.[10] In the 2006 consensus guidelines for the management of women with cervical intraepithelial neoplasia, cytologic follow-up is the only recommended management option, regardless of satisfactory colposcopy for women with CIN 1, especially in adolescents. Management for CIN 2 and 3 is basically the same, however options for the adolescent have been increased.[11] Women treated for CIN 3 should have regular surveillance for at least 25 years independently of their age, because of an increased risk of invasive cancer.[12] Emphasis has been placed on adenocarcinoma *in situ* and adenomatous and glandular atypical cytology because none of the diagnostic measures are precise, the invasive cancer is discovered late and it is increasing in younger women. The endocervix is difficult to evaluate because lesions can be in deep clefts, can be high in the canal and is multifocal. An excellent review of management including the Bethesda system of 2006 was published by the American College of Obstetricians and Gynecologists.[13] (see chapter by Wu M, cytology).

Discussion

Human papillomavirus (HPV) is required to initiate cervical neoplasia but there are other factors involved. Genotypes 16 and 18 are the leading oncogenic high-risk types. Although most sexually active adolescents and college students acquire HPV, there is spontaneous cure in 70% of oncogenic HPV and in 90% of low-risk HPV. The American College of Obstetricians and Gynecologists (ACOG) recommends cervical cancer screening to begin three years after the onset of sexual activity or at age 21. Of course, sexually transmitted diseases (syphilis, gonorrhea, AIDS, hepatitis etc.) should be considered as well as contraception. Women with negative cytology with oncogenic HPV should have both repeated in one year and if persistent have colposcopy "....regardless of the cytologic findings."[13] The ACOG advised that older women who are sexually active, have many partners and have had abnormal cytology continue to have routine annual cytology. A cytology report of atypical glandular cells (AGC) is more serious than atypical squamous cells (ASC). About 9%–23% with AGC have high-grade CIN, AIS, and 3%–17% have invasive cancer. In older women, the risk is higher. Because HPV testing, cytology and colposcopy are not sufficiently reliable, a cone or loop excision of the cervix might be required, especially with AGC-favor neoplasia. Long-term follow-up is necessary after treatment of CIN. The 2006 recommendation is not to treat CIN 1 initially, but to monitor it, regardless of colposcopy. The 2006 advice for women with repeated HSIL with inadequate colposcopy is to have a diagnostic excision.

Endocervical Preneoplastic and Neoplastic Changes

A report of atypical glandular cells presents a special and difficult problem in diagnosis and management and should be emphasized in this chapter. "Human papillomavirus testing, cervical cytology, and colposcopy are all poor at detecting glandular disease." Because of a high-risk of invasive cancer with cytologic AGC, favor neoplasia, diagnostic excision may be necessary.[13] (Comment: Before doing a conization with its hazards, one might consider using a technique which I have used.) A four quadrant microcervical punch biopsy is done. It almost never requires cervical dilatation. The cup removes a 1 mm–2 mm piece of tissue. Historically, prior to cervical colposcopy a four quadrant cervical portio biopsy had an 80% chance of detecting the source of the pathology. Since the endocervical canal diameter is much smaller than the cervical portio diameter the percent of the circumference of the endocervical canal sampled would be much greater and the theoretical chance of detecting endocervical pathology should approach 100%. I do the procedure just prior to endocervical curettage as an additional routine diagnostic test. It takes less than 3 minutes and is done without any anesthesia. It has the advantage of detecting an endophytic lesion. Whereas an endocervical curettage may be difficult with an irregular or curved canal and inadequate tissue be obtained, the biopsies can always retrieve tissue (Fig. 2).

An excellent review by Herzog and Monk on cervical adenocarcinoma was published in 2007.[14] The most common cervical cancer is squamous cell (SCC), while adenocarcinoma is second. Whereas the former has been declining (now 69.3%), the latter has been slowly rising (now 24.9%). In addition, adenocarcinoma *in situ* (AIS) and invasive adenocarcinoma tend to occur in women underage 50. Although SCC mortality has been declining adenocarcinoma has not, perhaps due to to the fact that Pap cytology is more reliable for the former. In addition, SCC is associated with HPV type 16 (50% to 60%), whereas the latter is associated with type 18 (40%–60%). Adenocarcinoma has a worse prognosis than SCC because of increased node metastases, deeper cervical invasion and probably because it is associated with type 18 HPV. Liquid based cytology is better than Papanicolau (Pap) cytology for glandular cell cytology. With atypical glandular cells (AGC) cytology there should be colposcopy, endocervical sampling and endometrial sampling for women aged 35 or over. An endocervical brush may improve cytology with AGC in the endocervix. Vaccination will prevent oncogenic HPV types 16 and 18 which cause 90% of oncogenic virus-induced adenocarcinoma.

An extensive literature review was published in 2006 on "Clinical significance of atypical glandular cells on cervical cytology".[15] The difficulties include continuing changes in nomenclature of histology and/or Pap cytology and quality of the laboratory, and follow-up methods. In 1988, the Bethesda system was developed by the National Cancer Institute to classify Pap cytology pathology. The term "atypical glandular cells of undetermined significance" (AGUS) was created and defined as something between benign reactive reaction and invasive adenocarcinoma. In 1991, it was modified by "favor reactive", "favor neoplasia", and "not otherwise specified" (NOS). In 2001, the words "AGUS" and "favor reactive" were cancelled. A new term was created "atypical glandular cells" (AGC). Atypical glandular cells (AGC) or atypical glandular cells of undetermined significance (AGUS) should be investigated by colposcopy with directed biopsy, endocervical curettage, and endometrial biopsy for patients over age

35 or at risk for endometrial cancer. In addition, pelvic examination (to rule out a vaginal or cervical lesion) and transvaginal ultrasound (to check the adnexa) are done.

Follow-up of AGUS found a 8.5% low-grade LSIL, 11.1% HSIL; 2.9% adenocarcinoma *in situ*; 1.4% endometrial hyperplasia; and 5.2% malignancy. The most common malignancies were endometrial adenocarcinoma (57.6%); cervical adenocarcinoma (23.6%); ovarian and fallopian tube carcinoma (6.4%); squamous cell carcinoma of the cervix (5.4%) and other (6.9%). A cytologic diagnosis of AGUS, favor a neoplastic process, or with a concurrent ASCUS (atypical squamous cells of undetermined significance) "... significantly increases the likelihood of a premalignant or malignant disease."[15] A cytologic diagnosis of AGUS-favor neoplasia implies a 21% risk of malignancy and a 13% chance of adenocarcinoma *in situ.* A cytologic diagnosis of AGUS and concurrent ASCUS implies a 34% risk of HSIL and a 21% prevalence of LSIL. If atypical glandular cells that favor a neoplasm are identified, as well as a concurrent ASCUS, or persistent atypical glandular cells, a cone biopsy should be done. If negative, consider breast and colon cancer screening. There is a possibility of a 4.7% false-negative rate.

Adenocarcinoma *in situ* (AIS) is a precursor to invasive adenocarcinoma. AIS is multifocal in half of the cases. AIS can be cured by simple hysterectomy or possibly by cone biopsy. Endocervical glandular dysplasia has an undefined behavior and existence. Microinvasive adenocarcinoma has many definitions, and clinical decision making is best guided by depth, horizontal extent and lymphatic or vascular invasion.[16] A review indicated that the incidence of malignant and premalignant endocervical glandular lesions is increasing. There are differences between UK terminology and the widely used World Health Organization classification.[17]

Atypical glandular cells (AGC) cytology confer a 38% risk of either preinvasive disease or carcinoma. The risk for the latter is increased for women age 40 or older. The recommended management for AGC includes colposcopy with or without biopsy, endocervical curettage and endometrial biopsy.[18] HPV DNA (Hybrid Capture 2) testing is recommended for all atypical glandular cell (AGC) cytology.

Interestingly, most high-risk HPV positive AGC cases were found to have high-grade squamous intraepithelial lesion (HSIL) rather than adenocarcinoma *in situ* (AIS).[19] Superficial endocervical adenocarcinoma *in situ* (SAIS) is confined to the surface mucosa or crypt openings. The mean age for SAIS is 26.7 years old versus 37.9 years old for AIS. SAIS is an early variant of AIS that occurs at a younger age, has variable atypia and arises adjacent to normal columnar epithelium. Diffuse p16 expression and integrated HPV pattern are the same as in extensive disease. Superficial AIS is suspected with endocervical columnar epithelium displaying segmental nuclear hyperchromasia with mitotic activity and is confirmed by biomarker staining (p16 and MIB-1). It may coexist with CIN and may arise in endocervical polyps.[20] Most cases of atypical glandular cells (AGC) on cytology are benign, nevertheless AGC requires a thorough clinical evaluation to investigate possible glandular neoplasia.[21]

Adenocarcinoma *in situ* (AIS) occurs in 1.25 cases/100,000 women while cervical intraepithelial squamous cell neoplasia (CIN) occurs in 41.4 cases/100,000. The incidence of AIS has been increasing perhaps due to better detection, a true rise, an increase in HPV 18 infection or the use of oral contraceptives. Sometimes AIS is discovered in a conization done for CIN. AIS is associated with invasive cancer in 38%. About 50% of women with AIS have simultaneous squamous cell cervical intraepithelial neoplasia (CIN) or cancers. It is thought that AIS progresses to adenocarcinoma in 5 to 13 years. Simple standard cervical cytology and colposcope-directed biopsy may overlook 60% of AIS. Endocervical curettage greatly increased the detection rate. Cold-knife conization can determine invasive disease and margin status.

AIS is difficult to manage conservatively because:

1. There are no clear features to monitor.
2. The lesion may be high in the endocervical canal, or in the deep endocervical clefts or be multifocal. Cervical Pap, endocervical cytobrush sampling and endocervical curettage each have a sensitivity of only about 50% for detection of AIS.
3. After conization, 9% still have residual AIS, or invasive adenocarcinoma, especially if there are positive margins. With the latter

58% of hysterectomy specimens have residual disease. The negative predictive value of ECC varies from 33% to 94%.

Extrafascial hysterectomy is the definitive therapy for AIS if there is no wish for pregnancy. For patients who wish further pregnancies and understand the risks, it is advised to have a second excision if the original one had positive margins or if the ECC was positive. Cervical cytology, colposcopy and endocervical sampling is done every six months indefinitely. The cytology of atypical glandular cells of cervical adenocarcinoma *in situ* resembles that of invasive adenocarcinoma but histologically there is no stromal invasion in AIS.[22]

Conization may not excise the entire transformation zone especially in pregnancy, when it is large or high in the endocervical canal, or deep in the cervical stroma or extending into the vaginal fornices. With a large high grade ectocervix lesions, colposcopy of the upper vagina is done. A deep cone of 2 cm or more may be done in postmenopausal women because the squamocolumnar junction is high in the endocervical canal. A vasoconstrictor injected into the cervix might distort the specimen. The residual upper endocervical canal is curetted. If there is abnormal glandular cytology or abnormal bleeding or high risk for endometrial cancer, an endometrial curettage is done. The configuration of the cone should be individualized.[23]

VAGINAL AND VULVAR CANCER

General Considerations

Vaginal intraepithelial neoplasia (VAIN) 1 involves the lower 1/3 of the epithelium, VAIN 2 the lower 2/3 and VAIN 3 involves more than 2/3. The incidence is 0.2 to 0.3 cases per 100,000 women in the US. The average age is 43 to 60 years old. It is associated with human papilloma virus (HPV). About 50%–90% of VAIN is associated with previous or present intraepithelial neoplasia or invasive carcinoma of the cervix or vulva. About 5% of women who have had a hysterectomy for CIN are found to have VAIN later.[23]

Since HPV infection of the cervix and CIN occurs in the majority of sexually active young adults most are suspect for VAIN and require vaginal inspection. Vaginal glandular intraepithelial dysplasia (atypical vaginal adenosis) is associated with exposure to diethylstilbestrol (DES) *in utero*. Vaginal neoplasia is rare, causing only 1% of gynecologic cancer. Vaginal intraepithelial neoplasia (VAIN) is reported similar to cervical intraepithelial neoplasia (CIN) since both are stratified squamous epithelium of vaginal mucosa. VAIN usually occurs in the upper vagina. It is believed that 1/2 to 2/3 of VAIN occur in women who previously had cervical or vulvar neoplasia. This suggests that the origin was in the cervix; however, it may be multicentric.

Diagnosis

Diagnosis is made by colposcopic guided biopsy since VAIN has the appearance of CIN.[24] Although VAIN is considered asymptomatic, there may be postcoital spotting or transvaginal discharge. There may be thickening or irregularity of the vagina by palpation. Ideally, colposcopy of the entire vagina should be done, however it is technically difficult and if a hysterectomy had been done the vault is distorted and irregular. Acetic acid washing causes VAIN to look flat or raised white areas with vascular punctation and well demarcated edges. In postmenopausal women, topical estrogen cream for several weeks may improve discovery of VAIN. Biopsies are done of suspicious lesions. Failure of estrogenic vaginal mucosa to take Schiller's (Lugol's iodine) staining may suggest VAIN. Despite the various modes of therapy (excision, ablation, radiation, topical 5-fluorouracil (5-FU)), there is a 20% recurrence rate.[25] Most authors recommend local excision of the focal lesions, followed by histologic examination. With multifocal lesions 5-FU is recommended.[26(a)] VAIN may be suspected with a current or past history of CIN or invasive cervical cancer, a previous hysterectomy with CIN, abnormal squamous cytology without a cervix or not explained by the cervix or small white patches. Pap cytology of the vagina can be done with testing for human papilloma virus HPV.

Management of VAIN

VAIN 1 and 2 are usually simply observed and not treated. VAIN 3 is treated.[25] The usual and best method is complete excision of a local lesion and histologic examination of the specimen. Laser and cryotherapy may damage the vaginal wall. Another treatment is weekly vaginal insertion of 5-fluorouracil cream at night for eight to ten weeks. It may cause scarring of the vagina. If VAIN is diagnosed after cervical radiation, biopsy is necessary to rule out vaginal cancer.[24] Vaginal intraepithelial neoplasia (VAIN) is less common than cervical intraepithelial neoplasia (CIN) because in the latter, in adolescent and young women, there are histological and molecular changes at the squamocolumnar junction (squamous metaplasia) while the vaginal mucosa is stable. Most cases of CIN in the young patients resolve spontaneously in one to three years. (Comment: It would be interesting to know whether the same happens to VAIN.) Patients who have been treated for intraepithelial or invasive cancer of the cervix or vulva should continue to have routine Pap cytology screening of the vagina.[24]

Vaginal Squamous Cell Carcinoma

Primary vaginal cancer is rare causing 0.3% of female genital malignancies. Most vaginal cancers are metastatic from the endometrium, cervix, vulva, ovary, breast, rectum and kidney.[26(c),27] Primary vaginal cancer is associated with HPV DNA 16/18. It is usually in the upper posterior 1/3 of the vagina and is most commonly squamous cell carcinoma. Between 3% and 7% of VAIN patients develop invasive carcinoma even after treatment.[26(c)] Most cases are over age 60, however it may occur between ages 35 to 90. The mean age is 60.[26(c)] The vaginal speculum blades may obscure the lesion.[27]

The risk factors for vaginal intraepithelial and invasive squamous cell cancer are similar to that of the cervical cancer — multiple sexual partners, early age of first intercourse, and smoking. About 1/3 had been treated for cervical neoplasia. It is also associated with HPV 16.[26(c)] The symptoms include vaginal bleeding or blood-tinged, watery or bad smelling discharge, vaginal mass, and urinary symptoms. In 20% malignant cells may be detected in cervical cytology.[26(c),27] Vaginal cancer may present as a mass; induration, exophytic or endophytic plaques; or ulcer. If there is abnormal cytology, or if the lesion is not visible, colposcopy of the cervix and vagina is done. Colposcopy and biopsy are facilitated by washing with diluted 4% acetic acid or Lugol's iodine stain. The upper vaginal biopsy might have to be done with a cervical punch biopsy instrument because it is too high for the standard Keyes punch biopsy which is used by hand and resembles a "cork borer" (Fig. 3).

Vaginal tumors are often multicentric. The extent of the cancer is evaluated by physical examination, surgical staging, cystoscopy, proctoscopy and imaging by magnetic resonance or computed tomography. The International Federation of Gynecology and Obstetrics stage 0 is carcinoma *in situ* (VAIN 3); stage I is carcinoma limited to the vaginal wall; stage II is carcinoma involving the subvaginal tissue but has not extended to the pelvic sidewall; stage III is when the carcinoma has extended to the pelvic sidewall.[26(c),27] (Comment: The vaginal biopsy should be deep enough to sample tissue under the vaginal wall.)

Other Vaginal Malignancies

Verrucous Carcinoma of Vagina

This is an unusual type of well differentiated squamous cell carcinoma. It is a large, warty cauliflower-like mass which usually grows and infiltrates locally but does not metastasize. It does not respond to radiation. Complete local resection usually cures this neoplasm.[27] (Comment: Rather than a biopsy, the surgeon should consider initial complete excision with a free border.)

Adenocarcinoma of Vagina

Most primary vaginal cancers under the age of 20 are adenocarcinomas. They may be associated with vaginal adenosis, Wolffian cell nests, periurethral glands and endometriosis. Clear-cell adenocarcinomas of the vagina are found in one out of a thousand of young women with intrauterine exposure to diethylstilbestrol (DES). It presents as anterior vaginal polypoid masses and may also be present in the cervix. The age range is 7–33 years old with a median age of 19. Exposed women should have their first gynecologic examination at menarche, ideally with colposcopy of the cervix and vagina, annual cytology of cervix and vagina and a one finger palpation.[27] (Comment: Since the original report of clear cell adenocarcinoma by Herbst in 1971, DES is no longer prescribed to prevent miscarriages.) Nevertheless, DES has been given to animals to fatten them up to one month before slaughter. This may explain the characteristic benign associated structural deformities of the cervix which I have observed in some young women whose mothers did not take DES, due to possible ingestion of DES with meat.

Primary Sarcoma of the Vagina

The most common of these rare sarcomas is rhabdomyosarcoma with a mean age of appearance at three years. It presents as a polypoid protruding mass resembling a cluster of grapes ("sarcoma botryoides") and bleeding. Since it is submucosal, early lesions require excision of the entire polypoid mass to make the diagnosis rather than excising only the superficial normal vaginal mucosa. Any polypoid protrusion however benign looking, whose origin is from the vagina above the hymen should be excised. Polyps of the hymen are usually benign.[26(c),27(a)] Although in the past years rhabdomyosarcoma (sarcoma botrioides) was fatal within two years except for unusual patients who had an early diagnosis and pelvic exenteration, in recent years with early diagnosis, local excision and chemotherapy, most patients are cured and retain fertility.

Malignant Melanoma of the Vagina

Malignant melanomas of the vagina are rare. They are usually discovered in Caucasian women with a mean age of 58 (range 28–83), in the distal anterior wall usually as a blue-black or black-brown mass, plaque or ulcer. They may be non-pigmented and are very aggressive.[27] (Comment: Because the cervix is the site of most pathological changes, clinicians tend to automatically insert a speculum into the vagina to examine the cervix with a bright light and often overlook the vagina.) Another problem is that some normal African-American women have benign patches of melanosis in the distal vaginal mucosa.

Vulvar Intraepithelial Neoplasia (VIN)

The International Society for the Study of Vulvar Diseases (ISSVD) created the classification for epithelial disorders.[28,29] The incidence of vulvar intraepithelial neoplasia (VIN) is increasing because of its prevalence in young women due to HPV infection so that at present, 75% of cases occur in young women. VIN in the young females is multifocal and associated with high risk HPV 16, 18 and 31 infections. Vulvar condyloma acuminata and VIN 1 are associated with low risk HPV 6 and 11 infections.

Diagnosis

There seems to be two types of vulvar intraepithelial neoplasia (VIN). The first type occurs in young women, age 15–27, with multiple, pigmented, warty and basaloid lesions (undifferentiated VIN), who are infected with HPV. Sometimes progression of VIN 2 and 3 might occur over 3–30 months with a median age of 9.5 months.[31] Older women (median age 66 years old) with differentiated VIN and positive p53 immunostaining have a predisposition to vulvar cancer in one localized area.

VIN 3 includes carcinoma *in situ*, Bowen's disease, and Bowenoid papulosis and has the potential to become invasive cancer. The basaloid type of VIN 3 displays a thickened epithelium with a flat, smooth surface. There is also a warty-condylomatous type which tends to occur in younger women with HPV infection. The differentiated (simplex) type of VIN 3 has a thick epithelium and parakeratosis with elongated rete ridges. It stains for p53, and is a precursor of HPV negative vulvar cancer.[29,30] It tends to occur in the older women. Clinically, half of the cases of VIN are asymptomatic. When symptoms are present, there may be pruritus, a visible lesion, a palpable abnormality, pain, burning or dysuria. Hyperkeratotic raised pigmented lesions are suspicious.[26(b)]

The epithelium of the embryonic cloaca becomes the epithelium of the cervix, vagina, anus, and lower 3 cm of rectal mucosa up to the dentate line. All these areas are sensitive to HPV infection and may have multicentric (involving more than one organ) lesion. About 60% with VAIN 3 or VIN 3 have preexisting or simultaneous CIN. Ten percent of CIN 3 lesions are associated with 3% of VAIN 3 and 7% with VIN 2 or 3. There may be a monoclonal high-grade VIN and VAIN lesion which originates in high-grade CIN or cervical cancer. Up to 2/3 of young women infected with HPV have multifocal or confluent areas of VIN. The lesions tend to occur in the interlabial grooves, posterior fourchette and perineum (not hair bearing areas).[26(b)] The lesions may be hyperpigmented, white, brown or red. Unifocal lesions tend to occur in postmenopausal women, are not related to HPV infection and are well differentiated histologically.

Physical examination include careful inspection and palpation for masses, ulceration or color changes, especially in non-hairy areas. The lesions may be raised, verrucous, and white but also red, pink, gray or brown. Macular lesions are on adjacent mucosal surfaces. There may be several patterns in the same patient.[29] The differential diagnosis include lichen sclerosus, lichen planus, condylomata acuminata and condyloma lata. Colposcopy or a magnifying glass may be helpful. Cotton balls soaked in 2%–5% acetic acid is applied for several minutes causing the VIN lesion to present as a well demarcated white lesion. Then 1% toluidine blue dye is applied for 2 minutes which is then washed off with 1% acetic acid. Abnormal areas will stain blue and should be biopsied. There may be false positives or false negatives in thick hyperkeratotic lesions. The Keyes punch biopsy is used. For hemostasis, use Monsel solution or silver nitrate stick.

Management

The treatment of VIN 3 is wide excision (1 cm margins) which is also used to discover any early invasive squamous cell carcinoma. The depth of the excision is 1 mm, and 3 mm in hairy areas. VIN 1 is not treated because it does not become malignant and is also controversial to diagnose histologically.[29,30,31] Topical imiquiniod cream (Aldara®) is being used experimentally for VIN 3.[29] If untreated, high grade VIN may continue, progress or resolve. Sometimes there is complete spontaneous regression in women under age 35 and also in pregnancy.[29,31]

Long-term follow-up after surgery is required because VIN may recur in 1/3 of cases regardless of the treatment used. About 4%–8% develop locally invasive cancer. The patient is seen every six months for two years, then annually, especially the patients with immunosuppression (HIV), high grade VIN, multifocal or multicentric disease, or positive margins on the surgical specimens.[26(b),29] Prophylactic vaccination could prevent 2/3 of vulvar, vaginal and perianal intraepithelial neoplasia in young women.

Discussion

The worldwide HPV associated VIN is increasing as well as invasive vulvar cancer. There are often delays in diagnosis. "The liberal use of biopsy is mandatory." This requires a high index of suspicion by a careful visual inspection.[30] A review of 405 cases of untreated VIN 2–3 found that the VIN mean age decreased from age 50 before 1980 to 39 in later years (up to 2003). Spontaneous clearing of VIN was found in 47% (mean age of 24.6) over a mean interval of 9.5 months.[31] Surgically treated VIN has a high rate of recurrence. VIN in women over age 30 has a significant risk for invasive cancer. In young women there has been a recent increase in incidence of VIN and VIN-related cancers, probably related to increasing early multiple partners, early sex activity, HPV infection increase and smoking.[29] HPV type 16 is found in 90% women with warty/basaloid VIN and is associated with multifocal and multicentric neoplasic lesions of cervix and vagina. More than 1/3 of cases had been treated for preinvasive or invasive neoplasia in the cervix or vagina. It was suggested that "sexual health screening, cervico-vaginal cytology and colposcopy should therefore be an integral part of the assessment and continuing care of women with VIN."[31] Spontaneous regression of cases of VIN was seen in young women with a history of genital condylomata acuminata, with multifocal, pigmented, papular lesions in the perineum, of mean age of 24, in Auckland, New Zealand natives, in 9.5 months. Therefore, it was recommended that women under the age of 30 with this lesion (previously called Bowenoid papulosis) can be closely observed without treatment for 12 months. However, in some young women (especially with HPV 16) it may progress into invasive cancer.[31]

There are two different types of invasive vulvar cancer in women who have been treated for VIN. In the first group, 2% of patients previously diagnosed with VIN had invasive cancer within 7 years (mean 2.4 years) after treatment, thought to be due to progression, inadequate treatment, invasion at the site of previous lesion, or previous positive surgical margins. In the second group, 1.8% of patients previously diagnosed with VIN, the invasion came many years (median 13.8 years) after treatment. Sometimes the cancer develops at some distance from the previously treated VIN lesion, possibly by new neoplastic change due to HPV field effect, especially at the urethra and anal margins.[26(b)]

Conclusion

The incidence of VIN increased by 410% between 1973 and 2000, from 0.56 to 2.86 per 100,000 women. There are two types of VIN: the type 1 pattern is usually diagnosed in young women (age 15–27) with HPV infection. It tends to be warty, basaloid and mixed (complex, undifferentiated). It may be also associated with smoking, previous cervical, vaginal or perianal cancer and immunosuppression and it may become invasive. The type 2 is VIN, differentiated type. It is associated with lichen sclerosus or squamous cell hyperplasia (lichen simplex chronicus), is more common in older women (median age 66) and with less or no association with HPV. It is also described as VIN, simplex (or differentiated) type — usually unifocal, seen as ulcer, warty papule or hyperkeratotic plaque. It may become invasive cancer in 9% of cases if untreated or 3.3% if treated. It may have a higher risk for cancer.[29,32]

The treatment of VIN is surgical resection of the lesion. Other destructive treatments do not have a pathology specimen to check for invasive cancer. There should be a 3 mm or greater depth to remove the hair follicles and a 1 cm margin around the VIN in the surgical specimen. Long-term follow-up is important, especially for immunosuppressed patients. The incidence of HPV related VIN is increasing together with invasive cancer in young women throughout the world. About 2.5%–7.0% of women no matter how treated for vulvar intraepithelial neoplasia (VIN) will develop invasive cancer.[26(b),33,34] In 2004, it was decided to avoid the diagnosis of VIN 1 and combine VIN 2 and 3. VIN 1 has histologic variability and may be an indication of acute HPV infection. VIN 2 and 3 have a high risk of invasive cancer and require excision. At present general population screening for VIN or invasive cancer "... is not recommended." (Nevertheless the vulva should always routinely be inspected.)[32] For patients with VIN or cancer careful periodic evaluation is recommended. It should be kept in mind that colposcopy may be difficult because of a large area and great variability of the vulvar lesions and that in hyperkeratinized lesions maybe topical acetic acid may take a long time to reveal abnormalities.

VULVAR CANCER

Vulvar cancer represents 5% of female genital cancers, much less than endometrial, ovary and cervix. About 90% of vulvar cancer is squamous cell carcinoma, originating from the keratinized skin. More than 20% of vulvar intraepithelial neoplasia (VIN) is associated with human papilloma virus (HPV) (usually younger women). Vulvar cancer usually occurs in postmenopausal women with a mean age of 65; however, the age of the patients may be going down to 55.

The risk factors include smoking, vulvar dystrophy (lichen sclerosus) and vulvar or cervical intraepithelial neoplasia, HPV infection, immunodeficiency and previous cervical cancer. Although the incidence of vulvar intraepithelial neoplasia (VIN) is increasing in young women, earlier detection and treatment keeps the incidence of vulvar cancer stable. The usual clinical picture is a unifocal vulvar plaque, ulcer or fleshy, nodular, warty mass on the labia majora. About 5% are multifocal. There may be a synchronous secondary CIN in 20% of cases.[33] The symptoms include (1) pruritus, especially with lichen sclerosus or squamous cell hyperplasia and (2) vulvar bleeding or discharge. Some are asymptomatic.[29]

Biospy is essential and best done from the center of the lesion. It should include some surrounding skin, underlying dermis and underlying connective tissue to determine the depth of stromal invasion. If there is no gross lesion, a suspicious colposcopy (done with 5% acetic acid which shows acetowhite areas with abnormal blood vessels) must be biopsied. The differential diagnosis includes seborrheic keratosis, lichen sclerosus, other dermatoses, condyloma acuminata, epidermal inclusion cysts, lentigo, hidradenoma, acrochordons and Bartholinitis. If these apparent conditions do not respond to treatment biopsy should be considered.

Over 90% of vulvar cancer is squamous cell carcinoma which is usually located on the labia or vestibule. There are two types:

1. The more common type is the differentiated, keratinizing, simplex type, occurring in older women, not associated with HPV but rather with chronic dystrophies.
2. Less commonly, the warty Bowenoid type is associated with HPV 16, 18 and 33, and occurs in younger women. The risk factors are those of HPV infection (early age at first sexual activity, multiple sex partners, HIV and smoking). These cancers usually are found in early stages.[32,33]

Some high grade VIN and VAIN may be monoclonal from CIN 3 or cervical cancer.

Other vulvar cancers are:

1. Malignant melanoma, the second most common, causing 5% of primary vulvar neoplasms and 3%–7% of all melanomas. It usually present in postmenopausal white women with a median age of 68 (range 10–99). Other skin melanomas usually develop before age 45. It is usually pigmented, arising *de novo* on the clitoris or labia minora. It can also develop from junctional or compound nevi.
2. Verrucous carcinoma is a variant of squamous cell cancer.
3. Basal cell carcinoma represents 2% of vulvar malignancies and usually presents in white women, is locally invasive and often associated with previous or simultaneous malignancy elsewhere.
4. Soft tissue sarcoma causes 1%–2% of vulvar malignancy.
5. Extramammary Paget's disease represents less than 1% of vulvar malignancies and is usually found in white women in their 60th and 70th decades. It usually causes pruritus, is multifocal, well demarcated and eczematoid. Invasive adenocarcinoma may be found in or underneath the lesion in 4%–17% of cases. There may also be a synchronous neoplasia in another site in 20%–30% of cases.
6. Bartholin gland adenocarcinoma is rare, involving patients with a median age of 57 (when inflammatory disease does not usually occur). It presents as a solid mass with deep infiltration and metastasizes readily. In women over 40, any mass in the Bartholin area should be biopsied.[26(b)]

Practical Clinical Evaluation

A basic evaluation of the vulva was published in "Vulvar Diseases" in 1983.[35] Heading the list of diagnostic equipment is well-trained eyes! Inspect the intertriginous area between the vulva and the thighs, the skin of the hairy areas, of the mons and labia majora, the interlabial sulci, lateral and medial surface of the labia minora, the prepuce and glans, and the vestibule up to the hymenal ring. The colposcope is of relatively little value in the initial examination because it would take too much time. A simple 2x or 4x magnifying glass at least three inches in diameter is excellent together with good lighting. A circular fluorescent light surrounding a large round magnifying lens is recommended.

A color photographic record of serial observation is very helpful especially when following an untreated patient with carcinoma *in situ*, vulvar dystrophies over a long time and to evaluate the effect of therapy on a lesion. The toluidine blue test is recommended. It is a nuclear stain. Diluted acetic acid bleaches any dye not bound to the nucleus. With normal skin keratin layer there are no surface nuclei and the dye is washed away. Nuclei are present on the surface in ulcers and parakeratosis representing an abnormality of squamous cell maturation when nucleated squames are present in the top epithelial layer. Parakeratosis may also be present in benign conditions with rapid cell turnover such as condylomata acuminata. Acetic acid by itself dehydrates cells so that area of increased density and atypia becomes white and opaque.

The skin must be clean when doing the test. One percent aqueous toluidine blue is applied with a large cotton swab and allowed to dry for 1 to 2 minutes. Then it is rinsed with 1% aqueous acetic acid. The skin is then examined with magnification and good light. Most early squamous neoplasms have a surface layer of hyperkeratosis or parakeratosis. The latter is detected by the stain. The vagina and the vestibule have non-keratinizing squamous epithelium; the outer layer containing nucleated squamous cells will stain positively with Lugol solution. Pap smear cytology of the vulva is not feasible.[35]

Gynecologists and most physicians are somewhat reluctant to managing vulvar problems. We were sparingly taught about it in medical school and during training as house doctors we were only briefly lectured on sexually transmitted diseases and the vulva. (We never learned about doing biopsies.) Even dermatologists are not well versed in vulvar problems. They rarely inspect the vulva and are taught that local factors (heat, humidity, friction) change the appearance of dermatoses such as psoriasis. Assuming that the gynecologist knows how to do it, in general one never regrets doing a biopsy but may often regret not doing it. Visual clinical diagnosis is often difficult. Failure of therapy is an appropriate reason to perform a biopsy.

Vulvar biopsies should be done liberally. Gynecologists should do more but have limited experience. It should be done for difficult diagnoses of benign conditions as well as to rule out malignancy, especially with hyperpigmented or exophytic lesions, changes in blood vessels appearance, or lesions which persist despite therapy. Before injecting local anesthesia with a 1 ml tuberculin syringe and fine #25 gauge needle, topical EMLA cream is used to numb the area.[32] Another topical is 4% liposomal cream or lidocaine-prilocaine which, however, take longer to act.[34] The standard vulvar "punch" biopsy is the Keyes 3 mm–5 mm instrument (Fig. 3) which resembles a "cork borer" and operates by twisting at a right angle to the skin surface. The entire thickness of the skin is bored out to check for invasion. The base is cut with fine scissors, the specimen is lifted with a fine forceps and placed on dry blotting paper for a moment to become adherent and orient the sectioning and then placed in a preservative — fixing solution and send to a dermato-pathologist or gynecologic pathologist.[32]

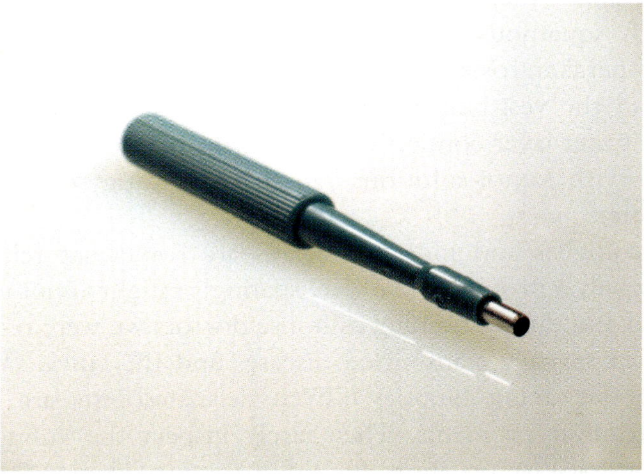

Fig. 3 The standard Keyes punch biopsy. It is a "cork borer" device which is rotated or twisted to the appropriate depth. The 3 mm–5 mm width is usually used.

Biopsies of ulcers are done at the edge, and for hyperpigmented areas in the widest part of the lesion. If there is suspicion of early vulvar squamous cell carcinoma, multiple biopsies are indicated because different areas may have different depths of invasion. If there is a palpable tumor, biopsies should include the center and surrounding area.[36] Ethyl chloride or other refrigerant spray is used for momentary local skin anesthesia but it is not used on the vestibule because its mucocutaneous surface is very sensitive. The biopsy site is cleansed with an alcohol wipe. The usual local anesthesia is 2% lidocaine (Xylocaine) injected with a 30-gauge needle, with or without epinephrine. With the latter it takes longer for the anesthetic to act but it lasts longer and improves hemostasis. The tissue to be biopsied is compressed between the thumb and index finger of the surgeon's hand while the other dominant hand rotates the Keyes punch into the subcutaneous fat. Monsel's solution or silver nitrate stick is used for hemostasis.

VIN lesions have usually a raised surface. About 2/3 retain 1% toluidine blue vital stain after being decolorized with 1% acetic acid. About 1/3 are pigmented and dark, but some are pink, white-gray or red. They may be macular, popular, single or multiple or confluent. There may be pruritus. They may also develop in the perianal skin and anal canal. Vulvar invasive cancer usually occurs on the labia majora or minora, is usually single with a papillomatous appearance or endophytic and ulcerated. Lichen sclerosus is a chronic inflammatory dermatosis with lymphocytic infiltration and fibrosis of the stroma and probably related to autoimmunity.[37] It may occur in one out of 30 women over 65 years old.

About 20% of lichen sclerosus (LS) occurs in prepubertal children. There is no association with malignancy in the child. The risk of vulvar and perianal cancer developing in elderly women with lichen sclerosus increases with age, from 2.0 to 25 per 100,000 at age 75. It is thought that squamous cell carcinoma of the vulva (SCCV) may present ten years after the onset of lichen sclerosus. Recurrent or metachronous SCCV in lichen sclerosus is suggestive of a "field effect". Most vulvar cancers in older women develop from differentiated VIN and are not related to HPV. The young women with HPV-associated

VIN have an undifferentiated VIN which may resolve without treatment or infrequently progresses to SCCV.

The older women with long-term chronic inflammation from lichen sclerosus or lichen simplex chronicus are at risk to develop SCCV.

Recommendations for following women with lichen sclerosus of the vulva:

1. Careful observation if there is difficulty in controlling symptoms or there is localized thickening of the skin.
2. Careful observation of women with previously treated vulvar squamous cell carcinoma associated with lichen sclerosus or vulvar intraepithelial neoplasia (VIN).
3. Careful observation if the biopsy is not positively diagnostic for differentiated VIN.

Vulvar biopsy or excision should be done liberally of any suspicious area.

There is a small risk that years after surgical construction of a vagina from split-thickness skin graft or a segment of ileum or colon, the neovagina may develop carcinoma *in situ* or squamous cell invasive carcinoma in the former and adenocarcinoma in the latter. The risk for neoplasia is increased after X-ray treatment or chronic treatment with podophyllin or with cauterization.[38]

REFERENCES

1. Creasman TW, Preinvasive disease of the cervix, in *Clinical Gynecologic Oncology*, 7th edn., PJ DiSaia, WT Creasman (eds.), Mosby–Elsevier Philadelphia, pp. 1–37, 2007.
2. Cervical Cancer Screening (PDQ^R) Health Professional Version. National Cancer Institute www.cancer.gov; last modified 4/10/2008.
3. Holschneider CH. Epidemiology, clinical features, and diagnosis of invasive cervical cancer, in *UpToDate*, Rose, BD (ed.), UpToDate, Waltham, MA, *http://www.uptodate.com*, 2008.

4. Feldman S, Goodman A, Tests for screening for cervical cancer: cervical cytology, human papillomavirus testing, and visual inspection, in *UpToDate*, BD Rose, (ed.), UpToDate, Waltham, MA, *http://www.uptodate.com*, 2008.
5. Wright T, Massad S, Dunton C, *et al.*, 2006 consensus guidelines for the management of women with cervical intraepithelial neoplasia or adenocarcinoma *in situ*, *Am J Obstet Gynecol* **197**:337–339, 2007.
6. Wright JD, Davila RM, Pinto KR, *et al.*, Cervical dysplasia in adolescents, *Obstet Gynecol* **106**:115–120, 2005.
7. Moore K, Cofer A, Elliot L, *et al.*, Adolescent cervical dysplasia: histologic evaluation, treatment and outcomes, *Am J Obstet Gynecol* **197**:141 e1–e6, 2007.
8. Solomon D, Stoler M, Jeronimo J, *et al.*, Diagnostic utility of endocervical curettage in women undergoing colposcopy for equivocal or low-grade cytologic abnormalities, *Obstet Gynecol* **110**:288–295, 2007.
9. Waxman AG, *OBG Management*, Nov:19 2007.
10. Spitzer M, Moore DH, Cervical neoplasia, in *Precis — An Update in Obstetrics and Gynecology. Oncology*, 3rd edn., The American College of Obstetricians and Gynecologists, Washington, DC, pp. 51–73, 2008.
11. Wright T, Massad S, Dunton C, *et al.*, The 2006 American Society for Colposcopy and Cervical Pathology — Sponsored Consensus Conference, *Am J Obstet Gynecol* **197**:346–358, 2007.
12. Strander B, Andersson-Ellstrom A, Milsom I, *et al.*, Long-term risk of invasive cancer after treatment for cervical intraepithelial neoplasia grade 3: population-based cohort study, *BMJ* **335**:1077, 2007.
13. Spitzer M, *OBG Management* Nov: 27 2007.
14. Herzog T, Monk B, Reducing the burden of glandular carcinomas of the uterine cervix, *Am J Obstet Gynecol* **197**:566–571, 2007.
15. Schnatz P, Guile M, O'Sullivan D, *et al.*, Clinical significance of atypical glandular cells on cervical cytology, *Obstet Gynecol* **107**:701–708, 2006.
16. Zaino RJ, Symposium, Part I: Adenocarcinoma *in situ*, glandular dysplasia and early invasive adenocarcinoma of the uterine cervix, *Int J Gynecol Pathol* **21**:314–326, 2002.
17. McCluggage WG, Endocervical glandular lesions: controversial aspects and ancillary techniques, *J Clin Pathol* **56**:164–173, 2003.
18. DeSimone CP, Day ME, Tovar MM, *et al.*, Rate of pathology from atypical glandular cell Pap tests classified by the Bethesda 2001 nomenclature, *Obstet Gynecol* **107**:1285–1291, 2006.

19. Saqi A, Gupta PK, Erroll M, *et al.*, High-risk human papillomavirus DNA testing: a marker for atypical glandular cells, *Diagn Cytopathol* **34**:235–239, 2006.
20. Witkiewicz A, Lee KR, Brodsky G, *et al.*, Superficial (early) endocervical adenocarcinoma *in situ*: a study of 12 cases and comparison to conventional AIS, *Am J Surg Pathol* **29**:1609–1614, 2005.
21. Wood MD, Horst JA, Bibbo M, Weeding atypical glandular cell look-alikes from the true atypical lesions in liquid-based Pap tests: a review, *Diagn Cytopathol* **35**:12–17, 2007.
22. Holschneider CH, Cervical adenocarcinoma *in situ*, in *UpToDate*, BD Rose (ed.), UpToDate, Waltham, MA, *http://www.uptodate.com*, 2008.
23. Hoffman M, Mann W, Procedures for cervical conization: technique and outcome, in *UpToDate,* BD Rose (ed.), UpToDate, Waltham, MA, *http://www.uptodate.com*, 2008.
24. Bosquet J, Cliby W, Vaginal neoplasia, in *Precis, an Update in Obstetrics and Gynecology, Oncology*, 3rd edn., The American College of Obstetricians and Gynecologists, Washington, DC, pp. 47–50, 2008.
25. Holschneider CH, Berek JS, Vaginal intraepithelial neoplasia, in *UpToDate*, BD Rose (ed.), UpToDate, Waltham, MA, *http://www.uptodate.com*, 2008.

26(a). Creasman TW, Preinvasive disease of the vagina and vulva and related disorders, in *Clinical Gynecologic Oncology*, 7th edn., PJ DiSaia PJ, WT Creasman (eds.), Mosby–Elsevier Philadelphia, pp. 37–54, 2007.

26(b). Stehman FB, Invasive cancer of the vulva, in *Clinical Gynecologic Oncology*, 7th edn., PJ DiSaia, WT Creasman (eds.), Mosby–Elsevier Philadelphia, pp. 235–264, 2007.

26(c). Slomovitz BM, Coleman RC, Invasive cancer of the vagina and urethra, in *Clinical Gynecologic Oncology*, 7th edn., PJ DiSaia, WT Creasman (eds.), Mosby–Elsevier Philadelphia, pp. 265–282, 2007.

27. Elkas JC, Berek JS, Vaginal cancer, in *UpToDate*, BD Rose (ed.), UpToDate, Waltham, MA, *http://www.uptodate.com*, 2008.

27(a). Altchek A, Vaginal Bleeding in the child, in *Pediatric, Adolescent and Young Adult Gynecology*, A Altchek, L Deligdisch (eds.), Wiley–Blackwell Oxford, 2008, (in press).

28. Saunders A, Kueck A, Haefner H, Classification of vulvar intraepithelial neoplasia, *Female Patient* **33**:62–66, 2008.

29. Holschneider CH, Berek JS, Vulvar intraepithelial neoplasia, in *UpToDate*, BD Rose (ed.), UpToDate, Waltham, MA, *http://www.uptodate.com*, 2008.
30. Joura E, Epidemiology, diagnosis and treatment of vulvar intraepithelial neoplasia, *Curr Opin Obstet Gynecol* **14**:39–43, 2002.
31. Jones R, Rowan D, Stewart A, Vulvar intraepithelial neoplasia, aspects of the natural history and outcome in 405 women, *Obstet Gynecol* **106**:1319–1326, 2005.
32. Naumann RW, Cancer of the vulva, in *Precis, An Update in Obstetrics and Gynecology. Oncology* 3rd edn., The American College of Obstetricians and Gynecologists, Washington, DC, pp. 37–46, 2008.
33. Elkas JC, Berek JS, Clinical manifestations, diagnosis, pathology, and staging of vulvar cancer, in *UpToDate*, BD Rose (ed.), UpToDate, Waltham, MA, *http://www.uptodate.com*, 2008.
34. Diagnosis and management of vulvar skin disorders. In *Obstetrics and Gynecology*, Vol III, ACOG Practice Bulletin, November **3**:1243–1253, 2008.
35. Friedrich EG, Jr., Vulvar disease, in *Series Major Problems in Obstetrics and Gynecology*, 2nd edn., W.B. Saunders, Philadelphia, 1983.
36. Tyring SK, Vulvar squamous cell carcinoma: guidelines for early diagnosis and treatment. *Am J Obstet Gynecol* **189**:S17–S23, 2003.
37. Jones R, Scurry J, Neill S, *et al.*, Guidelines for the follow-up of women with vulvar lichen sclerosus in specialist clinics, *Am J Obstet Gynecol* **198**:496 e1–e3, 2008.
38. Idrees M, Deligdisch L, Altchek A, Squamous papilloma with hyperpigmentation in the skin graft of the neovagina in Rokitansky syndrome. Literature review of benign and malignant lesions of the neovagina, *J Pediatr Adolesc Gynecol*, 2008 (in press).

CHAPTER 4

EARLY DIAGNOSIS OF ENDOMETRIAL CANCER

Liane Deligdisch

INTRODUCTION

Endometrial cancer is the most common malignant tumor of the female pelvis in the US and in most parts of the Western world. Its high incidence is related to the increased longevity, high fat diets, hormone replacement therapy, and prolonged estrogenic stimulation, both exogenous and endogenous (of which obesity is the most common). It is the fifth most common cancer of women in the US. Hormone therapy is widely used throughout the world and the histopathologic changes of the uterus, especially of the endometrium in women treated with hormones encompass a variety of morphologic features which are often difficult to interpret. The assessment of such changes in terms of precancerous potential is challenging since the endometrium is one of the most sensitive target tissues to hormone stimulation and can display structural features suggestive of, but not necessarily representing endometrial neoplasia.

Endometrial carcinogenesis is generally considered to be related to metabolic and hormonal anomalies. Other factors are also involved, operating at a molecular genetic level that were recently explored and seem to involve different carcinogenic pathways.

The prognosis of endometrial carcinoma, as in most cancers, is closely related to the early diagnosis either of precancerous lesions or of early invasive cancer, the survival rates being very different from the cases detected in late stages.

The precursors of endometrial carcinoma consist of endometrial hyperplasia, especially atypical glandular hyperplasia or endometrial intraepithelial neoplasia (EIN) and endometrial *in situ* carcinoma (EIC). Early endometrial carcinomas are endometrioid and non-endometrioid.

PRECURSORS OF ENDOMETRIAL CARCINOMA

The endometrium is endowed with a remarkable capacity to translate hormonal stimulation into structural changes due to the presence of receptors in the nuclei and the finely tuned mechanism of steroid receptor binding to the cellular cytoplasmic organelles and their transfer to the nuclear receptor sites.

Estrogenic stimulation is translated by the target cells in the endometrial glands into epithelial proliferation, which takes place during the reproductive period in life, followed by secretory changes induced by the progesterone secreted by the postovulatory corpus luteum. Continuous unopposed estrogen secretion elicits a continuous proliferation of the endometrial tissue, especially its glandular compartment, with hyperplastic changes that may increase in severity from simple, cystic, to complex, and atypical.

The diagnosis of endometrial hyperplasia is based on histopathologic examination. With the increasing degree of severity of the hyperplasia, the reversibility of these changes decreases. Simple, cystic, and even complex glandular hyperplasia often revert to normal under progesteronic stimulation. Complex glandular hyperplasia with atypia may progress to endometrial carcinoma and is therefore considered a premalignant lesion.

Endometrial hyperplasia is seen most often in peri and postmenopausal women with progressively failing ovulation. But it can also be present in younger women. It is associated most often with obesity and/or polycystic ovarian disease, causing anovulatory cycles, and occasionally, with ovarian sex cord stromal tumors. In most cases in perimenopausal women, hypersecretion of steroid hormones by the ovary and/or adrenal cortex is converted to estradiol, estrone, and estriol, of which estradiol is the most stimulating because of its abundant receptor sites in the nuclei of the endometrial tissue. In postmenopausal women, the androgenic hormones secreted by the ovaries and adrenal cortices can be converted into estrogens as well and continue the estrogenic stimulation of the endometrium. Obesity, diabetes, and other metabolic diseases may enhance the extragonadal endogenous estrogen production by aromatization.

In addition to the endogenous hyperestrogenic stimulation, the effect of estrogenic substitution therapy used frequently for alleviating menopausal symptoms represents a common cause of endometrial hyperplasia. Less commonly, young women who are treated with estrogens for premature ovarian failure or congenital sexual gonadal maldevelopment such as Turner's syndrome may develop endometrial hyperplasia and neoplasia.

The addition of progesterone to the estrogen therapy is meant to imitate the natural effect of ovulation on the endometrium. However, this combined therapy does not always produce the expected effect of inhibiting all proliferation, probably because of the irregular distribution of progesterone receptors in the postmenopausal endometrium.[2]

Endometrial hyperplasia is often associated with irregular vaginal bleeding, which is fortunate because it brings the patient to medical attention. Actually, any postmenopausal bleeding should be suspected as due to neoplastic changes unless proven otherwise, therefore endometrial biopsy is mandatory. At biopsy, it turns out that vaginal bleeding is not due to cancer in about two thirds of the cases. However, bleeding does not always occur and sometimes endometrial hyperplasia and even neoplasia are detected fortuitously, at sonograms or hysteroscopic examination. The hyperplastic changes may involve the endometrium diffusely or regionally as is the case with endometrial polyps.

Endometrial polyps represent focal lesions of the endometrium and are most often benign. They are composed of endometrial glands, stroma, and thickened blood vessels in various proportions. While the glands are often inactive, similar to those seen in the basal endometrial layer, and cystic with benign epithelial lining, hyperplastic and neoplastic changes can occur in endometrial polyps. They may represent precancerous lesions. The surgical removal of endometrial polyps and their histological examination is mandatory. Their development involves a monoclonal proliferation of endometrial stromal cells.[3] Both glandular and stromal cells in the polyp have to be examined for possible precursor or overt malignant changes.

Pathology

On gross examination, the endometrial cavity containing hyperplastic tissue may be thickened to various degrees, uniformly or with polypoid structures protruding into the cavity. In postmenopausal women, endometrial hyperplasia may also be found in a thin, grossly atrophic-appearing endometrium. The histologic diagnosis of endometrial hyperplasia is based on architectural and cytologic criteria classically divided into a three-tier system that was first described in 1947 by SB Gusberg as adenomatous hyperplasia (mild, moderate, severe) and then by the WHO in 1994 as simple, complex, and atypical hyperplasia.[1] A recent trend is to classify endometrial hyperplasia into benign and potentially precancerous (endometrioid and EIN). The basic question is whether there is a continuity between the hormonally induced exaggerated endometrial hyperplasia and its neoplastic transformation into an independently growing tumor tissue. The continuous unopposed (by progesterone) estrogenic stimulation may elicit continuous endometrial proliferation resulting in simple, cystic, and complex glandular hyperplasia. Simple glandular hyperplasia consists of glandular proliferation at the detriment of the stroma, thus increasing the proportion between glands and stroma that is normally 1/1. The glands appear crowded and display dilatation often

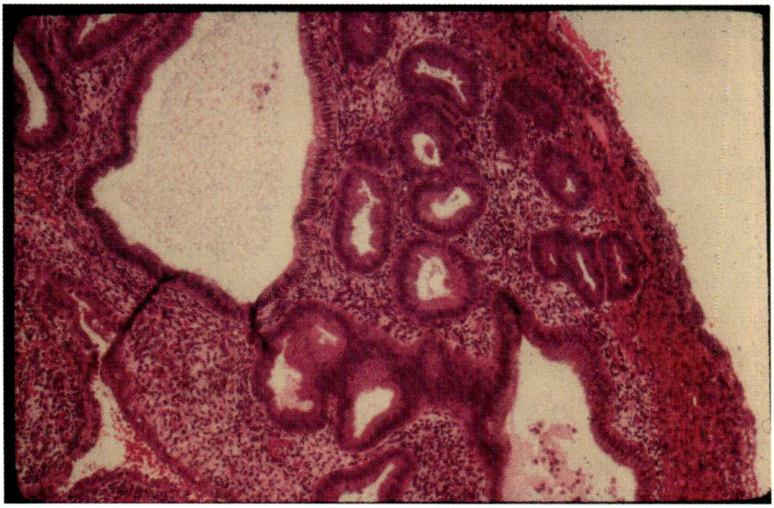

Fig. 1 Endometrial simple glandular-cystic hyperplasia in a 51 years old peri-menopausal woman with persistent estrogen effect. Hematoxylin/eosin, orginal magnification 100×.

forming cystic structures and outpouching into the adjacent stroma (Fig. 1). The epithelial cells lining the glands are tall columnar and pseudo-stratified. Their nuclei are round to oval, hyperchromatic with a thickened nuclear membrane, and a variable number of mitoses which are generally symmetrical, similar to those seen in the normal proliferation phase. Complex glandular hyperplasia represents a more advanced stage, probably resulting from a more prolonged or more intense estrogenic stimulation. It is characterized histologically by a complex glandular pattern with branching, irregular outlines, and papillary infoldings that compress the surrounding stroma, thus increasing the glandular crowding and the stroma becomes considerably diminished (Fig. 2). Frequently, there is also a breakdown of the stroma and vascular microthrombosis with hemorrhage. The glandular lining often is piled up to form a stratified layer. The cells exhibit a variable amount of mitotic activity, and occasionally undergo squamous metaplasia that may fill the glandular lumen with polygonal immature uniform squamous cells which represent "squamoid morules" (Fig. 3).

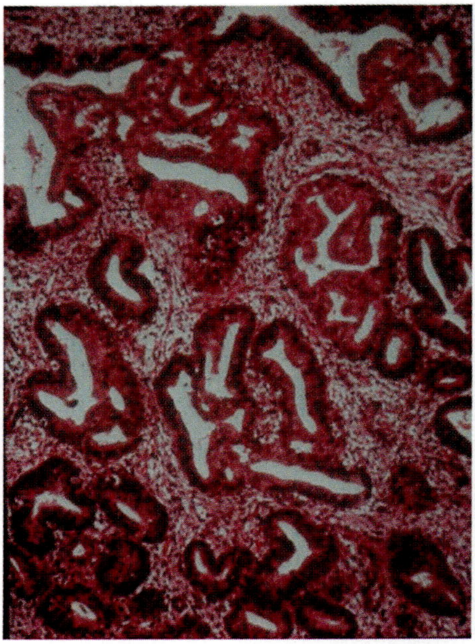

Fig. 2 Endometrial complex glandular hyperplasia resulting from prolonged estrogen effect. Glands are crowded with complex lumina, stroma is diminished. Hematoxylin/eosin, orginal magnification 100×.

The most important diagnostic issue for endometrial hyperplasia is the identification of atypical lesions. Histologically, atypia consists of architectural and cytologic changes bearing the significance of a certain degree of "commitment" to progress towards malignancy. The reversibility of atypical hyperplasia after progesterone therapy, as opposed to simple, cystic, and complex glandular hyperplasia, due to the down regulation of estrogen receptors by progestins,[2] is questionable. The data in the literature mention a 25%–40% progression to adenocarcinoma of lesions diagnosed as atypical complex glandular hyperplasia.[1]

Endometrial atypical glandular hyperplasia consists of marked glandular crowding, with a back-to-back configuration and nuclear changes involving an increased nuclear-cytoplasmic ratio, coarse chromatin clumping, prominent nucleoli, and an irregular thickened

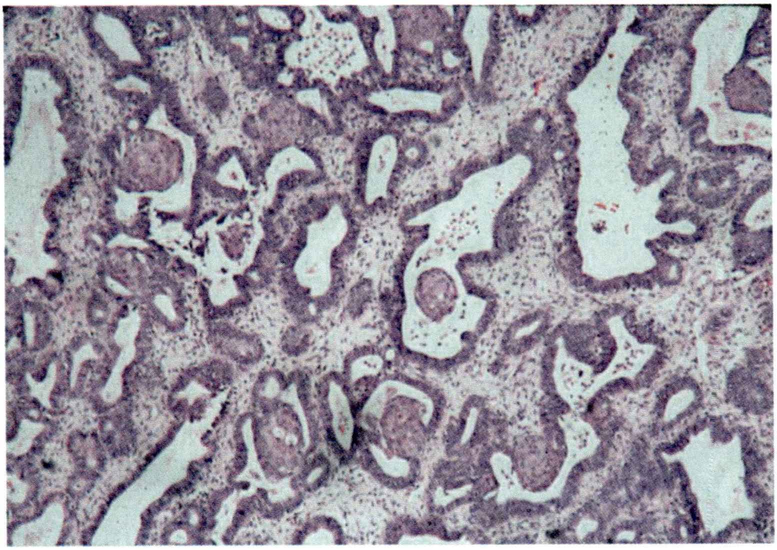

Fig. 3 Endometrial complex glandular hyperplasia with squamoid morules. Hematoxylin/eosin, orginal magnification 40×.

nuclear membrane (Fig. 4). Stratification and mitotic activity are variable. Glandular crowding with stromal breakdown, in the absence of cytologic changes, are not diagnostic for severe/atypical hyperplasia.

Recently, a new classification of endometrial hyperplasias into benign endometrioid and endometrial intraepithelial neoplasia (EIN) has been proposed.[3] EIN was defined as a separate category of monoclonal premalignant lesion, different from the benign endometrial hyperplasia. EIN was assumed to infer a 45-fold higher long term cancer risk as compared to the polyclonal benign hyperplasia which is associated with prolonged estrogen effect and has a two- to ten-fold increased risk for endometrial carcinoma.[3,4] The two lesions often coexist, with EIN lesions displaying clearly atypical nuclear characteristics. They represent localized monoclonal outgrowths of mutated endometrial cells with an atypical architectural and cytologic configuration to be recognized when compared with the background source polyclonal field.[3] Molecular biology studies identified a frequent (63%) inactivation of the PTEN tumor suppressor gene[5] suggesting a

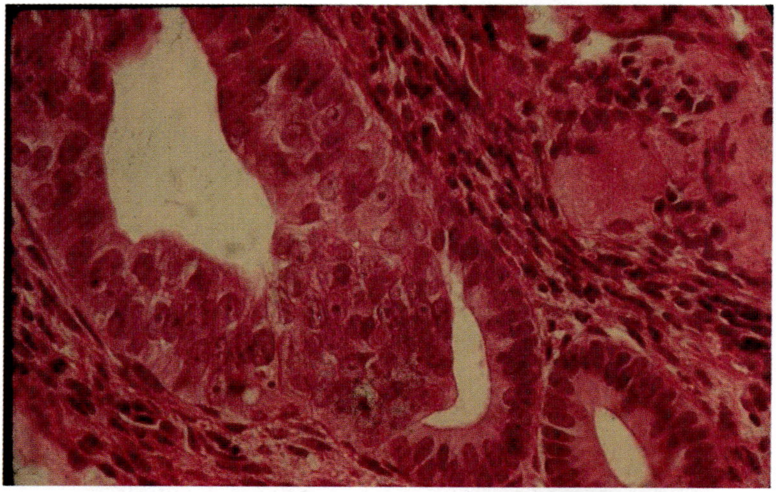

Fig. 4 Endometrial atypical glandular hyperplasia (EIN). The endometrial gland is partially filled with atypical epithelial cells, piled up, with loss of polarity, displaying increased nuclear-cytoplasmic ratio and prominent nucleoli. Hematoxylin/eosin, orginal magnification 400×.

premalignant potential of this lesion. The hormonal risk factors are the same for EIN and benign hyperplasia, with estrogens acting as promoter and progestins as protectors. High levels of nuclear estrogen and progesterone receptors are found in EIN lesions, and unopposed estrogens may act as positive selection factors for previously mutated cells allowing further clonal expansion. Genetically intact endometrial glands shut down the PTEN expression on progesterone exposure.[3]

It should be mentioned that the histological appearance at the diagnosis of an endometrial biopsy from a patient with EIN treated with progesterone may be heavily modified and difficult to interpret due to the non-proliferating appearance of the glands, showing secretory changes and the stromal decidual reaction. Hyperplastic lesions may persist, however, in a deceptively quiescent appearing endometrium.

Associated histologic changes often noted in endometrial hyperplasia of various degrees of severity are metaplasias (changes into different mature tissue patterns), most commonly tubal and occasionally eosinophilic, clear cell or mucinous metaplasias, all of which are probably related to estrogenic and progesterone stimulation. In the stroma, there may be aggregates of foamy histiocytes with cytoplasmic vacuoles containing lipid droplets that are actually deposits of steroids reflecting a local deposit of excessive steroid hormones. These "foamy" histiocytes are seen more often in advanced degrees of endometrial hyperplasia and in endometrial carcinoma. Neither the metaplastic epithelial changes nor the stromal foam cell reaction bear a prognostic significance in terms of precancerous change.

A very different type of endometrial clearly precancerous lesion is the endometrial intraepithelial carcinoma (EIC), characterized by markedly atypical epithelial cells lining the surface and glands, without apparent stromal invasion of a usually atrophic endometrium. Papillary structures may protrude from the surface or into the glands (Figs. 5–7). The atypical epithelial cells display enlarged irregular nuclei with a granular and vesicular chromatin pattern and enlarged eosinophilic or amphophilic nucleoli. EIC can be seen in endometrial polyps and has a different immunoreactivity than endometrial hyperplasia, including EIN. In EIC, there is an immunohistochemical overexpression of p53 protein (Figs. 7 and 8) and a loss of heterozygozity for chromosome 17p. EIC is also encountered in a different clinical setting. Being relatively independent from hormonal influences, it is considered as a precursor of endometrial serous adenocarcinoma, a non-endometrioid variant of endometrial carcinoma which also expresses immunoreactivity for p53 mutation proteins.

The natural history of EIC is that of a more aggressive lesion, being a precursor of a non-endometrioid uterine cancer (uterine serous papillary carcinoma) similar in many ways to the ovarian serous carcinoma with a proclivity to extend to the peritoneal cavity and pelvic organs.

CLASSIFICATION OF ENDOMETRIAL CARCINOMA

Endometrial carcinomas (EC) are classified into two major groups based on histopathologic, pathogenetic, and clinical characteristics:

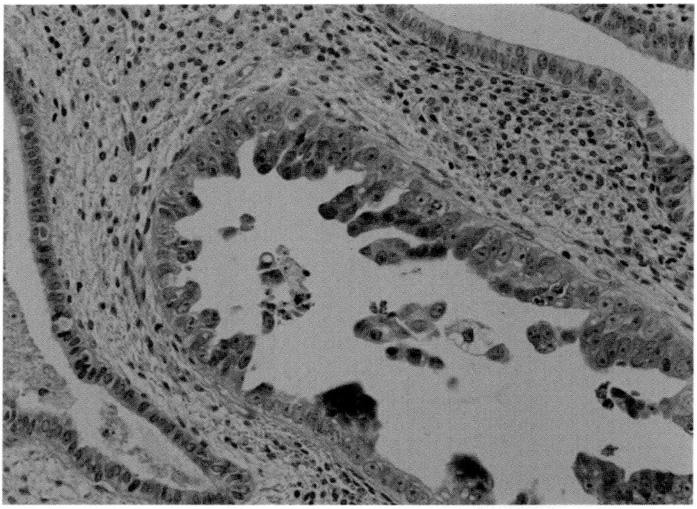

Fig. 5 Endometrial intraepithelial carcinoma (EIC) in a 72 years old patient with metastatic spread to pelvic lymph nodes and peritoneum. Hematoxylin/eosin, orginal magnification 100×.

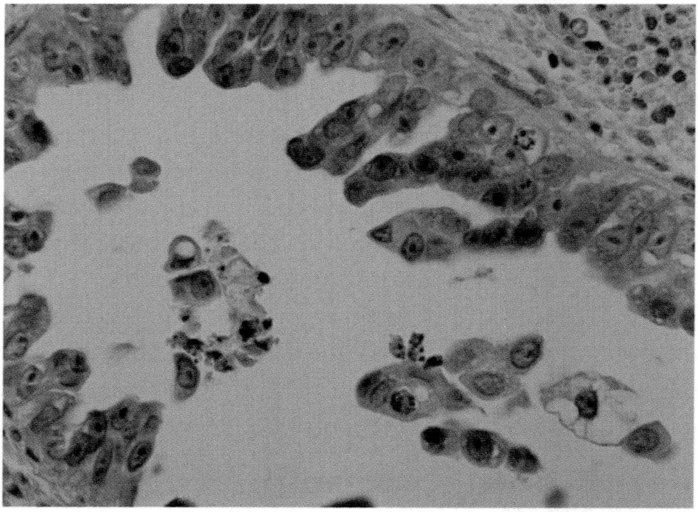

Fig. 6 Same patient as in Fig. 5. Note severely atypical nuclei with prominent nucleoli, papillary proliferation and detached clusters of tumor cells. Hematoxylin/eosin, orginal magnification 400×.

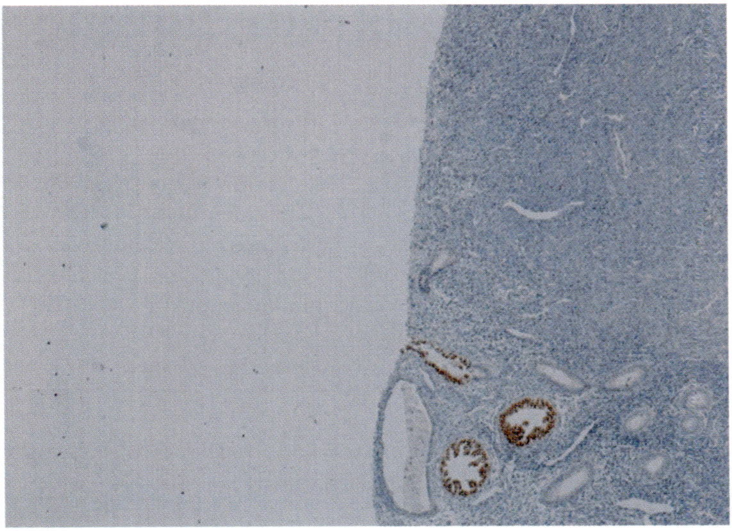

Fig. 7 Endometrial intraepithelial carcinoma (EIC) positive immune reaction to p53 mutation. Despite the focal endometrial lesion there were metastases in the peritoneum and pelvic lymph nodes 40.

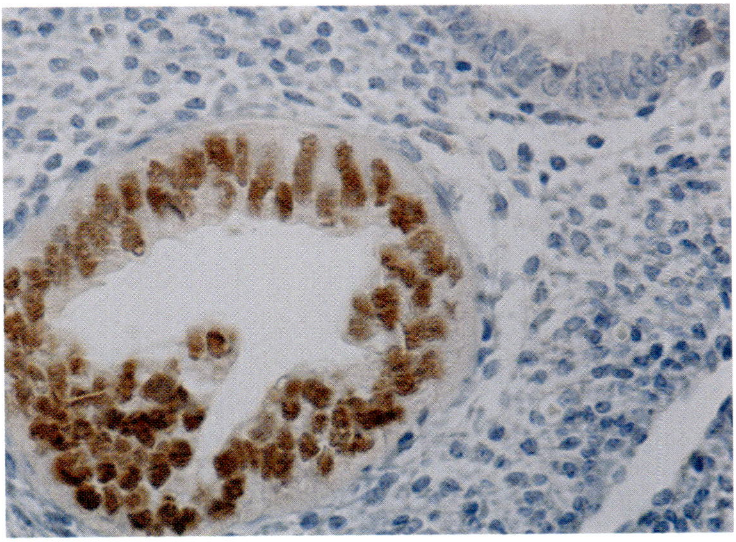

Fig. 8 EIC with positive stain for p53 mutation proteins.

Table 1. Pathogenetic and Clinical Classification of Endometrial Carcinoma

Type I	Type II
Unopposed estrogen effect	Hormonal-independent
Peri-menopausal and post-menopausal	Post-menopausal
Precursor: Atypical glandular hyperplasia and intraepithelial neoplasia (EIN)	Precursor: Endometrial intraepithelial carcinoma (EIC)
Variable myometrial invasion, often focal	Myometrial invasion, often deep
Endometrioid histologically	Non-endometrioid histologically
PTEN and K-ras mutations	p53 mutations
Favorable prognosis	Poor prognosis
Various degrees of differentiation	Poor differentiation

endometrioid and non endometrioid EC (Table 1). Overlapping of those characteristics in individual patients is of course possible. Endometrioid adenocarcinoma is more often diagnosed early.

EARLY ENDOMETRIAL CARCINOMA

The high risk for developing endometrial carcinoma in women exposed to continuous estrogenic stimulation is similar to that for endometrial hyperplasia which can be considered as a precursor especially the atypical glandular hyperplasia (EIN). Progression from hyperplasia to carcinoma is not always predictable only from histologic criteria. Hormonal therapy with substitution estrogen therapy and tamoxifen therapy for breast carcinoma may have a profound influence on the natural history of endometrial carcinogenesis.[2,6]

A relatively less common group of endometrial carcinomas arise in a non-hyperestrogenic clinical context, independently from risk factors such as obesity, nulliparity, chronic anovulation or exogenous hormone intake. These cancers are usually non-endometrioid and seen in older patients as compared to the endometrioid carcinomas.[7]

Tamoxifen (a non-steroidal synthetic triethylene estrogen derivative) has been widely and successfully used in the adjuvant therapy and prophylaxis of breast cancer. Tamoxifen binds to the estrogen receptors in a manner similar to that of estradiol and induces the binding of the tamoxifen/receptor complex to the nuclear DNA, resulting in a decrease of available unbound receptors. It is still considered as an important adjuvant therapeutic agent for this cancer, based on its antiestrogenic effect on the breast tissue. The effect of tamoxifen therapy on the endometrium is more complicated. A majority of patients do not develop abnormal changes and endometrial biopsies of about 60% of patients from a large cohort displayed normal cyclic and atrophic changes. However, endometrial polyps were found in a larger proportion (about 24%) and endometrial carcinoma, mostly seen in the polyps, was diagnosed in 4.7% of the cases. Interestingly, the endometrial cancers (33 out of 700 patients treated with Tamoxifen) were non-endometrioid (Figs. 9 and 10) in about two thirds of the cases. They were mostly associated with atrophic glands, therefore are not characteristic for a hyperestrogenic milieu.[6] The estrogenic agonist/antagonist effect of Tamoxifen on

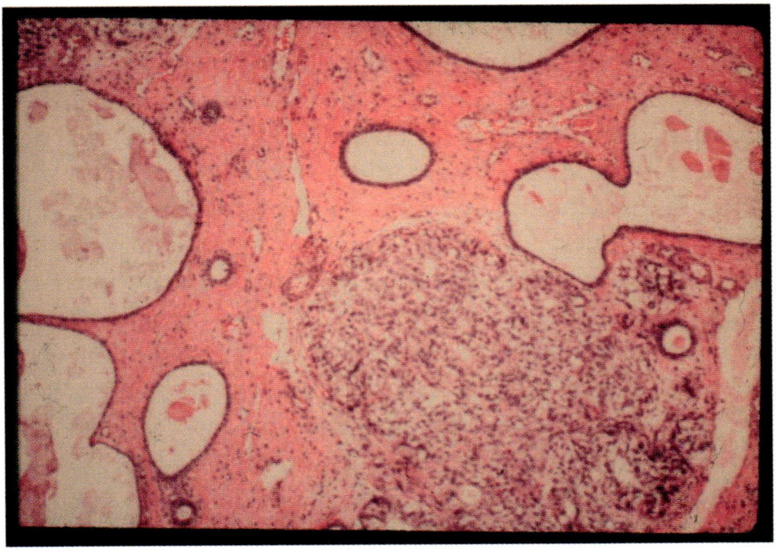

Fig. 9 Endometrial polyp in a 57 years old patient treated with Tamoxifen for breast carcinoma. Cystic atrophic glands and non-endometrioid clear cell adenocarcinoma (right lower quadrant). Hematoxylin/eosin, orginal magnification 100×.

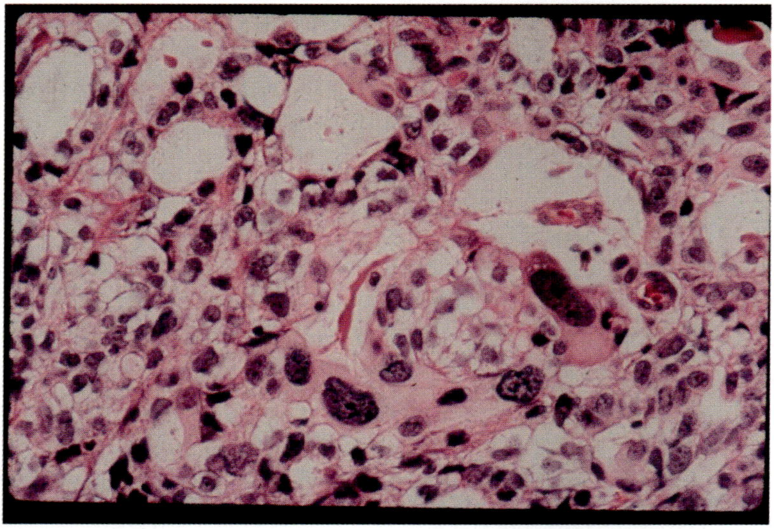

Fig. 10 Same patient as in Fig. 9. Clear cell adenocarcinoma with marked nuclear atypia. Hematoxylin/eosin, orginal magnification 400×.

the uterus by eliciting both myometrial (leiomyomas, adenomyosis) and endometrial (polyps) abnormal proliferation and even cancer has resulted in the recent recommendation to replace this drug with other antiestrogenic agents. An early diagnosis of endometrial neoplasms, including EIN, EIC, and overt carcinoma is possible by screening the patients treated with Tamoxifen with sonograms and endometrial biopsies.

Early endometrial cancer is considered to be an endometrial neoplasm confined to the uterus, Stage I, with or without invasion of the adjacent myometrium. Endometrial carcinoma confined to the endometrial layer represents Stage Ia; invading the inner half of the myometrium is Stage Ib; and invading the myometrium beyond the inner half is Stage Ic. Invasion of the cervix uteri represents a more advanced stage (Stage II); extension to the pelvis and vagina represents Stage III; and to the bladder and rectum, Stage IV (FIGO classification).

Endometrioid adenocarcinomas represents the majority of endometrial carcinomas in the developed countries, where they are also diagnosed in Stage I (confined to the uterine corpus) in about 75% of cases. Histologically, they are composed of glandular structures resembling the normal endometrial tissue from which they originate. Non-endometrioid histologic variants may coexist in up to 10% of the tumor volume.

While most patients are peri and postmenopausal, endometrioid adenocarcinomas can be diagnosed in younger women. They are usually but not always associated with polycystic ovarian disease and with other conditions leading to anovulation. Most often in younger women, EC is well differentiated and non-invasive.

The majority of endometrial carcinomas are manifested by vaginal bleeding and can be diagnosed in the early stages as opposed to non-endometrioid carcinomas which may be diagnosed only in later stages when they are spread beyond the uterus and even beyond the pelvic-abdominal cavity.

An early diagnosis of endometrial cancer is possible and more likely in the endometrioid variant, due to the frequent association with endometrial hyperplasia of all degrees which is symptomatic, the patients presenting with vaginal bleeding. Hyperplasia and carcinoma often coexist and represent indications for hysterectomy even if the proportion of overt carcinoma admixed with hyperplasia is low in the examined endometrial tissue. Hysterectomy is also indicated in atypical endometrial hyperplasia or EIN, especially in postmenopausal women.

PATHOLOGY OF ENDOMETRIAL CARCINOMA

Gross examination reveals a shaggy often polypoid surface with hemorrhagic and necrotic areas in the more advanced cases. The tumor expansion is more often exoplytic than infiltrative but can be both. The uterus is usually enlarged but sometime small uteri may harbor diffuse and infiltrative tumors. The neoplasm may be diffuse or localized to one or more areas, mostly protruding into the endometrial cavity and often with myometrial invasion. Many endometrial carcinomas are confined to the endometrial lining. Extension into the lower uterine segment is common but the endocervical canal is involved only in 20% of the cases.

Histopathologic examination should define the grade of differentiation of the tumor based on architectural and cytological criteria.

The histologic architecture of endometrial carcinoma derives from the glandular structures lining the uterine cavity. The more similar the tumor is to the normal glands, the better the differentiation. The glands are closely packed, with little or no intervening stroma and lined by atypical epithelial cell often piled up in multiple layers (Fig. 11). In Grade 1 EC 95% or more of the tumor has a glandular pattern; in grade 2, 6%–50% is composed of solid masses of tumor cells; and in grade 3, more than 50% of the tumor is composed of solid masses. The solid masses of tumor cells should not be represented by squamoid cells which represent squamous metaplasia and are often seen in better differentiated tumors.

The nuclei generally correlate with the architectural pattern being less atypical in the well differentiated tumors. However, in the presence of grade 3 nuclei (markedly enlarged, with irregular coarse chromatin, pleomorphic in shape and with multiple prominent nucleoli), the

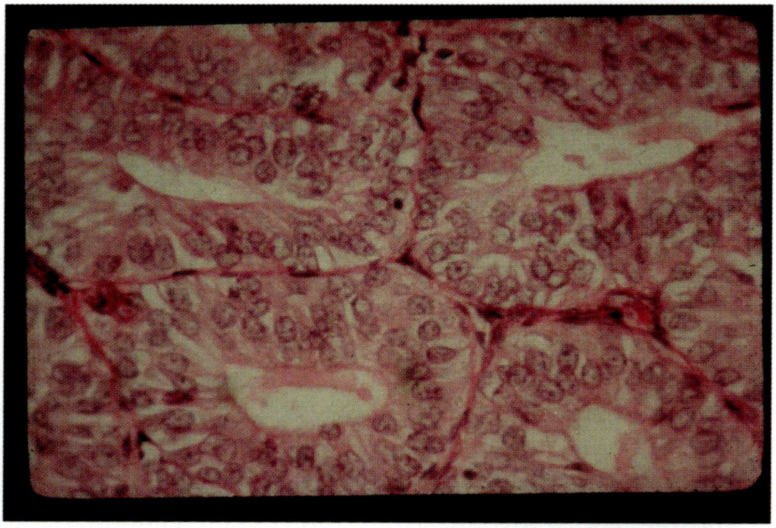

Fig. 11 Well differentiated (Grade 1) adenocarcinoma, endometrioid type. Back-to-back glands lined by a stratified epithelium. Hematoxylin/eosin, orginal magnification 400×.

better differentiated adenocarcinoma (grade 1 or 2) should be upgraded to grade 3.

The same tumor often displays various degrees of differentiation in different areas. Discordance between the grade of differentiation of an endometrial carcinoma from endometrial curettage to that seen in the hysterectomy specimen is not very unusual due to sampling.

Early endometrial carcinoma is often associated with endometrial hyperplasia of all degrees of severity, and especially with atypical complex hyperplasia (or EIN).

Endometrioid EC are the most common early endometrial carcinomas, with a polypoid or diffuse exophytic expansion and no or just local myometrial invasion. Also often seen in early endometrial adenocarcinoma is an associated adenomyosis with areas of endometrial glandular hyperplasia and even neoplastic changes confined to the adenomyotic area, with diminished or absent stroma. Because these changes are early neoplastic rather than invasive infiltrating, they represent a challenging dilemma for the patients' management. Most of such cases, however, are treated as infiltrating carcinomas to the myometrium, despite their origin in adenomyotic foci to which they are confined.

HISTOLOGIC PATTERNS OF ENDOMETRIAL CARCINOMAS (TABLE 2)

Endometrioid Adenocarcinomas Histologic Variants

Endometrioid adenocarcinomas composed of glandular structures somewhat analogous to normal endometrial glands can present villous infoldings lined by epithelial cells similar to those lining the glands, with rather bland nuclei. This represents the **villoglandular** endometrial carcinoma which is a variant of a low grade endometrioid adenocarcinoma. It should not be confused with papillary carcinoma which represents a non-endometrioid uterine carcinoma. **Secretory carcinomas** may be seen along with low grade endometrioid adenocarcinomas. The glandular structures display

Table 2. Pathologic Classification of Endometrial Adenocarcinoma

Endometrioid adenocarcinoma	Non-endometrioid carcinoma
Villo-glandular adenocarcinoma	Serous carcinoma
Secretory adenocarcinoma	Clear cell carcinoma
Ciliated (with tubal metaplasia) carcinoma	Papillary carcinoma
Squamous differentiation in adenocarcinoma	Mixed types and MMMT
Mucinous adenocarcinoma	Undifferentiated

an epithelial lining with vacuolated cytoplasm representing secretory changes, often due to progesterone therapy, with glycogen vacuoles in a subnuclear location reminiscent of normal post ovulatory changes (Fig. 12).

These features should not be interpreted as clear cell carcinoma, which is a non-endometrioid carcinoma characterized by atypical, often hobnail-shaped cells.

Squamous differentiation in endometrioid carcinoma occurs very frequent, and the grading of these tumors is that of the glandular

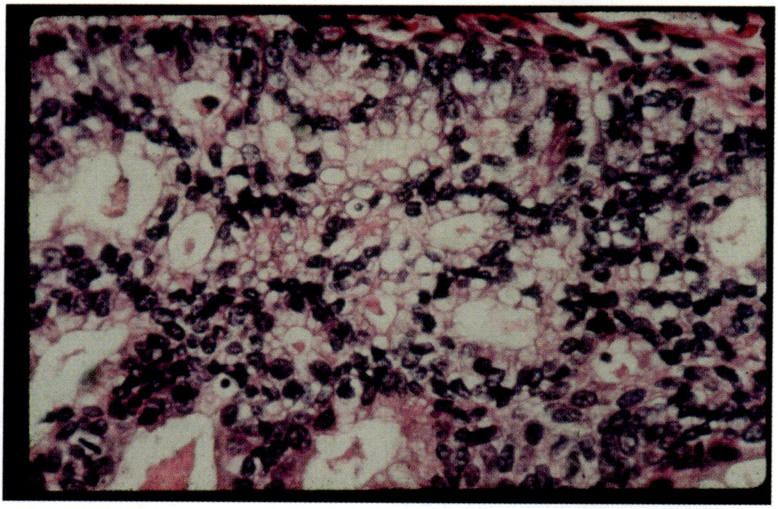

Fig. 12 Endometrial adenocarcinoma, endometrioid type, treated with progesterone (megace) for six months. Subnuclear vacuoles similar to secretory changes in a crowded glandular pattern. No mitotic activity is noted. Nuclei are relatively small and quiescent. Hematoxylin/eosin, orginal magnification 100×.

component rather than of the squamous elements. Squamous metaplasia of the endometrium is associated with estrogen effect and consists of "morules" similar to those seen in endometrial hyperplasia, or diffuse sheets with keratinized areas replacing the glandular structures.

Mucinous and **ciliated** endometrial carcinoma are less common, are usually well differentiated (Grade 1) and diagnosed in Stage I as most endometrioid carcinomas. Their origin in the endometrium on biopsy has to be confirmed because mucinous adenocarcinomas usually originate in the endocervix.

Non-Endometrioid EC

These tumors are less commonly seen than endometrioid EC. The histologic variants are serous, papillary and clear cell carcinomas.

Serous carcinomas were described also as **papillary** carcinomas because of their similarity to ovarian serous papillary carcinomas. They are a group of highly aggressive tumors. Most patients in this group are elderly.[7] Clinically, they do not have the classical endogenous risk factors (obesity, hyperestrogenism nulliparity etc.), neither were they likely to have been treated with estrogens. Cervical cytology may detect abnormalities more often in this group than in endometrioid EC. The uteri tend to be smaller and atrophic, sometimes with polypous growths that are partially benign, containing EIC and/or early serous carcinomas.

Histologically, these tumors have glandular, papillary, and solid patterns. The cells are often hobnail-shaped with clear cytoplasm and atypical nuclei. The papillary fronds resemble those of ovarian serous carcinomas (Fig. 13). Multinucleated and bizarre-shaped nuclei are also present. Mitotic activity is high and abnormal. Psammoma bodies are also encountered. The adjacent endometrium is often atrophic and endometrial hyperplasia is unusual. EIC and minimal serous carcinoma represent the early stages of these tumors which can, however, metastasize to early to the ovary and peritoneum by exfoliation and implantation (Fig. 7).

Clear cell carcinomas are infrequent EC, also seen more often in older women. The tumor cells are mostly large containing glycogen-rich

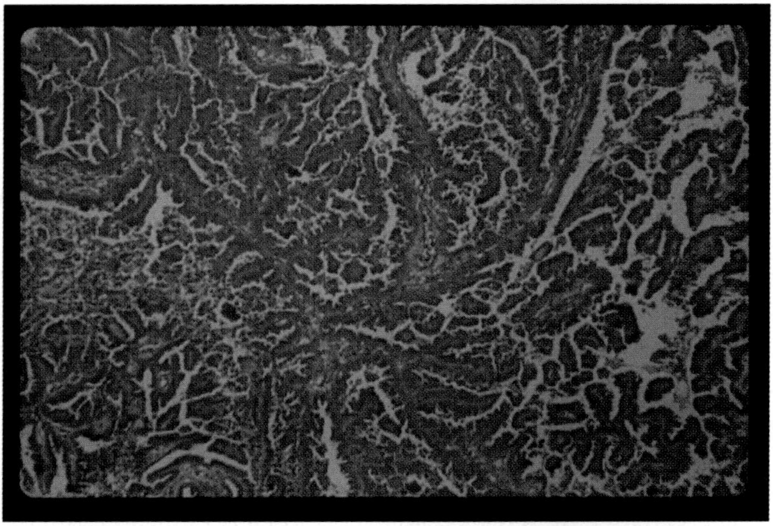

Fig. 13 Non-endometrioid serous papillary endometrial carcinoma, histologically similar to ovarian serous papillary carcinoma. Hematoxylin/eosin, orginal magnification 40×.

cytoplasmic vacuoles with pleomorphic nuclei and high mitotic activity (Fig. 14). They are often mixed with serous carcinomas, tend to be invasive into the myometrium, and metastatic to the regional lymph nodes.

Malignant mixed mullerian tumors (MMMT), also seen in elderly patients, are composed of malignant epithelial and stromal elements. They are uncommon tumors with occasional early stage presentation in endometrial polyps.

MOLECULAR BIOLOGY OF ENDOMETRIAL CARCINOMA

Estrogen and progesterone receptors (ER/PR) are present in most endometrial cancers, being higher in the endometrioid adenocarcinomas of low grade (Fig. 15). It is generally considered that ER/PR receptor positivity is predictive of responsiveness to progesterone therapy and has prognostic significance.[8–10]

For the evaluation of the biological behavior of EC, the immune reactivity to various markers for proliferation, apoptosis, tumor suppressor

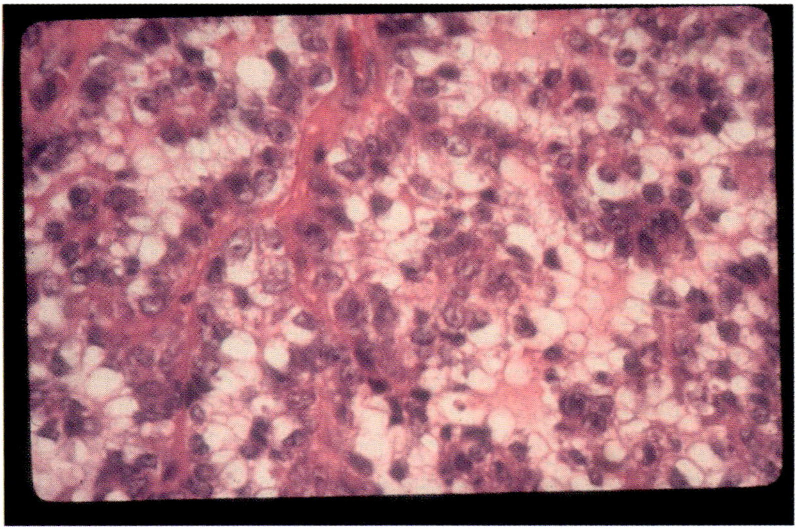

Fig. 14 Non-endometrioid endometrial clear cell carcinoma in a 69 years old patient. Hematoxylin/eosin, orginal magnification 400×.

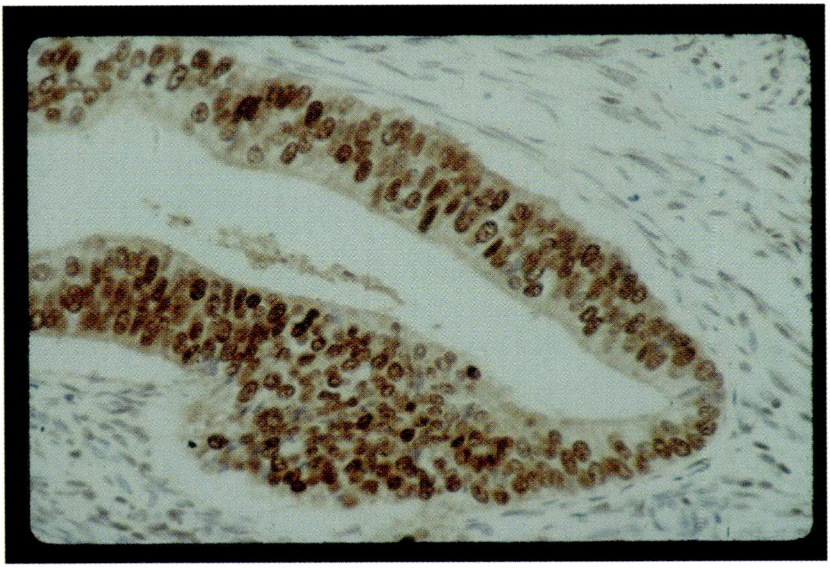

Fig. 15 EIN with positive stain for estrogen receptors, 100×.

genes and oncogenes, such as *BCL-2*, *MIB-1*, *HER2*, and especially *p53* and *K-ras* have yielded results suggestive of a correlation with metastatic potential and survival.[1]

Molecular genetics has confirmed the classification of EC into two broad groups, endometrioid, and non-endometrioid, based on pathologic, clinical, epidemiological and histochemical features.[11] The most commonly altered gene in endometrioid carcinoma is the *PTEN* tumor suppressor gene mutated in 30%–50% of endometrioid carcinomas and in 20% of endometrial hyperplasias. The inactivation of this gene seems to be involved in the early carcinogenesis of endometrioid EC. It is a marker for detecting endometrial glands predisposed to progress to malignancy.

Mutation of the *p53* tumor suppressor gene is seen in more advanced grades of endometrioid EC (G2, G3) and therefore may play a role in the progression and not in the initiation of this tumor.[12]

Microsatellite instability, related to a DNA mismatched repair system that results in an increased rate of mutations leading to neoplastic proliferation of the cells, has been found in both endometrial carcinoma and hyperplasia (and in hereditary non-polyposis colorectal carcinoma). Other oncogenes such as *K-ras*, *Her2/Neu*, *bcl-2*, and *3 catenins* have been found mutated in various proportions in EC.[1]

In non-endometrioid EC the mutation of *p53* is found in about 75% of serous endometrial carcinomas, in their early stages accounting for its aggressive behavior, as compared to endometrioid EC in which *p53* mutations occur more often later, in G2-G3 lesions.

This marker can be considered as an indicator of aggressive EC. K-ras and PTEN are rarely found in serous EC. Clear cell EC are non-endometrioid EC that tend to be high-grade and deeply invasive, presenting in advanced stages in which *p53* mutations are less frequently expressed than in serous EC.[13]

CONCLUSIONS

Endometrial carcinoma is the most common gynecologic cancer in the USA and in many other countries. Its incidence has increased because of the increase of risk factors such as longevity, obesity, nulliparity, hormone replacement therapy. Fortunately, most cases can be and actually are diagnosed relatively early in their development and can be cured by surgical and adjuvant therapies. The mortality due to this neoplasm is relatively low, about 7000 for approximately 40,000 new cases in the USA (estimated for 2006, American Cancer Society). An early diagnosis is possible due to the frequent association of EC with endometrial hyperplasia, especially atypical hyperplasia which is associated with the same risk factors as most endometrial cancers. These cancers are most often histologically endometrioid adenocarcinomas. They usually become symptomatic with irregular vaginal bleeding and especially postmenopausal bleeding. Patients receiving hormone replacement therapy for postmenopausal symptoms and Tamoxifen therapy against breast cancer, as well as those with certain predisposing hereditary conditions, should be screened with sonography, hysteroscopy, and especially endometrial biopsies. The smaller group of patients without clinical risk factors and without clinical symptoms such as vaginal bleeding, increased uterine volume who are also generally older and less likely to have frequent gynecologic check-ups, often present in later stages of the disease, with involvement of pelvic, abdominal and distant organs by the tumor. Predictably, there is a higher mortality in this group of patients in whom the histopathologic diagnosis is more often that of non-endometrioid adenocarcinoma. The challenging question is that of an early diagnosis of EC in women who are elderly, not obese, often multiparous, with no history of hormone intake, often from a social-economical deprived background, unlikely to have frequent gynecologic examinations. The pathologic findings that are revealing in such cases are precancerous lesions without endometrial hyperplasia and occasionally abnormal Pap smears. Endometrial intrauterine carcinoma (EIC) may be seen in atrophic polyps or adjacent to atrophic endometrium. Unfortunatelly, invasive non-endometrioid EC is not often diagnosed in its early stages because of the absence of clinical risk factors and often, the absence of symptoms (vaginal bleeding, tumor mass). These mostly type 2 EC are often diagnosed in a late stage by the time they become symptomatic. The natural history of the non-endometrioid EC is somewhat similar to that of ovarian serous carcinoma, the early diagnosis of which is still elusive.

REFERENCES

1. Ronnett B, Zaino RJ, Ellenson LH, *et al.*, Endometrial carcinoma, in *Blanstein's Pathology of the Female Genital Tract*, 5th edn., Springer Verlag, New York, Berlin, Heidelberg, pp. 533–537, 2002.
2. Deligdisch L, Hormonal pathology of the endometrium, *Mod Pathol* **13**(3):285–294, 2000.
3. Mutter GL, Zaino RJ, Baak JP, *et al.*, Benign endometrial hyperplasia sequence and endometrial intraepithelial neoplasisa (review), *Int J Gynecol Pathol* **26**:103–114, 2007.
4. Mutter GL, Duska L, Crum CP, Endometrial intraepithelial neoplasia, in Crum CP, Lee K (eds.), *Diagnostic Gynecologic and Obstetric Pathology*, Philadelphia PA Saunders, pp. 493–518, 2005.
5. Mutter GL, Lin MC, Fitzgerald JT *et al.*, Altered PTEN expression as a diagnostic marker for the earliest endometrial precancers, *J Natl Cancer Inst* **92**:924–930, 2000.
6. Deligdisch L, Kalir T, Cohen CJ, *et al.*, Endometrial histopathology in 700 patients treated with Tamoxifen for breast cancer, *Gynecol Oncol* **78**:181–186, 2000.
7. Deligdisch L, Kase N, Bleiweiss I, Endometrial cancer in elderly women: a histologic and steroid receptor study, *Gerontology* **46**:17–21, 2000.
8. Fukuda K, Mori M, Uchiyama M, *et al.*, Prognostic significance of progesterone receptor immunohistochemistry in endometrial carcinoma, *Gynecol Oncol* **69**:220–225, 1998.
9. Ramirez PT, Frumovitz M, Bodurka DC, *et al.*, Hormonal therapy for the management of grade I endometrial adenocarcinoma: a literature review, *Gynecol Oncol* **95**:133–138, 2004.
10. Montz FJ, Bristow RE, Bovicelli A, *et al.*, Intrauterine progesterone treatment of early endometrial cancer, *Am J Obstet Gynecol* **186**(4): 651–657, 2002.
11. Deligdisch L, Holinka CF, Endometrial carcinoma? Two diseases, *Cancer Detection and Prevention* **10**:237–246, 1987.
12. Tashiro H, Isacson C, Levine R, *et al.*, p53 mutations are common in uterine serous carcinoma and occur early in their pathogenesis, *Am J Surg Pathol* **150**:177–185, 1997.

13. Baak JP, Mutter GL, Robboy S *et al.*, The molecular genetics and morphometry-based endometrial intraepithelial neoplasia classification system predicts disease progression in endometrial hyperplasia more accurately then the 1994 World Health Organization classification system, *Cancer* **103**:2304–2312, 2005.
14. Sherman ME, Sturgeon S, Brinton LA, *et al.*, Risk factors and hormone levels in patients with serous and endometrial uterine carcinomas, *Mod Pathol* **10**:963–968, 1997.

CHAPTER 5

EARLY DIAGNOSIS OF OVARIAN CANCER

Liane Deligdisch

INTRODUCTION

Ovarian cancer is not the most common gynecologic cancer but it is the most lethal. Despite recent progress in the identification of risk factors, chemotherapy and cytoreductive surgery, the high lethality due to this neoplasm still represents a major public health problem.

There were about 165,000 cases of ovarian cancer annually, worldwide, and about 23,000 new cases in the US in 2007. It is the sixth most common cancer in women in the US. Ovarian cancer results in more deaths than all the other gynecologic cancers combined.

Only a small percentage of the cases are known to be related to an inherited mutated gene while most cases are considered to be sporadic, with mostly unknown risk factors. There is no implementation of a systematic screening for ovarian cancer at the present time; such screening for other malignancies, especially for cervical cancer, resulted in spectacular declines in their morbidity and mortality.

The high mortality due to ovarian cancer is related to the fact that the vast majority of cases (70%–75%) are diagnosed in late stages of the disease, when the tumor is spread beyond the ovary (ies) and the pelvis. The reason for this is the paucity or absence of specific clinical symptoms during the early stages of the tumor.

RISK FACTORS, GENETIC RISK

Non-Hereditary Risk

The incidence of ovarian cancer is considerably higher in industrialized countries in which there is high consumption of animal fat. This was evident in women who immigrated from countries with low incidence of ovarian cancer such as Japan to the US.

A controversial but much studied risk factor is ovarian epithelial injury by chemical carcinogens such as talcum powder or asbestos fibers. The injuries due to incessant ovulation that elicits a defective DNA repair may result in mutations leading to ovarian cancer. The use of fertility drugs with subsequent hyperovulation may promote an enhancement of errors in DNA replication and repair. There is no consensus on this subject because of a number of conflicting reports about the relationship between the effect of fertility drugs and ovarian cancer.[1]

Conversely, it seems that high parity, lactation, tubal ligation and the use of oral contraceptives have a significant protective effect, especially the latter. The low risk to develop ovarian cancer in women using contraceptives is related to the suppression of ovulation and thus the decrease of pituitary stimulation of the ovary by gonadotropins. Progestins were also shown to induce cell apoptosis in monkeys, thus having a protective effect.[2]

Hereditary Risk

Approximately 10% of ovarian carcinomas are related to mutations in specific inherited genes, namely *BRCA1* and *2*. These genes are also responsible for greatly increasing the risk of early-onset breast cancer. Mutations of other genes responsible for hereditary colorectal cancer and endometrial cancer may also be involved in some cases of ovarian cancer.

The risk of developing ovarian cancer due to mutations of *BRCA1* and *2* is about 28% to 44% by the age of 70.[3] Women already diagnosed with breast cancer due to the mutations of these genes have a ten-fold increase in their risk of ovarian cancer compared to other women with early onset breast cancer.[4]

Mutations of *BRCA1* and *2* genes confer cancer risk in autosomal dominant fashion, with offsprings having an equal chance of either being at greatly increased risk of cancer or being at the general population risk.

Most hereditary ovarian cancers are invasive serous papillary carcinomas (OSPC). The mutated suppressor genes *BRCA1* and *2* are also identified in families with tumors of other sites, often with one or more relatives diagnosed with breast cancer before the age of 50, or less commonly, with colorectal or endocervical cancer diagnosed before the age of 50.

Assessment of family history can identify the possibility of one's hereditary risk of ovarian cancer but cannot confirm whether the woman herself is at risk (Table 1).

OVARIAN DYSPLASIA

The histologic identification of precursors of epithelial cancer has contributed significantly to the screening for gynecologic cancers of the breast, cervix, and endometrium. The concept of a preinvasive oncogenic transformation of epithelial tissues, as a result of hormonal influences in endometrial or breast neoplasms, or as a result of infectious (viral) factors in cervical cancer, and the identification of actual tissue change precursors of malignancy has resulted in spectacular decreases

Table 1. Hereditary Ovarian Cancer

About 10% of invasive serous papillary carcinomas.
Hereditary breast/ovarian cancer (HBOC syndrome) have *BRCA1* and *2* gene mutations.
Germplasm BRCA1 gene mutations: 70%.
Germplasm BRCA2 gene mutations: 20%.
Highly penetrant autosomal dominant mutations.
HBOC associated with 75%–90% hereditary ovarian and 30%–70% breast cancer.

in morbidity and mortality of numerous malignant tumors. Histologic changes that do not represent overt malignancy but are related to an abnormal proliferation that increases in severity and/or may become invasive neoplasms are generally designated as dysplastic (bad molding in Greek). Dysplastic changes may also be seen in the vicinity of invasive neoplasms in many epithelial tissues such as colon, larynx, vocal cords, skin (dysplastic nevi and melanomas). In the female genital tract, the diagnosis of cervical dysplasia represents the most common, and the best example of a successful prevention of cancer by identifying and removing its precursors. It should be mentioned that the progression from dysplasia to overt cancer is unpredictable and related to mostly poorly understood factors of host defense. However, it is reasonable to assume that the more severe the degree of dysplastic change, the more likely the transformation to overt cancerous tissue.

Ovarian dysplasia has first been described in identical twin sisters of women diagnosed with ovarian cancer who underwent prophylactic oophorectomy.[5] The histologic examination of the grossly normal appearing ovaries revealed abnormal epithelial stratification, lack of polarity of the ovarian surface epithelium, and enlarged nuclei with a coarse chromatin texture (Fig. 1).

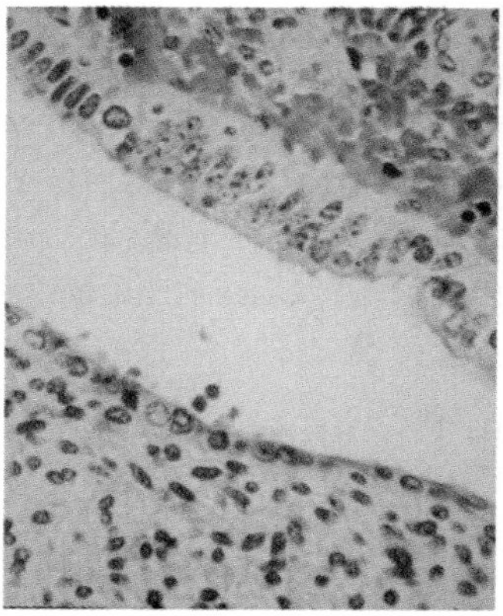

Fig. 1 Dysplastic ovarian epithelium diagnosed in an identical twin sister of a woman diagnosed with ovarian carcinoma. Note stratification, loss of polarity and coarse chromatin network. Hematoxylin/eosin, orginal magnification 100×.

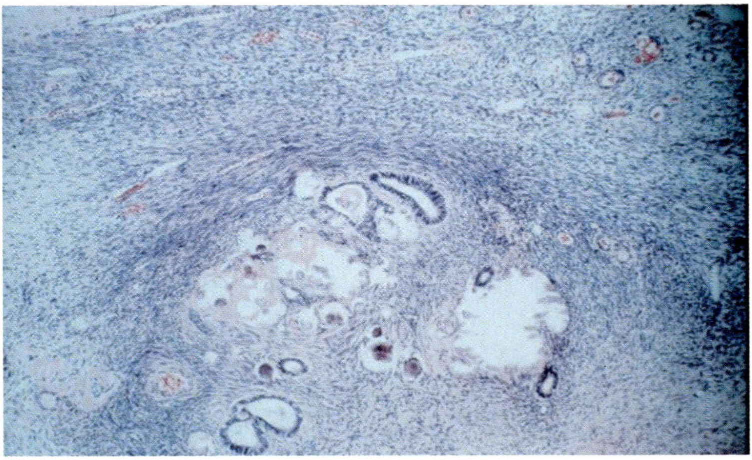

Fig. 2 Ovary "at risk": multiple small ovarian cysts and psamomma bodies in the ovarian cortex. Hematoxylin/eosin, orginal magnification 40×.

The surface epithelium of the ovary is an extension of the peritoneal mesothelium. It is the site of origin of the vast majority of ovarian epithelial tumors (ovarian carcinomas).

Invaginations of the surface epithelium often create inclusion cysts with papillary proliferation into the cysts. Most ovarian serous cystadenocarcinomas originate from such cysts and present at a late stage with solid and cystic components and most often, extension to the peritoneum. Precursors of serous papillary carcinomas are not easily identifiable because of the hidden location of these intraovarian cysts often of microscopic dimensions (Fig. 2).

Dysplastic changes of the ovarian surface epithelium and of the lining of these cysts were identified in two clinical settings:

(1) In apparently normal ovaries, often removed from women with family history of ovarian and/or breast cancer (incidental dysplasia).
(2) In the vicinity of overt invasive cancer (adjacent dysplasia). Since the histologic characteristics of these dysplastic changes were rather subtle and somewhat subjective, computerized image analysis was

used to validate the histological changes that turned out to be intermediate between normal and malignant ovarian epithelium by using morphometric assessments of architectural (crowding and stratification) and cellular (nuclear profiles) characteristics of normal cancerous and dysplastic cells (Figs. 3–6).

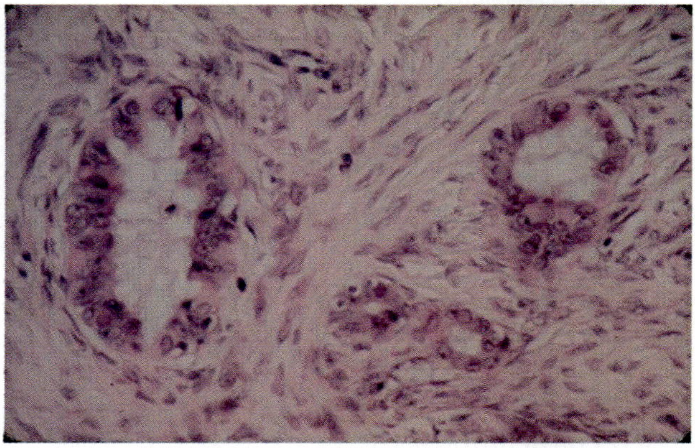

Fig. 3 Ovarian dysplasia: epithelial inclusion cysts with increased nucleo-cytoplasmic ratio, piling up of epithelial cells with loss of polarity. Hematoxylin/eosin, orginal magnification 400×.

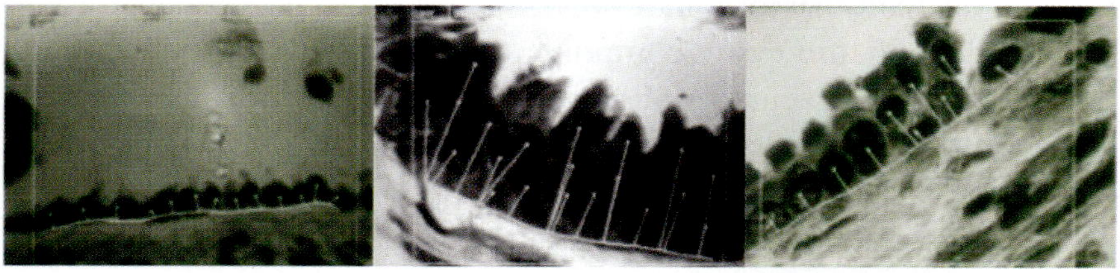

(a) (b) (c)

Fig. 4 (a) Morphometry of normal ovarian surface epithelium. Cells are at regular intervals and equal distance from basement membrane, as demonstrated by lines tracing the shortest distance from the center of nuclei to the basement membrane. (b) Morphometry of ovarian epithelial cancer cells: irregular high stratification and crowding as demonstrated by lines traced by computer from the center of nuclei to the basement membrane. (c) Morphometry of ovarian dysplasia: epithelial cells demonstrate cell density and stratification intermediate between normal and cancer.

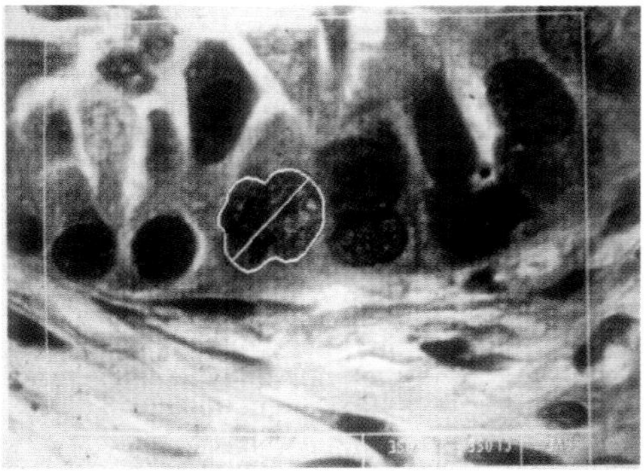

Fig. 5 Morphometric evaluation of nuclear surface, perimeter, and diameter of a dysplastic cell.

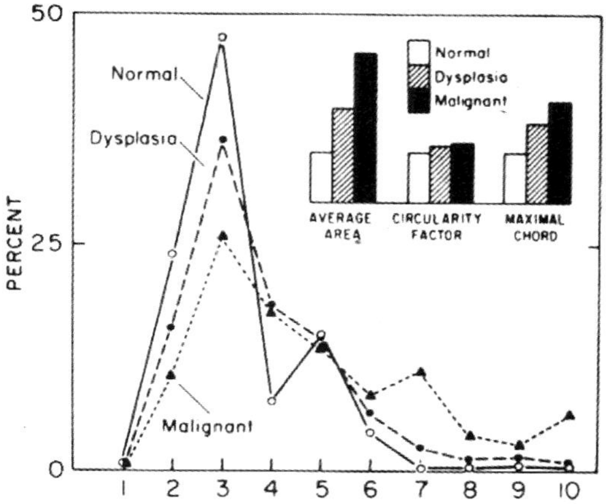

Fig. 6 Diagram of nuclear profiles. Normal nuclei distribution: 10 μm–35 μm. Malignant nuclei: 10 μm–100 μm. Dysplastic nuclei: Intermediate.

The architectural characteristics (crowding and piling up of epithelial cells) and nuclear profiles (area and diameter as well as texture) were evaluated by morphometric measurements and evaluated by statistical methods that also included neural networks.[6–8]

The objective methods of quantifying subtle differences in the tissue structure of dysplastic ovarian epithelium yielded accurate values characterizing tissue and cell changes intermediate between benign and malignant ovarian epithelium (Table 2). Interestingly, the histologic changes of incidental dysplasia diagnosed in grossly normal appearing ovaries were similar to the histologic changes in dysplastic epithelium adjacent to overt ovarian carcinoma, as measured with the most discriminating methods of multivariate statistical analysis and neural networks (Fig. 7).[8]

At the present time, there is no screening program for ovarian cancer. Serum tumor markers have not proven to be sensitive or specific enough for an early ovarian cancer screening. With the advent

Table 2. Criteria for Diagnosis of Ovarian Dysplasia

Architectural: Stratification, crowding, loss of polarity.
Cytological: Cellular atypia, enlarged nuclei and increased nucleo-cytoplasmic ratio, prominent nucleoli, changes in chromatin pattern (nuclear texture).
Morphometric data evaluated by statistical and artificial neural network analysis for validation.

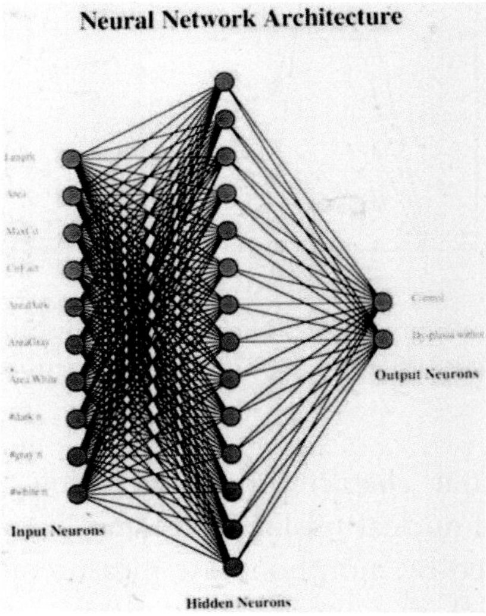

Fig. 7 Neural network architecture. Dysplastic nuclei in incidental dysplasia are indistinguishable from those of adjacent dysplasia.

of advanced laparoscopic techniques, the ovary becomes more accessible and asymptomatic precursors or low-stage ovarian cancer may be detected more readily. The routine histologic descriptions and the measurements performed by interactive methods of computerized image analysis have revealed changes that are recognizable and reproducible by the practicing pathologist. The structural changes of the ovarian epithelial tissue diagnostic for dysplasia were correlated with antigenic expression of certain tumor markers, such as p53 and Ki67.[9] More tumor marker studies are presently studied in order to gain an insight into the molecular biologic events occurring in histologically and morphometrically identified ovarian dysplastic changes.

PROPHYLACTIC OOPHORECTEMY AND THE OVARY AT RISK

The most effective prevention of ovarian carcinoma is prophylactic oophorectomy (PO), which is now considered a valid option for women at risk for ovarian cancer. PO is recommended for carriers of *BRCA1* and *2* mutations offering them a dramatic 90%–98% chance of reduction of ovarian and peritoneal cancer risk, and a 50% reduction of later breast cancer hazard.[10,11] Other potential benefits include the discovery of an occult ovarian cancer[12,13] and the possibility of studying pathobiological changes that may represent potential precursors of ovarian neoplasm in these ovaries "at risk".[9,14,15]

The prophylactically removed ovaries are generally described as grossly and most often microscopically normal. A number of recent studies, however, have challenged the notion of "normal" by submitting the grossly normal appearing ovaries to a thorough histologic analysis consisting of multiple sections of the organ; examination of histologic changes associated with neoplastic and preneoplastic features; morphometric studies including a novel approach of a tri-dimensional assessment of nuclear texture; and immunohistochemical identification of tumor markers using microdissection.[9,14]

A "cancer prone" phenotype has been described in ovaries removed by PO. It consists of inclusion cysts, surface papillomatosis, epithelial hyperplasia and deep invaginations of the surface epithelium into the ovarian stroma.[15]

The study of nuclear texture by computerized image analysis revealed changes in the size and texture of the ovarian surface epithelial nuclei in a statistically significant high proportion of ovarian tissue removed by PO from Ashkenazi Jewish women. These females also have genetic mutations predisposing to breast/ovarian carcinoma.[14] The nuclear texture analysis is based on the autocorrelation procedure which is a powerful discriminant especially when combined with nuclear measurements illustrated by three-dimensional images. These images represent the relationship between neighboring pixels. Normal nuclei with a homogenous chromatin network generate a flat surface reflecting the homogeneity of the nuclear chromatin. The nuclei of cancer cells with their characteristic irregularly clumped chromatin reflecting the out of control DNA replication have a markedly non-homogenous tri-dimensional image. In dysplastic nuclei, the tri-dimensional image is intermediate, that is less homogenous than the normal and less irregular than the carcinoma nuclei (Figs. 8(a)–(c)).

The size of the nuclei correlates with their texture being also intermediate for the dysplastic cells (31 μm versus 18 μm for normal and 51 μm for cancer cell nuclei).

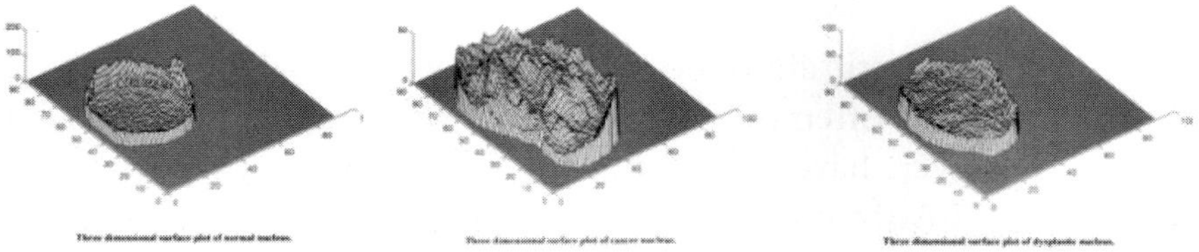

(a) (b) (c)

Fig. 8 (a) Tri-dimensional image of normal ovarian epithelial nucleus: flat surface reflects homogenous texture. Area: 18 μm. (b) Tri-dimensional image of malignant nucleus: high spikes and deep depressions due to markedly irregular chromatin texture. Area: 51 μm. (c) Dysplastic nucleus: irregularity of the tri-dimensional image is intermediate between benign and malignant. Area: 31 μm.

Further studies of prophylactic oophorectomy specimens identified a number of histologic changes significantly more common when compared to oophorectomies performed for reasons unrelated to ovarian carcinoma risk.[9]

These histologic changes include the following: deep invaginations of the surface epithelium into the ovarian hyperplastic cortical stroma; multiple, often clustering, epithelial inclusion cysts; and psammoma bodies (concentric calcifications around a proteinaceous central body) often seen in ovarian serous papillary carcinomas and considered to represent a "burnt-out" papillary proliferation. Surface papillations, hyperplasia of the surface epithelium and of the epithelium lining the inclusion cyst, and the presence of dysplastic changes of this epithelium (piling up, loss of polarity, nuclear size increase and irregular texture) are histologic changes that are found in the "ovaries at risk" removed by PO in significantly higher proportion than in control ovaries (Fig. 9). Immunohistologic analysis revealed a significantly higher immunoreactivity for tumor markers such as p53, MIB-1 (Ki67)

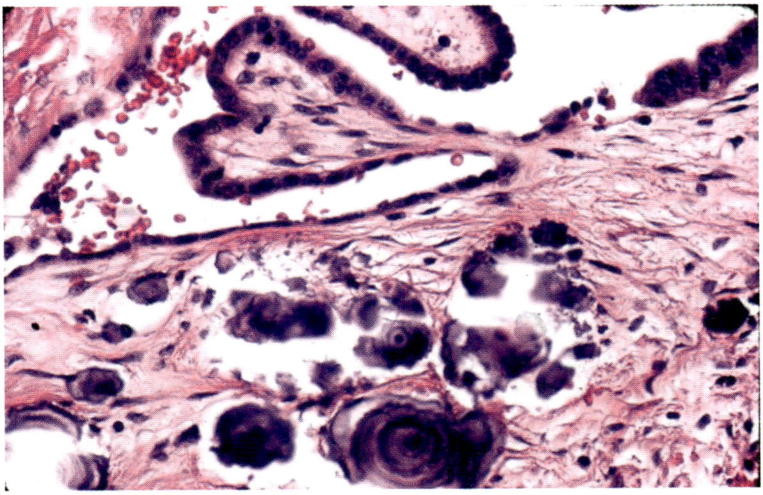

Fig. 9 Papillations next to psammoma bodies (concentric calcifications) often encountered in "ovaries at risk". Hematoxylin/eosin, orginal magnification 400×.

and Ca 125 in the ovarian tissue removed by PO as compared to the control specimens.[9]

The abnormal histologic, morphometric and immunohistologic findings in apparently normal ovaries removed by PO justify more detailed studies of this tissue. The thorough examination of multiple ovarian sections from PO specimens may occasionally reveal unsuspected, clinically silent, cancer tissue, associated with dysplastic epithelium (Fig. 10).

Overexpression of Ki67 proliferation marker (Fig. 11) and of the p53 tumor suppressor gene product (Fig. 12) in the ovarian epithelium suggest a proliferation abnormality and the loss of cell cycle control, clonal expansion and acquisition of potential invasive growth properties. Since it is unlikely that multiple mutations of such occur within the same cell cycle within the same cell, it is reasonable to assume the existence of preneoplastic changes in the ovarian epithelium.[10] Recent reports of morphometric studies of nuclear abnormalities in "high-risk" ovaries support their significance for early detection and prevention of ovarian cancer.[16,17]

With the advent of laparoscopy, the ovaries become more accessible for study; the analysis of structural and molecular changes in the "ovaries at risk" may offer an unique insight into the early preneoplastic changes of these tissue (Tables 3 and 4).

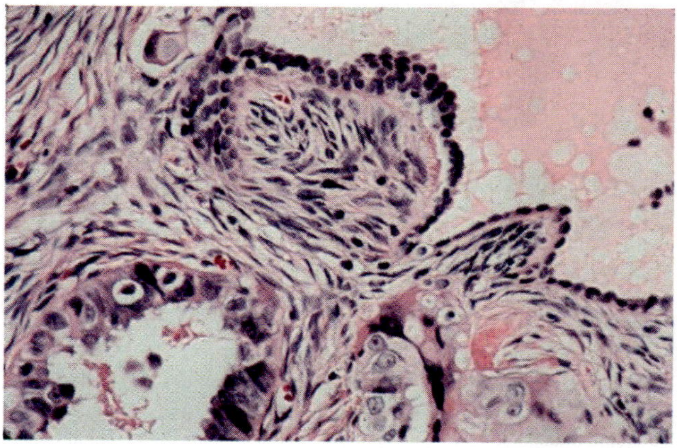

Fig. 10 Normal ovarian surface epithelium (above), dysplastic changes (left lower corner) and frankly malignant tissue (carcinoma, right lower corner). Hematoxylin/eosin, orginal magnification 100×.

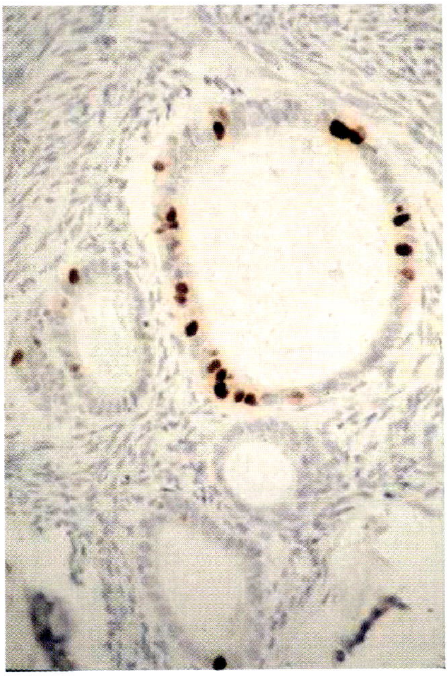

Fig. 11 Ki67 immunopositivity of ovarian epithelial inclusion cysts in "ovary at risk." Hematoxylin/eosin, orginal magnification 100×.

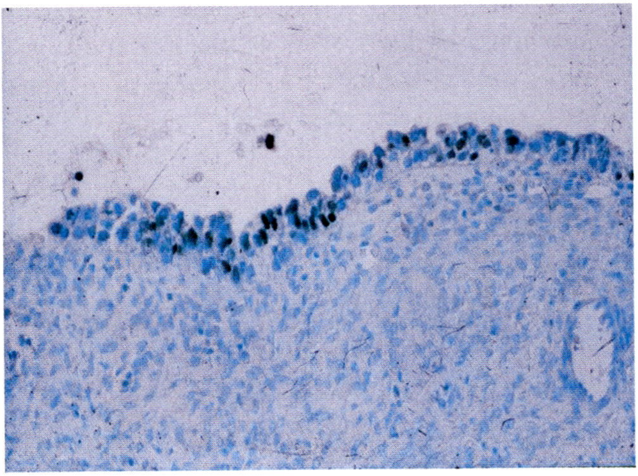

Fig. 12 p53 immunopositivity of ovarian surface epithelium in "ovary at risk".

Table 3. Prophylactic Oophorectomy

Most effective way to prevent ovarian cancer in women at high risk.
Most commonly found structural alterations: epithelial invaginations, surface papillations, psammoma bodies, epithelial stratification, ovarian dysplasia (cancer-prone phenotype) and occasional "silent" carcinoma.
Most common biologic/molecular changes: increased expression of MIB-1, Ca 125, p53.
Ovarian carcinogenesis requires multiple mutations leading to the loss of cell cycle control, clonal expansion and invasive growth.
Prophylactic oophorectomy specimens may reveal cancer precursor changes.

Table 4. "High Risk" Ovarian Study

Multiple sections of entire ovarian and fallopian tube specimens necessary.
Occasional occult carcinoma.
Precursor lesions of ovarian carcinoma significantly more common in PO specimens.
Identification of subtle morphologic features of "preneoplastic phenotype".
Validation by morphometry and metabolic/molecular biology.

Prophylactic oophorectomy (PO) is performed along with bilateral removal of the fallopian tubes (prophylactic salpingo-oophorectomy, PBSO) in order to remove potential precursors of fallopian tube carcinoma. An occasional carcinoma *in situ* or overt early carcinoma is discovered in the specimens of PBSO in women at risk as well as in the control population. Since primary fallopian tube carcinomas are rare, their precursors are assumed to be unusual findings. However, atypia of the fallopian tube mucosal epithelium is not unusual. The progression of such atypical changes reminiscent of dysplasia to overt carcinoma is possibly hindered by still poorly understood host defense mechanisms in the fallopian tube.

STAGE I OVARIAN CARCINOMA

Only a minority of ovarian cancers of epithelial origin are diagnosed in early stages, when confined to one or both ovaries. The prognosis changes dramatically for ovarian cancers diagnosed in late stages. In about 75% of Stage I ovarian carcinomas the prognosis is 80%–90% five year survival. The prognosis for Stage III/IV ovarian carcinoma is only 30% five year survival.

The high lethality of ovarian carcinoma diagnosed in late stages is due to a paucity of symptoms in the majority of cases. Most ovarian carcinomas are classified histologically as serous papillary adenocarcinomas (OSPC, 46%) and present most commonly as bilateral ovarian cystic and solid neoplasms with the involvement of the peritoneum by tumor masses that often exceed the volume of the ovarian tumors. It is amazing how often large masses of tumor contained in the abdominal cavity are asymptomatic, or are manifested only by vague upper gastrointestinal symptoms such as bloating and nausea. Symptoms often appear with the advent of ascites that occurs in late stages of the disease.

Ovarian carcinomas histologically diagnosed as non-serous, include mucinous, endometrioid and clear cell carcinomas. These are generally less frequent than their serous papillary (OSPC) counterparts. When considered in all stages: they are 20% mucinous, 28% endometrioid and 6% clear cell carcinomas. These tumors are more often unilateral and are less often associated with peritoneal tumor involvement at the time of diagnosis. Their prognosis does not differ much when diagnosed at the same stage as the OSPC. However, they are more frequently diagnosed in early stages, due to their association with pathologic findings that are symptomatic. Endometrioid and clear cell carcinomas of the ovary are often associated with endometriosis, especially endometriotic ovarian cysts and pelvic endometriosis. The patients harboring these non-serous ovarian carcinomas are usually younger and often present with symptoms of infertility, irregular vaginal bleeding and hormonal disturbances associated with hyperestrogenism such as endometrial polyps, adenomyosis, and uterine leiomyomas. Endometrial hyperplasia of various degrees of severity and endometrial carcinomas are not infrequently diagnosed in patients with ovarian carcinoma. It is not very uncommon to find an ovarian neoplasm that has been clinically silent, only to be discovered at surgery performed for endometrial/uterine pathology that was manifested clinically by abnormal vaginal bleeding or pelvic pain.[18]

Ovarian endometriosis is a very common disorder and fortunately only rarely associated with ovarian cancer. Patients suffering from symptoms due to endometriosis are often diagnosed with ovarian endometriotic cysts, which are occasionally lined by an atypical endometrioid epithelium. An adjacent overtly neoplastic endometrioid and/or clear cell carcinoma is identified in some cases which came to medical attention due to symptomatic endometriosis (Fig. 13).

It was reported that 30%–40% of ovarian endometrioid and clear cell carcinomas contain identifiable areas of endometriosis.[19] The atypical areas of endometriosis adjacent to carcinoma (Fig. 14) share some immune-phenotypical characteristics with the malignant tissue such as bcl-2 and p53 altered proteins (Fig. 15).

Bax, MMP-9 and PTEN have been reported as positive in cancer associated endometriosis along with the high positivity of the cancerous tissue for the same markers.[19] Ovarian endometrioid and clear-cell adenocarcinomas are not infrequently associated with simultaneous primary endometrial carcinomas. They are often diagnosed in Stage I, are unilateral and despite the concomitant primary endometrial carcinoma, their prognosis is generally more favorable than that of ovarian serous papillary carcinomas.[20]

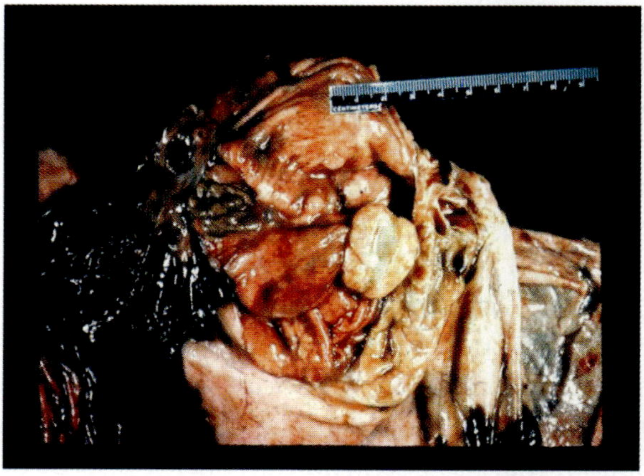

Fig. 13 Ovarian endometriotic cyst with solid nodule representing a clear cell carcinoma.

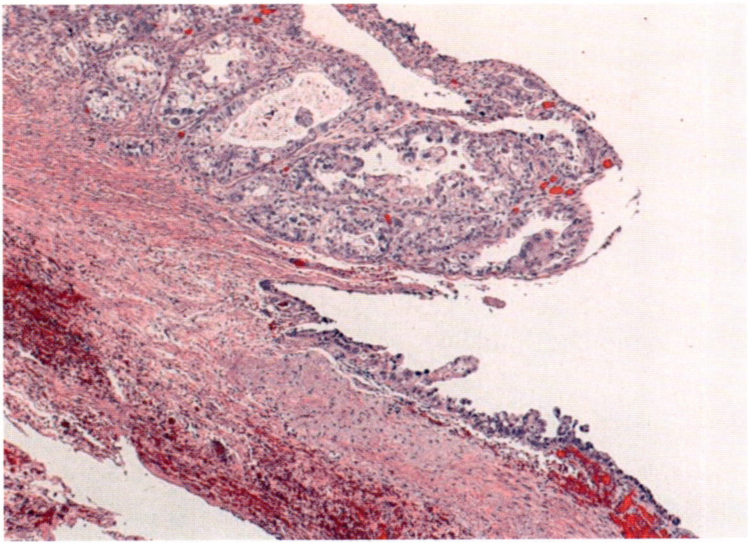

Fig. 14 Endometrioid adenocarcinoma (left) adjacent to atypical endometriosis (right) Hematoxylin/eosin, orginal magnification 40×.

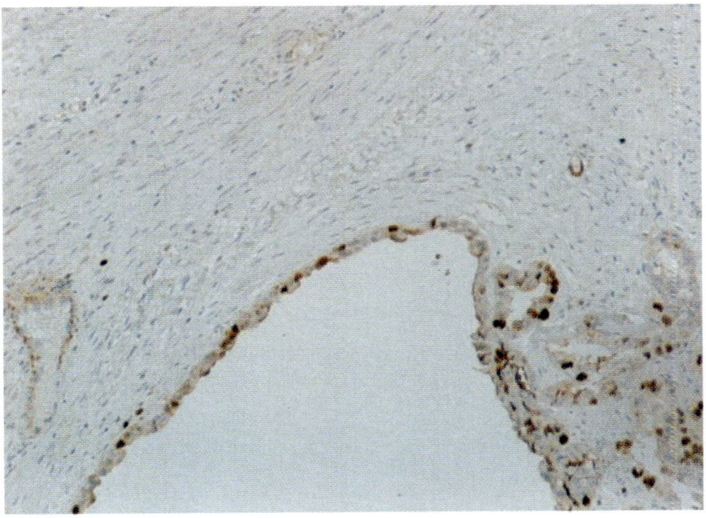

Fig. 15 Immunoreactivity to PTEN similar in endometrioid adenocarcinoma and adjacent endometriosis.

These findings are suggestive of biological alterations taking place in the endometriotic tissue adjacent to malignancy, reminiscent of the dysplastic ovarian epithelium adjacent to ovarian serous papillary carcinoma, both representing early manifestations of preinvasive ovarian cancer, involving two different carcinogenetic mechanisms (Table 5).

Indeed, serous papillary ovarian neoplasms are different from non-serous carcinomas in a number of ways, clinically, histologically and biologically. The biological markers are different as well, with p53 being the most reliable for OSPC and PTEN for endometrioid and clear cell carcinomas (Table 6).

Table 5. Ovarian Carcinoma Adjacent to Endometriosis

Carcinoma arising from ovarian endometriosis is more common than from other locations of endometriosis.
Clear cell and endometrioid carcinoma associated with endometriosis in 30%–40%.
Atypical epithelial changes at the transition between endometriosis and carcinoma.
Abnormal immunoreactivity: bcl-2, p53 altered proteins, Bax, MMP-9, PTEN in a typical endometriosis.
Ovarian endometriosis associated with cancer with potentially precancerous biological activity?

Table 6. Ovarian Carcinoma and Carcinogenesis

Serous papillary	Endometrioid, clear cell
Most frequent	Less frequent
70%–80% diagnosed Stage III, with peritoneal involvement	Often diagnosed in Stage I, rare peritoneal involvement
Mostly bilateral	Mostly unilateral
Older patients	Younger patients
Breast Ca hx, *BRCA1* and *2* mutations	Hyperestrogenism: Endometriosis, infertility, endometrial pathology
Precursor: ovarian dysplasia, precancerous phenotype, often identified in prophylactic oophorectomy specimens	Precursor: Endometriosis, atypical, clear cell carcinoma *in situ*
Tumor markers: p53, Ca 125, MIB-1	Tumor markers: Bax, MMP-9, PTEN, Bcl-2

In terms of early diagnosis, ovarian carcinomas diagnosed in Stage I are, as mentioned, rare, and their histologic distribution is fundamentally different from that of ovarian carcinomas of all stages. While in all stages, OSPC are by far the most common, in Stage I, they represent a minority of cases, which is less than a third as recently reported.[21] Mucinous carcinomas are rather rare primary ovarian neoplasms but they are more often diagnosed in Stage I. Endometrioid carcinomas are the most common ovarian carcinomas diagnosed in Stage I. This is due to their association with symptomatic pathologic findings such as endometriosis manifested by pelvic pain, compression of neighboring organs, and endometrial hyperplasia or neoplasia manifested by abnormal vaginal bleeding (Table 7).

The OSPC diagnosed early represent uncommon situations when sonograms performed for various reasons, often in patients with breast cancer histories who are under close surveillance, reveal clinically silent ovarian tumors. It should be emphasized, however, that despite the lack of a screening program for ovarian carcinoma and the lack of adequate tumor markers (CA 125 is neither sensitive

Table 7. Stage I: Ovarian Carcinoma

Different histopathologic distribution of Stage I compared to all stage ovarian carcinoma: predominant non-serous ovarian carcinomas in stage I versus predominant serous in all stages.
Different clinical settings in Stage I ovarian carcinoma: frequent hyperestrogenic, younger patients with history of endometriosis, infertility, endometrial pathology.
Non-serous ovarian cancers more often diagnosed early due to symptomatic pelvic masses and/or vaginal bleeding.
Endometriosis: A potential cancer precursor?
Serous carcinomas mostly asymptomatic; early diagnosis in patients closely followed for breast cancer history.
Occasional early diagnosis of asymptomatic ovarian cancer at hysterectomy for symptomatic associated neoplasm.
Essential clinical pathological and biological (immunological, genetical) differences between serous and non-serous ovarian carcinomas.
Different natural history.

nor specific enough for an early ovarian carcinoma diagnosis) a combination of vaginal ultrasound, serum tumor markers and especially a thorough clinical examination and history including the search for paraneoplastic syndromes may disclose the presence of early stage OSPC, especially in the group of genetically high-risk patients.[22,23]

A separate group of ovarian neoplasms often diagnosed in Stage I are the so called borderline ovarian tumors which are still the object of controversial opinions in terms of diagnostic criteria, biological behavior and clinical management. They are generally seen in patients younger than those with invasive carcinomas. Histologically, they are most often serous papillary, followed in frequency by mucinous, endometrioid and rare clear cell carcinomas of borderline malignancy (or low malignant potential). Their biological behavior is less aggressive than that of invasive tumors and the survival is markedly higher. Histologically, these tumors are characterized by lack of invasion of the ovarian parenchyma and mild to moderate nuclear atypia with a relative low mitotic activity. Their biological characteristics, as demonstrated by molecular biology studies, are different from those of the invasive ovarian carcinomas.[24] These tumors are often associated with implants of the peritoneum, non-invasive or invasive, the latter having a more ominous prognosis.[25] The five-year survival of borderline ovarian tumors is generally good, especially for those diagnosed in Stage I, which is close to 95%. Borderline ovarian tumors recur often at variable time intervals and the recurrent tumors are histologically similar to the primary. Recurrences of tumors with a frank invasive histological pattern probably represent invasive ovarian carcinomas that were not diagnosed initially as such. Borderline ovarian serous tumors are presently classified into atypical proliferative and micropapillary variants, the latter being more often associated with peritoneal implants and having a more ominous prognosis.[26] While most borderline ovarian tumors recur as borderline, some may progress to a low-grade serous papillary adenocarcinoma with micropapillary features.[27,28] Their long time survival is more favorable than that of the common variety of invasive ovarian serous papillary carcinomas.[29–31] While the precursor of the low-grade serous papillary carcinoma seems to be the serous borderline ovarian tumor, the precursor of the more common high grade ovarian serous carcinoma is to be searched in the subtle changes of the ovarian surface epithelium described as ovarian dysplasia.

CONCLUSIONS

The present knowledge of early ovarian carcinogenesis is quite limited as compared to that of other gynecologic malignancies. Despite numerous ongoing studies, not much progress has been obtained in the past decades in terms of early diagnosis of this highly lethal cancer. No prevention and no screening program are presently implemented. Only a minority of women are known to be at risk because of genetic mutations while the majority of ovarian cancer patients represent sporadic cases. Chemotherapy regimens offer longer remission periods and are presently better tolerated than in the past. However, the main task for the future is the discovery of preventive measures and of diagnostic tools for early stage diagnosis. Diagnosing and removing precursors of cancer by identifying dysplastic tissues obtained by biopsies and by cytologic screening for cervical neoplasms, or by endometrial curettings for endometrial hyperplasia, resulted in spectacular decreases in the morbidity and mortality due to these cancers. Unfortunately, these models could hardly be applied to ovarian cancer at the present time.

The progress made in the laparoscopic technology, the discovery of reliable tumor markers, the identification of patients with genetic risk, as well as patients with past histories of breast cancer, endometriosis, endometrial hyperplasia and neoplasia may contribute to the early diagnosis and possibly to a systematic detection of precancerous changes of the ovaries.

REFERENCES

1. Piver MS, Frank TS, Epidemiology of ovarian cancer, in *Diagnosis and Management of Ovarian Disorders*, 2nd edn., A Altchek, L Deligdisch, N Kase (eds.), Publ Academic Press — Elsevier Science, Amsterdam, London, New York, Tokyo, pp. 209–217, 2003.

2. Rodriguez GC, Walmer DK, Cline M, *et al.*, Effect of progestin on the ovarian epithelium of macaques: cancer prevention through apoptosis? *J Soc Gynecol Invest* **5**:271–276, 1998.
3. Whittemore AS, Gong G, Itnyre J, Prevalence and contribution of BRCA1 mutations in breast cancer and ovarian cancer: results from three US population-based case-control studies of ovarian cancer, *Am J Hum Genet* **60**:496–504, 1997.
4. Stratton JF, Gayther SA, Russel P, *et al.*, Contributions of BRCA1 mutations to ovarian cancer, *N Engl J Med* **336**:1125–1130, 1997.
5. Gusberg SB, Deligdisch L, Ovarian dysplasia: a study of identical twins, *Cancer* **54**:1–4, 1984.
6. Deligdisch L, Gil J, Characterization of ovarian dysplasia by interactive morphometry, *Cancer* **63**:748–755, 1989.
7. Deligdisch L, Miranda C, Barba J, *et al.*, Ovarian dysplasia: nuclear texture analysis, *Cancer* **72**:3253–3257, 1993.
8. Deligdisch L, Einstein AB, Guera D, *et al.*, Ovarian dysplasia in epithelial inclusion cysts: a morphometric approach using neural networks, *Cancer* **75**:1047–1054, 1995.
9. Schlosshauer P, Cohen CJ, Penault-Llorca F, *et al.*, Prophylactic oophorectomy: a morphologic and immunohistochemical study, *Cancer* **98**:2599–2606, 2003.
10. Altcheck A, Clues to tumors: new concepts of symptoms, signs, syndromes, paraneoplastic syndromes and predisposition to ovarian cancer, in *Diagnosis and Management of Ovarian Disorders*, 2nd edn., A Altchek, L Deligdisch, N Kase (eds.), Publ Academic Press — Elsevier Science, Amsterdam, London, New York, Tokyo, p. 231–269, 2003.
11. Kauff ND, Satagopan JM, Robson ME, *et al.*, Risk-reducing salpingo-oophorectomy in women with a BRCA1 or BRCA2 mutation, *N Engl J Med* **346**:1609–1615, 2002.
12. Rebbek TR, Lynch HT, Neuhausen SL, *et al.*, Prophylactic oophorectomy in carriers of BRCA1 and BRCA2, *N Engl J Med* **346**:1616–1622, 2002.
13. Lu KH, Garber JE, Cramer DW, *et al.*, Occult ovarian tumors in women with BRCA1 or BRCA2 mutations undergoing prophylactic oophorectomy, *J Clin Oncol* **18**:2728–2732, 2000.
14. Deligdisch L, Gil J, Kerner H, *et al.*, Ovarian dysplasia in prophylactic oophorectomy specimens: cytogenetic and morphometric correlations, *Cancer* **86**:1544–1550, 1999.

15. Salazar H, Godwin AK, Daly MB, *et al.*, Microscopic benign and invasive malignant neoplasms and a cancer-prone phenotype in prophylactic oophorectomies, *J Nat Cancer Inst* **88**:1810–1820, 1996.
16. Brewer MA, Ranger-Moore J, Baruche A, *et al.*, Exploratory study of ovarian intraepithelial neoplasia, *Cancer Epidemiol Biomarkers Prev* **14**:299–305, 2005.
17. Chêne G, Penault-Llorca F, LeBouëdec G, *et al.*, Ovarian epithelial dysplasia: myth or reality? *Gynecol Obstet Fertil* **36**:800–807, 2008.
18. Walsh C, Holschneider C, Heang Y, *et al.*, Coexisting ovarian malignancy in young women with endometrial cancer, *Obstet Gyencol* **106**:693–699, 2005.
19. Ogawa S, Kaku T, Amada S, *et al.*, Ovarian endometriosis associated with ovarian carcinoma: a clinical-pathologic and immunohistochemical study, *Gynecol Oncol* 77:298–304, 2000.
20. Irving JA, Catasus L, Bussaglia E, *et al.*, Synchronous endometrioid carcinomas of the uterine corpus and ovary: alteration in the beta-catenin (CTNNB1) pathway are associated with independent primary tumors and favorable prognosis, *Hum Pathol* **36**:605–619, 2005.
21. Deligdisch L, Penault-Llorca F, Schlosshauer P, *et al.*, Stage I ovarian carcinoma: different clinical pathologic patterns, *Fertil Steril* **88**:906–910, 2007.
22. Goff BA, Mandel L, Muntz HG, *et al.*, Ovarian carcinoma diagnosis, *Cancer* **89**:2068–2075, 2000.
23. Fishman DA, Cohen LS, Is transvaginal ultrasound effective for screening asymptomatic women for the detection of early-stage ovarian carcinoma? *Gynecol Oncol* 77:347–349, 2000.
24. Seidman JD, Kurman RJ, Ovarian serous borderline tumors: a critical review of the literature with emphasis on prognostic indicators, *Hum Pathol* **31**:539–557, 2000.
25. Slomovitz BM, Caputo TA, Gretz HF, *et al.*, A comparative analysis of 57 serous borderline tumors with and without a non-invasive micropapillary component. *Am J Surg Pathol* **26**:592–600, 2002.
26. Prat J, De Nictolis M, Serous tumors of the ovary (borderline tumors and carcinomas) with and without micropapillary features, *Int J Gynecol Pathol* **27**:725–736, 2003.
27. Singer G, Oldt R III, Cohen Y, *et al.*, Mutations in B-Raf and K-ras characterize the development of low-grade ovarian serous carcinoma, *J Nat Cancer Inst* **95**:484–486, 2003.

28. Diebold J, Seemuller F, Lohrs U, K-ras mutations in ovarian and extraovarian lesions of serous tumors of borderline malignancy, *Lab Invest* **83**:251–258, 2003.
29. Trimble CL, Kosary C, Trimble EL, Long time survival and patterns of care in women with ovarian tumors of low malignant potential, *Gynecol Oncol* **86**:34–37, 2002.
30. Berchuk A, Iversen ES, Lancaster JM, *et al.*, Patterns of gene expression that characterize long-term survival in advanced stage serous ovarian cancers, *Clin Cancer Res* **11**:3686–3690, 2005.
31. Kurman RJ, Visvanathan K, Roden R, Le-Ming Shih, Early detection and treatment of ovarian cancer: shifting from early stage to minimal volume of disease based on a new model of carcinogenesis, *Am J Obstet Gynecol* **198**:351–356, 2008.

CHAPTER 6

EARLY DIAGNOSIS OF OVARIAN AND ENDOMETRIAL CANCER: A CLINICIAN'S VIEW

Albert Altchek

OVARIAN CANCER

Risk Factors

Although ovarian cancer is not the most common gynecologic cancer it causes the most deaths because about 75% are discovered in an advanced stage. Most ovarian cancers are epithelial serous papillary carcinomas. About 85% of ovarian cancer is sporadic, occurring at random. About 10%–15% of patients have an inherited higher risk for ovarian cancer, mainly because of the associated *BRCA1* and *BRCA2* gene mutations.[1] Women with *BRCA1* or *2* mutations have a 50%–80% lifetime risk of breast cancer. Those with *BRCA1* have a 30%–40% additional risk for ovarian cancer, and with *BRCA2* have a 15%–25% risk for ovarian cancer. There is also some increased risk for pancreatic, gallbladder and stomach cancers.

About 16% of hereditary (and presumably ovarian) cancer patients do not have the usual *BRCA1* and *2* mutations. There are innumerable mutations of *BRCA* genes. Most are unique and exist in one family. Because of the "founder effect", certain groups have common mutations. Three "founder mutations" are found in 1/40 Ashkenazi Jews in the US. Other "founder" mutations are found in the French Canadians and in Iceland.[2] A smaller number have predisposing syndromes, such as hereditary nonpolyposis colorectal cancer (HNPCC) (Lynch syndrome 2).[3] There may be synchronous primary cancers of the ovary and endometrium. Five percent of women with endometrial cancer may have simultaneous ovarian cancer (usually endometrioid) and 10% of those with ovarian cancer have endometrial cancer. (See section on endometrial cancer.) The patients with hereditary nonpolyposis colorectal cancer (HNPCC, Lynch syndrome 2) have a 40%–60% risk of colorectal cancer, a 40%–60% risk of endometrial cancer and a 5%–10% risk of ovarian cancer. There are mutations in the mismatch repair genes *MSH 2*, *MSH 1* and possible *MSH 6*. There is a risk of gastrointestinal, pancreatic, upper urinary tract and brain cancers.

Risk reducing hysterectomy and bilateral salpingo-oophorectomy at age 30 resulted in a life expectancy of 79.88 years, while surveillance resulted in a life expectancy of 79.31 years and annual examination of 77.41 years. There is a small reduction in endometrial and ovarian cancer and improved survival with prophylactic surgery which should be offered as an option.[3–6] Another approach is annual colonoscopy at age 25 and annual endometrial sampling starting at age 25–35. There is no reliable ovarian screening. At the time of colorectal surgery, consideration is given for total hysterectomy and bilateral salpingo-oophorectomy. The colon cancer usually occurs in the right colon at an average age of 44, with a life time risk of 80%. The mean age of endometrial cancer in patients with HNPCC is 48 and of ovarian cancer age 42.

The main significant risk factors for ovarian cancer are *BRCA1* and *2* mutations and family history of breast and ovarian cancer even without *BRCA* testing, and even with negative (partial) *BRCA* testing for the usual three mutations in the US, rather than the complete genome (which is very expensive to do) if the patient had a localized ancestry elsewhere. Liberal genetic counseling is encouraged with any question of family history. Protective factors include oral contraceptives (OC) and parity. The former gives long term protection of 0.7 relative risk (RR) for two years of OC and 0.5 RR for five years of OC. Other risk reducing factors are tubal sterilization and hysterectomy. Factors which may cause an increase in ovarian cancer risk include family history, early menarche, late menopause, infertility and advancing age.[7] Before age 30, epithelial cancer is rare even in hereditary cancer families. Regarding genetic aspects, the main ovarian cancer risk factor is having one first degree relative with it, giving a risk odds ratio of 3.1. The BRCA*1* and *2* autosomal dominant mutation inheritance can be transmitted through both maternal and paternal heritage. The risk of inheritance of the individual is 50%, however, not all women at risk will develop cancer because of incomplete penetrance.[8] With *BRCA1* and *2* mutations, the ovarian cancers are more likely to be serous papillary adenocarcinoma, rather than mucinous or borderline. In addition, fallopian tube and primary peritoneal papillary serous carcinomas are associated with *BRCA* mutations as well as the serous endometrial carcinoma.[1] Even with prophylactic salpingo-oophorectomy there is a small chance of later primary peritoneal cancer with the same histology as ovarian serous cancer. Clues to a familial predisposition to ovarian cancer include a family history of ovarian or breast cancer, especially at an early age (such as the fourth decade and progressive reduction of age with each succeeding generation) in first degree relatives, in Ashkenazi Jewish families, a second cancer in the opposite breast, a family history of various cancers, and previous breast cancer. Family history may not be reliable with small families, adoptions and lack of family history (such as due to the holocaust in Jewish families).

Early Detection

The overwhelming problem for early discovery of ovarian cancer is that the ovary is not accessible without surgery (laparoscopy or laparotomy) which has a small risk and it is not feasible to do repetitively. The other gynecologic malignancies are in accessible areas — the cervix, vagina and vulva, and even the uterus by endometrial biopsy and hysteroscopy. There is a new concept of early detection — shifting from early stage to minimal volume of disease. Most serous ovarian carcinomas even at their earliest stage are thought to be probably not confined to the ovary. A new model divides ovarian cancer into two types.[9] Type I is slow growing, confined to the ovary at diagnosis and develops from precursor lesions (so-called borderline tumors). Type I includes low-grade micropapillary serous carcinoma, mucinous, endometrioid and clear cell carcinomas. These tumors are genetically stable and have gene mutations such as *KRAS*, *BRAF*, *PTEN* and *beta-catenin*. Type II is rapidly growing, highly aggressive and lacking well defined precursor lesions. Ovarian dysplasia is a subtle change, identified adjacent to the invasive cancer or incidentally in prophylactic oophorectomy specimens. Most cases are diagnosed at an advanced stage at or soon after inception and include high grade serous carcinoma, malignant mixed mesodermal tumors (MMMT) and undifferentiated carcinomas. They have *TP53* mutations and genetic instability. Most cancers are type II.

This classification, however, does not address the histogenesis of the tumors in type I which have different phenotypic characteristics (serous, mucinous, clear cell carcinomas) and are evolving from different precursor lesions such as clear cell and endometrioid from endometriosis. For example, it should be mentioned that endometrioid adenocarcinoma while in many cases diagnosed in stage I and of relatively low malignant potential, is often highly aggressive and rapidly metastatic, thus belonging rather to type II. A more rational approach to early detection should be focused on low volume (to make de-bulking easier) rather than low stage.[9]

Screening

Screening the general population (average risk) for ovarian cancer is not feasible and is not recommended. Since the incidence is low (40 per 100,000) any screening test would have poor positive predictive value (PPV). For example, although transvaginal ultrasound has up to 100% sensitivity and 98% specificity, the PPV is only 1% when it is used alone. False-positive screening results in unnecessary surgery with its risks, costs and emotional disturbances. Rapid cancer growth requires frequent testing.[10] Even intensive screening of high risk women has been a failure and therefore such women are offered prophylactic risk reduction salpingo-oophorectomy.[6]

Symptoms

Despite the name "the silent killer", experienced gynecologists have long noticed a non-specific "dyspepsia" or undiagnosed gastrointestinal symptoms which often preceded the correct diagnosis. This was emphasized by the late Dr. Hugh R. K. Barber of Lenox Hill Hospital in New York City, who created a triad index of suspicion for ovarian epithelial cancer: over age 40, history of ovarian dysfunction and infertility and vague abdominal discomfort and mild digestive symptoms which persist (dyspepsia, flatulence and distension after eating).[11]

A retrospective study by an in-person interview by trained interviewers found that 92% of 166 women with ovarian cancer had four months of symptoms before the diagnosis of advanced cancer was made. The symptoms were 71% pelvic discomfort, 47% bowel irregularity, 37% urinary frequency and/or urgency and 53% other symptoms. The short time period suggested rapid growth. These symptoms are often found in the normal population. The delay in diagnosis faulted the patient, physician and was system-related.[12]

An interesting but overlooked study of the Mayo Clinic Gastroenterology Research Unit described a paraneoplastic gastrointestinal motor dysfunction associated with distant malignant tumors which caused similar symptoms reported prior to discovery of cancer. One of their cases was ovarian papillary serous adenocarcinoma. They recommended serologic tests for paraneoplastic antibodies, gastric emptying tests and esophageal screening tests.[13] Goff *et al.* reported a large retrospective study of 1,725 women with ovarian cancer and found that 97% with advanced stage and 89% with early stage had symptoms an average of three months before seeing a doctor. The most common symptoms were abdominal and gastrointestinal and were often diagnosed as stress, irritable bowel syndrome and depression.[14] To differentiate these symptoms from non-specific complaints, the ovarian cancer patients had frequent symptoms (20 to 30 times a month), which were severe and of recent onset. The emphasis was on frequency, severity and duration of symptoms. Forty-four percent of cases had a triad of bloating, increased abdominal size and urinary urgency. The most recent report emphasized and condensed it to pelvic/abdominal pain, increased abdominal size/bloating, and difficulty eating/feeling full. A consensus statement in 2007 indicated the following symptoms were a cause for concern: bloating, pelvic or abdominal pain, difficulty in eating or feeling full quickly and urinary symptoms. These symptoms are even more of concern if they are new, persistent and frequent (almost daily) for a few weeks. Other symptoms are less helpful because they occur in the general population with the same frequency: fatigue, indigestion, back pain, pain with intercourse, constipation and menstrual irregularity.[10]

The practical problems are that the symptoms are not gynecological, are often present in the general population and would require testing in a large number of women. It would increase medical costs. Patients are often late in seeking medical care. Physicians would have to spend time with gastroenterological testing. In addition, there is no proof that early cancer could be discovered earlier and mortality be reduced. Theoretically earlier diagnosis with smaller tumor bulk which is readily removed would improve prognosis.[14] Based on health insurance claims data, ovarian cancer related symptoms were most pronounced in the 2–3 months prior to diagnosis. For most of the preceding nine months the symptoms were similar to those in normal women.[15]

The retrospective vague symptoms several months before the discovery of ovarian cancer implies that the cancer might have been detected in an early stage and would have resulted in a cure or significant improvement in survival. This has not yet been verified although it seems logical.[16] Retrospective history taking of women with ovarian cancer of advanced and early disease discloses that months before diagnosis there were continuous symptoms of bloating, increase of the abdomen, pain, fatigue, indigestion, dyspepsia, urinary frequency or incontinence, and sometimes weight loss (or weight gain from ascites).[17] These retrospective histories do not readily translate to practical clinical care since the symptoms are non-specific and common and would require significant use of medical resources and costs which might not be endorsed by Health Maintenance Organizations (HMO) and/or society. Retrospective investigation suggests that women between ages 40 and 69 with continuous gastrointestinal complaints (vague discomfort, dyspepsia, mild digestive disturbance) for several months that have not been diagnosed, should be investigated for ovarian cancer. These symptoms are often associated with non-specific functional disturbances. Because the ovary is mobile early cancer may not cause symptoms or only non-specific symptoms. "These vague symptoms frequently either are ignored by the patient or are not recognized as potential signs and symptoms of ovarian cancer by her physician."[17]

When to Operate

The three standard methods to discover ovarian cancer are not reliable. They are physical examination, serum CA 125 and transvaginal ultrasound. Standard textbooks reflect the general pessimism of early detection "...the diagnosis of early ovarian cancer is more a matter of chance than a triumph of the scientific method."[17]

Paraneoplastic syndromes are rare. Ovarian cancer (high grade serous) is a leading cause of neurologic paraneoplastic syndromes, especially subacute cerebellar degeneration. Circulating antibodies to tumor antigens by coincidence attack the Purkinje cells. The symptoms include unsteady gait, ataxia, dysarthria, nystagmus, dysphagia, vertigo, headache and diplopia.[1] Symptoms of advanced disease include abdominal pain, bloated feeling, gastrointestinal or urinary disturbances, ascites, irregular or postmenopausal vaginal bleeding.[17] With advanced disease, the patient has a typical large abdomen and thin extremities and face. The only certain method of diagnosis is to obtain the ovarian cancer tissue. This requires surgery, laparoscopy and/or laparotomy and the clinical decision to operate.

Most ovarian enlargements of premenopausal women are benign. Indications for surgery include a CA 125 level of over 200 units/ml, ascites, metastases and family history of first degree relatives with ovarian or breast cancer.[17] Postmenopausal women with simple unilocular cysts, 8 cm–10 cm or less, normal CA 125 and negative family history may be managed by observation.[17] Comment: Many gynecologists would be concerned by cysts larger than 5 cm.

On physical examination in advanced cases usually there is a palpable abdominal mass and clinical ascites, although symptomatic and stage III tumors may have not be detectable on physical examination. There may be a fluid wave, shifting dullness, enlargement of an umbilical hernia and bowel tympany in the anterior midline in the supine position. An umbilical lymph node may be present. A large ovarian cyst (with mucous or serous fluid) may give a fluid wave but without shifting dullness or umbilical herniation and the bowel has lateral tympany. The upper abdomen may have a solid irregular feel of "omental cake" due to metastases. There may be a partial bowel obstruction or ileus and pleural effusion. A bimanual recto-vaginal examination is done, with an empty bladder and rectum. On examination, colorectal cancer or diverticulitis abscess may simulate ovarian cancer. Benign ovarian tumors are usually mobile, smooth, cystic, unilateral and less than 10 cm in diameter. Benign mucinous cystadenomas may be huge. Malignant tumors are usually solid, fixed, irregular, nodular, shoddy, bilateral (especially the serous) large and have cul-de-sac nodularity. Infrequently, there is inguinal and supraclavicular adenopathy, pleural effusion, skin and lung metastases. Less common are hormone-producing tumors causing amenorrhea, masculinization, precocious puberty and abnormal bleeding. Ovarian tumors may be metastatic from the gastrointestinal tract, pancreas or breast and are usually bilateral.

The serum marker CA 125 test fails to detect half of the early cases with an upper normal of 35 units/ml, although it is usually positive with a high level in advanced or recurrent disease. There may be a false negative with cancer and a false positive without cancer, especially in menstruating women. False positives may occur with uterine myomas (fibroids), endometriosis, ovarian mature cystic teratomas (dermoid cyst), pelvic inflammatory disease and functional ovarian cysts. False positives may occur in 3% of women without malignancy. CA 125 may be elevated with non-gynecologic cancer such as pancreas. CA 125 is more reliable in the postmenopausal women. A rising level may be more ominous then one high level. Some consider the upper normal to be about 64 units/mL.[9,17–19] Performing transvaginal ultrasound in women with elevated CA 125 did not reduce mortality. In a group of over 8000 women, six cases were discovered, three being late stages.[17] Using CA 125 and transvaginal ultrasound has resulted in unnecessary surgery without detecting early cancer. The Prostate, Lung, Colon and Ovary Cancer Screening Trial recommended that the normal CA 125 level was up to 65 units/ml. It also indicated that 7 cm or larger lesions had a 26% risk of cancer but small lesions had only a 1.5% risk.[17]

The transvaginal ultrasound is more precise than physical examination and serum CA 125. It cannot detect any ovarian tumors until they enlarge and therefore may miss stage I. The characteristic suspicious signs of cancer include enlargement of the ovary, thick irregular walls, solid and liquid areas, septation, inner and outer surface papillations, and characteristic Doppler color blood flow pattern of enlarged irregular vessels with low pressure. There may be free intraperitoneal fluid. This classic description is often not present. A hemorrhagic corpus luteum of the ovary may mimic carcinoma and therefore the ultrasound should be repeated in young menstruating women after about six weeks to look for resolution. Thus, for the young woman there are frequent false-positives.

Ovarian cysts in the postmenopausal women are taken more seriously. Prior to ultrasound it was assumed that the post-menopausal ovary was quiescent. When the ultrasound became available and described small unilocular thin-walled cysts, many women were taken to surgery. Experience has changed this approach. It is now realized that about 14% of normal postmenopausal women have such cysts which may come and go or may persist. At present, with no other indications for surgery such women are usually simply observed with serial ultrasound and serum CA 125. The post-menopausal ovarian cyst is reminiscent of the functional ovarian cyst of the prepubertal and peripubertal functional ovarian cyst which is usually of no significance and simply observed with serial transvaginal ultrasounds. There have been ongoing studies of serial serum CA 125 which if increasing represents an indication for transvaginal ultrasound, but this has not been productive to date. Similarly, many tumor marker panels, serum proteomics, and immuno-proteomics have been investigated but generally without success.

Annual transvaginal ultrasound screening of the general population is not effective. The positive predictive value for transvaginal ultrasound (TVU) was 1.0% and for CA 125 was 3.7% when done individually. When done simultaneously, it was 23.5% when both were abnormal. Serial serum markers have been better than a single CA 125.[17] The general consensus is that screening for ovarian cancer for the general population is not recommended.[17] Despite intensive monitoring of high risk women at six months intervals by examination, serum CA 125 and transvaginal ultrasound a significant number of ovarian cancers are not discovered until at an advanced stage.[6,17]

At the present time, the usual recommendation for high-risk women is prophylactic salpingo-oophorectomy after childbearing and after age 35. Even with this, with serial sectioning of the ovaries, about 1%–3% of patients will reveal asymptomatic microscopic ovarian or distal fallopian tube (near the fimbriated end) adenocarcinoma.[6,17] The prophylactic surgery was originally described as prevention of ovarian cancer. At present it is referred to as "risk reduction" of ovarian cancer because in subsequent years there may be a primary peritoneal cancer with the histology of ovarian serous papillary carcinoma. The reason is that the epithelial covering of the ovary is contiguous and embryologically related with the peritoneum. For unknown reasons, the ovarian stroma may be involved in its surface epithelium becoming malignant while the peritoneal lining is less often the primary site of malignancy. The fallopian tube being close by may also get the same stimulus from the ovary.[17]

Infrequently the primary peritoneal cancer precedes the ovarian cancer and the ovaries are found to be normal. Although fallopian tube adenocarcinoma is rare, in patients with *BRCA* mutations it may be as high as 3% as demonstrated on histological serial sections from specimens obtained by prophylactic bilateral salpingo-oophorectomy (pB50), which is a 120 times increase compared to the general population.[18] In half of the cases of tubal carcinoma there was vaginal postmenopausal bleeding due to blood leaking from the tube to the uterus. This possibility should be considered when a dilatation and curettage of the uterus or endometrial biopsy are negative. There may also be colicky pelvic pain. Watery or bloody vaginal discharge occurs in 25%. Cervical cytology may contain tubal malignant cells in 10%–20% cases. There may be a high CA 125 as well.

The primary peritoneal cancer is seen in patients with *BRCA1* and *2* mutations as are the ovarian and tubal carcinomas. The possibility of early stage I ovarian carcinoma should be considered in the evaluation of women with endometriosis, infertility and history of breast cancer especially with pelvic pain or masses or vaginal bleeding from endometrial pathology.[20] Ovarian serous papillary carcinoma may present with a unilateral asymptomatic pelvic mass while nonserous carcinomas may present with pelvic pain or abnormal bleeding with or without a pelvic mass. In a report of 76 cases of stage I ovarian cancers, 29% were serous papillary carcinomas and 71% were nonserous carcinoma, composed of 40 endometrioid, ten clear cell and four mixed endometrioids and clear cell carcinomas. The stage I serous carcinoma cases had a history of breast carcinomas and *BRCA* mutations and had been carefully followed. The endometrioid carcinomas were associated with endometriotic ovarian cysts, endometrial carcinoma and endometrial hyperplasia and/or polyps due to hyperestrogenism. Although serous ovarian carcinoma is the most frequent type of cancer, when stage I early ovarian cases were studied it was found to be due to nonserous in over 2/3. The ovarian cancer was discovered because of associated symptoms of pelvic pain with endometriosis and/or adnexal masses or vaginal bleeding from endometrial pathology. The serous papillary carcinomas of ovary were more often asymptomatic and diagnosed in follow-up examinations after breast cancer. Of the 54 nonserous carcinomas the largest group was 40 endometrioid carcinomas which developed in ovarian endometriosis and 13 with synchronous endometrioid endometrial carcinoma.[20] Although endometriosis is common, only few patients develop endometrioid ovarian carcinoma. Nevertheless, ovarian endometriosis, pelvic pain, infertility and endometrial pathology (hyperplasia, polyps, carcinoma) suggest that ovarian endometriomas should be carefully examined for microscopic transformation into endometrioid carcinoma.[20]

The referral guidelines published by the American College of Obstetricians and Gynecologists (ACOG) and the Society of Gynecologic Oncologists (SGO) about when to refer a patient with a pelvic mass to a gynecologic oncologist perform well in predicting advanced stage ovarian cancer. The guidelines "perform poorly" for finding early stage cancer especially in premenopausal women due to absence of early markers and signs of cancer.[21] At laparoscopy the surgeon should view the surface topography of the ovary. Even if of normal size, deep cortical invaginations of the surface lining, multiple cysts and calcifications (psammoma bodies) should be viewed as suspicious. In perimenopausal women during laparoscopy for other reasons it would be reasonable to open the ovary or use an intraoperative probe sonogram to look for a small carcinoma in the ovary.[22] Although ovarian carcinoma is considered a surface tumor it originates in the inclusion cysts of the cortex resulting from invagination of the surface epithelium.

There are experimental *in vivo* surface ovarian stains and lights to attempt to detect small surface carcinomas.[17] In analogy with the detection of cervical dysplasia, ovarian dysplasia may require the identification of grossly visible changes leading to laparoscopically directed ovarian biopsies. There is a suggestion that ovarian dysplasia can be predicted by CA 125. "The odds ratio for dysplasia was six for women with CA 125 of 14 units/ml or higher, suggesting that this cutoff value may be taken as an additional parameter toward decision making in women considering pBSO."[23] There are many suggestions for developing new serum tests for ovarian cancer including small protein molecules (*proteomics*), *immunoproteomics*, abberant DNA methylation and biomarker panels.

A CA 125 stimulation test has been suggested.[22] A case report of a positive (abnormal) small mass in the ovary in a postmenopausal woman by 18-fluorodeoxyglucose (FDG) positive emission tomography (PET) computed tomography (CT) was followed 13 months later by a large cystoma with foci of primary ovarian adenocarcinoma. The patient had a breast cancer and was *BRCA2* positive. The positive scan could have been an early asymptomatic ovarian cancer or premalignant change. It is known that a FDG PET-CT is positive in advanced and recurrent ovarian carcinoma because of malignant cell uptake of tagged glucose. It is logical that premalignant change or dysplasia would also have an increased metabolism and also pick up glucose.[24] FDG-PET can detect recurrent ovarian cancer but has a high rate of false negative findings for microscopic or cystic lesions.[25] Investigation in deciding whether an adnexal mass is malignant or not is being done with PET-CT scanning with injected contrast which concentrates in cells with rapid metabolism.

New Ideas

There are ongoing investigations for early diagnosis of ovarian cancer in circulating aberrant DNA methylation epigenetic changes;[26] specific peptide signature changes;[27] genomics, transcriptomics, and proteomics;[28] a novel algorithm for group biomarkers identification using gene expression data which are involved in pathways related to different types of cancer development and stages of disease claiming a specificity greater than 99% and sensitivity equal to 100% for early detection;[29] a comprehensive identification of serum proteins involved in both humoral and cell-mediated immunity against ovarian cancer (immunoproteomics);[30] the possibility of serological screening with serum biomarkers (proteins and autoantibodies);[31] new improvements in proteomics using mass spectroscopy and genomic databases;[32] the elevated serum macrophage migration inhibitory factor (MIF) secreted by ovarian cancer cells;[33] and short term *in vitro* cultures of ovarian serous papillary carcinoma production of a group of RNA gene expression profiling biomarkers.[34] An interesting report indicated that there is an increase in general solid cancer incidence in atomic bomb survivors exposed *in utero* or as young children.[35]

ENDOMETRIAL CANCER

The most common gynecological cancer occurs in the endometrium. There are two types.

Types of Endometrial Carcinoma

The more common type I endometrial carcinoma tends to occur in younger women compared to type II, is associated with prolonged estrogen stimulation, obesity, history of anovulatory oligomenorrhea, polycystic ovarian syndrome, nulliparity, late menopause (an average at age 52), estrogen producing ovarian neoplasms, perimenopausal estrogen replacement therapy without progestin, Tamoxifen to prevent breast cancer, and diabetes, hypertension and hypothyroidism.

Type I is histologically endometrioid and associated with genetic mutations of *K-ras*, *PTEN* and *MLH 1* genes.[36] Type II endometrial carcinoma is histologically non-endometrioid, high grade, and aggressive papillary-serous or clear cell carcinoma. It tends to occur in older, thin, postmenopausal women with surrounding atrophic endometrium, and without excess estrogen. Prognosis is worse than in the common type I endometrial carcinoma. Type II endometrial carcinoma occurs in a higher percent age of African–American women.[36] "Most cases of endometrial cancer are diagnosed as a result of symptoms reported by patients, and a high proportion of these cases are diagnosed at an early stage and have high rates of survival."[37] "Although the incidence of endometrial cancer is lower among black women, mortality is higher. The National Cancer Institute initiated a Black/White Cancer Survival Study and concluded that higher grade and more aggressive histologies appear to be related to excess risk of advanced stage disease for black women."[37] The above suggests that black women in the USA may have a higher incidence of type II endometrial carcinoma. Type II is associated with aneuploidy, allelic imbalance, mutation in *p53* and *erb-B2* overexpression.[36]

There are two hereditary syndromes for endometrial carcinoma: (1) Lynch II syndrome, now often referred to as hereditary non-polyposis colorectal cancer syndrome (HNPCC).[3–5,38] (2) Site-specific uterine cancer syndrome, associated with a DNA mismatch repair.[37]

Who is at Risk for Endometrial Cancer?

Endometrial cancer is erroneously thought to be only a post-menopausal problem. Although the median age is 61, most patients with endometrial adenocarcinoma are between the age of 50 and 59. In about 5% it occurs before the age of 40 and 20%–25% occur before menopause. Especially in nulliparous women, women who took oral contraceptives in younger years had a 0.5 relative risk of developing endometrial carcinoma.[39] There is an emphasis on risk factors of abdominal obesity, nulliparity and late menopause.[39]

Routine screening for endometrial carcinoma in the general population is not cost effective. Nevertheless, the following represents high risk factors:

1. Postmenopausal uterine bleeding.
2. Bleeding between menstrual periods.
3. Anovulatory, obese women with polycystic ovarian syndrome.
4. Women over 70, thin, nulliparous, diabetic.
5. Stenotic cervix, especially with a distended uterine fundus in a postmenopausal woman.
6. Continuous estrogen hormone replacement therapy without progestin. Postmenopausal women who are on estrogen and progestin may still get endometrial cancer similar to the general population but less than those only on estrogen alone.[37]
7. Ovarian tumors discovered by coincidental ultrasound.
8. Tamoxifen therapy, used after treatment or prevention of breast cancer. Although Tamoxifen is anti-estrogenic for the breast, it may be an estrogenic agonist for the endometrium and uterus and may cause endometrial polyps, hyperplasia or carcinoma, as well as endometriosis.
9. Women with hereditary nonpolyposis colon cancer (HNPCC, Lynch syndrome II). In half of the cases, the endometrial or ovarian cancer appears before the colon cancer in the early 40s,

with the colon cancer (mean) 11 years later. In 14% of cases the gynecologic and the colon cancer appeared simultaneously.[38] Therefore, women with colon cancer especially right sided should have an endometrial biopsy and transvaginal ultrasound. HNPCC is rare, occurring in only 1%–5% of all colorectal cancers but carries a 40%–55% lifetime risk of colon cancer.

10. The finding of endometrial cells in the Pap cytology of the cervix in women over age 40 is considered suspicious by some, sufficient to do an endometrial biopsy.
11. The finding of endometrial abnormal serous papillary or clear cells on cervix cytology suggests type II endometrial cancer.
12. Fluid in the endometrial cavity.
13. Thick endometrium in postmenopausal women of over 4 mm–5 mm; or over 11 mm in premenopausal women.
14. Endometrial polyps.
15. Local site of bleeding in atrophic endometrium, especially in elderly thin women.
16. Bleeding after endometrial ablation.
17. Endometrioid ovarian carcinoma.

Genetic consultation is recommended for patients who have a greater than 20%–25% risk of having inherited predisposition to endometrial, colorectal and related cancers (Tables 1 and 2).[5]

For the following a lower threshold of risk is considered because of lack of history:

— only few female relatives;
— adoption;
— hysterectomy and/or oophorectomy at a young age in many family members.[5]

Genetic consultation problems include false negatives, uncertainties of genetic variations and emotional distress. Fortunately, apparently there has not been discrimination for health insurance or employment and a positive genetic test without symptoms is not considered a preexisting condition.[5] Women with autosomal dominant

Table 1. From Lancaster *et al.*, 2007

Patients with greater than approximately 20%–25% chance of having an inherited predisposition to endometrial, colorectal and related cancers and for whom genetic risk assessment is recommended.

Patients with endometrial or colorectal cancer who meet the revised Amsterdam criteria as listed below:

- ○ At least 3 relatives with a Lynch/HNPCC-associated cancer (colorectal cancer, cancer of the endometrium, small bowel, ureter, or renal pelvis) in one lineage.
- ○ One affected individual should be a first degree relative of the other two.
- ○ At least 2 successive generations should be affected.
- ○ At least 1 HNPCC-associated cancer should be diagnosed before age 50.

- Patients with synchronous or metachronous endometrial and colorectal cancer with the first cancer diagnosed prior to age 50.
- Patients with synchronous or metachronous ovarian and colorectal cancer with the first cancer diagnosed prior to age 50.
- Patients with colorectal or endometrial cancer with evidence of a mismatch repair defect (i.e. microsatellite instability (MSI) or immunohistochemical loss of expression of *MLH 1*, *MSH 2*, *MSH 6* or *PMS 2*).
- Patients with a first or second degree relative with a known mismatch repair gene mutation.

mutations in the DNA mismatch repair genes (*MLH 1*, *MSH 2* or *MSH 6*) clinically present as Lynch/hereditary non-polyposis colorectal cancer (HNPCC) syndrome, also known as Lynch syndrome II.

There is an about 40%–60% lifetime risk for endometrial and colorectal cancer and a 9%–12% lifetime risk of ovarian cancer. Under the age of 21, these cancers are very rare and to avoid emotional disturbances, it is generally recommended that genetic counseling and testing to be deferred until after age 21.[5] The endometrial cancer may occur years before the colon cancer, and the gynecologic cancers usually occur 15 years earlier than the sporadic cancers. Although HNPCC associated endometrial cancer is only 5%–10% of all endometrial cancers, in women with HNPCC who had more than one cancer in their lifetime, over 50% had an endometrial or ovarian cancer as their "sentinel" cancer.[40] Prophylactic total hysterectomy and bilateral salpingo-oophorectomy is a recommended option for

Table 2. From Lancaster *et al.*, 2007

Patients with greater than approximately 5%–10% risk of having an inherited predisposition to endometrial, colorectal and related cancers and for whom genetic risk assessment may be helpful:

- Patients with endometrial or colorectal cancer diagnosed prior to age 50.
- Patient with endometrial or ovarian cancer with a synchronous or metachronous colon or other Lynch/HNPCC-associated tumor* at any age.
- Patients with endometrial or colorectal cancer and a first degree relative with a Lynch/HNPCC-associated tumor* diagnosed prior to age 50.
- Patients with colorectal or endometrial cancer diagnosed at any age with two or more first or second degree relatives† with Lynch/HNPCC-associated tumors*, regardless of age.
- Patients with a first or second degree relative† that meets the above criteria.

* Lynch/HNPCC-related tumors include colorectal, endometrial, stomach, ovarian, pancreas, ureter and renal pelvis, biliary tract, and brain (usually glioblastoma as seen in Turcot syndrome) tumors, sebaceous gland adenomas and keratoacanthomas in Muir–Torre syndrome, and carcinoma of the small bowel.

† First and second degree relatives are parents, siblings, aunts, uncles, nieces, nephews, grandparents and grandchildren.

HNPCC syndrome after childbearing.[40] "Women should be offered surveillance with ultrasound and endometrial sampling from age 25–35, although there is no data to suggest that this will improve survival if endometrial cancer is diagnosed by these means."[39]

Other authors recommend annual endometrial biopsy starting at age 35. We concur with annual routine transvaginal ultrasound to check the endometrium and do an endometrial biopsy. For any unusual bleeding, the endometrial biopsy is done immediately. This approach should discover early endometrial carcinoma and improve clinical results.[39] Women with hereditary non-polyposis colorectal cancer syndrome (HNPCC), also referred as Lynch syndrome II, have a 40%–60% lifetime risk for colon cancer and for endometrial cancer, and a 12% lifetime risk for ovarian cancer. Some series report a 60% risk of endometrial cancer and a 34%–54% of colon cancer. The patients who develop endometrial or ovarian carcinoma first, had a mean age of 44. Those who developed colon cancer first, had a mean age of 40.

There may be other extracolonic cancers aside from endometrial and ovarian malignancies such as small bowel and ureteral/renal pelvis neoplasms. The risk of developing a second, metachronous cancer is 25% in the 10 years following and 50% in the 15 years following the initial cancer. If colorectal cancer comes first, the patient should be warned of the risk for a later endometrial cancer and *vice versa*. In a large series with HNPCC who developed two primary cancers, endometrial/ovarian cancer was the "sentinel cancer" preceding the development of colon cancer.[38]

Endometrial Sampling

Endometrial sampling is the "gold standard" to evaluate abnormal uterine bleeding in women for whom endometrial hyperplasia or carcinoma is a possibility. Office endometrial biopsy is usually done without or with minimal dilatation of the cervix, without anesthesia and usually with minimum cost or danger. It requires less than 3 minutes. Compared to other diagnostic methods (dilatation and curettage of the uterus, hysteroscopy and/or hysterectomy), Pipelle sampling was more sensitive for detection of endometrial cancer and atypical hyperplasia. The Pipelle detection rate for endometrial cancer was 99.6% (postmenopausal) and 91% (premenopausal). The detection rate for atypical hyperplasia was 81%. The specificity of all endometrial biopsy devices was 98% to 100%. Less than 5% had insufficient or no samples.[37] Endometrial biopsy is more reliable when the pathology affected half or more of the endometrium. Another problem is when the carcinoma is present only in an endometrial polyp. Endometrial cancer type II develops as a *de novo* cancer in one site as a focal lesion in a field of atrophic endometrium. All postmenopausal uterine bleeding requires investigation regardless of the amount.

If the endometrial biopsy is non-diagnostic, or if there is insufficient tissue, or if bleeding persists and there is a suspicion of carcinoma, consider a repeat endometrial biopsy, transvaginal ultrasound, dilatation and curettage of the uterus and hysteroscopy. Endometrial cancer is unusual if the endometrium is less than 4 mm thick (postmenopausal).

Table 3. Women who should undergo evaluation for endometrial hyperplasia or endometrial cancer,[5] from *Lancaster JM et al.*

1. Over age 40 years with abnormal uterine bleeding.
2. Under age 40 years with abnormal uterine bleeding and risk factors (e.g. chronic anovulation, obesity, Tamoxifen therapy, diabetes, family history of endometrial/ovarian/breast/colon cancer).
3. Failure to respond to medical treatment of abnormal uterine bleeding.
4. Women with uterus *in situ* receiving unopposed estrogen replacement therapy.
5. Presence of atypical glandular cells on cervical cytology.
6. Presence of endometrial cells on cervical cytology in a woman ≥40 years of age.
7. Women with hereditary non-polyposis colorectal cancer.

If saline infusion sonography shows a focal lesion, consider hysteroscopy. In asymptomatic postmenopausal women if the endometrium is 11 mm or more thick, there is a 6.7% risk of cancer, while only 0.002% if the thickness is less than 11 mm.[37] The transvaginal ultrasound may reveal an adnexal cause for bleeding such as ovarian or tubal carcinoma or an estrogen producing ovarian neoplasm. Endometrial biopsy is indicated in asymptomatic postmenopausal women who have a cervix Pap cytology reporting endometrial cells or glandular abnormalities.

Reliability of Endometrial Biopsy

For the more common endometrial cancer type I associated with anovulation, persistent estrogenic effect and endometrial hyperplasia, the endometrial biopsy is relatively reliable because of the global reaction of the endometrium. For the less common type II, aggressive, localized endometrial carcinoma developing *de novo* in a field of atrophic endometrium, the endometrial biopsy is less reliable. The reason is that only 5%–15% of the endometrium is obtained. Therefore, if suspicious bleeding persists after a negative pathology report consider dilatation and curettage of the uterus, and hysteroscopy. Another problem is an endometrial polyp which may be too large to be removed or be sampled by endometrial biopsy and may continue to bleed.

The endometrial biopsy is unable to sample myometrium and therefore cannot give information about myometrial invasion. A review of outpatient endometrial biopsies in women with abnormal uterine bleeding for the diagnosis of endometrial cancer showed there was a high overall accuracy when an adequate specimen is obtained. A positive test result is more accurate for ruling in disease than a negative test for ruling it out. If abnormal uterine bleeding persists further evaluation is needed.[41] The endometrial biopsy is the preferred initial investigation.

Hazards of Endometrial Biopsy

As women are living longer, with the tendency to have few or no children, the cervical canal may become stenotic and fibrotic. The fundus becomes smaller and has a thin wall. With obesity, even with a rectovaginal examination it is difficult to know the location of the fundus — anteflexed, anteverted; retroflexed, retroverted; or lateral displacement. Sometimes the location of the cervix gives a clue since an anterior pointing cervix suggests a retroflexed or retroverted fundus. If there is an endometrial carcinoma deep in the myometrium, the fundus is fragile. All these factors increase the risk of inadvertent perforation of the uterus by a preliminary sound or dilator when dilating the external os, endocervix or internal os of the cervix. The endometrial biopsy instrument might be advanced through the perforation and take a specimen from the peritoneal cavity.

Adequate Specimen

As with the introduction of all new procedures, the original studies are done by cautious, single experts with good results including no complications and adequate tissue. Many hospital residents are insufficiently taught how to do a difficult endometrial biopsy or difficult dilatation and curettage of the uterus. Nurse practitioners also require training. Most gynecologists use a sterile disposable Pipelle type flexible narrow plastic tube with a solid plunger core which gives a gentle suction as it is withdrawn while the tube is still in the uterus.

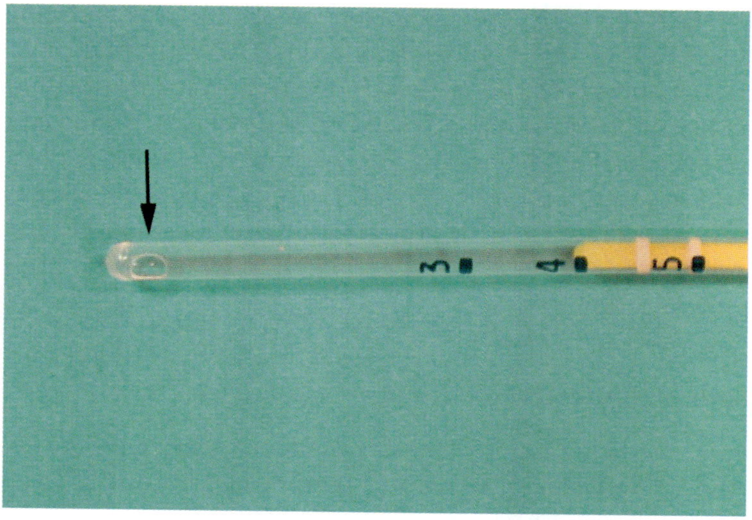

Fig. 1 Type of plastic Pipelle type endometrial biopsy (sampler) which has a flexible plastic outer sheath 3.1 mm in diameter and a 2.4 mm side opening near the tip.

Usually a tenaculum and dilator is not necessary (Fig. 1). There are multiple variations of the device. Some have a syringe attached for suction. The Vabra endometrial biopsy tube is metalic and narrow and a suction pump is attached. The disadvantage is that there may be a perforation of the uterus and bowel injury. Slightly curved, wide, rigid plastic tubes attached to a suction machine should not be used for endometrial biopsy. It requires cervical dilatation, causes pain and is used for early pregnancy termination or incomplete spontaneous abortion. The clinician and pathologist should understand that the usual endometrial biopsy instrument cannot remove a large endometrial polyp. Only the endometrium is sampled. The histologic sections will not indicate if there is myometrial invasion but can indicate endometrial neoplasia. This would be a sufficient reason to do a hysterectomy at which time myometrial invasion could be diagnosed.[39] The endometrial stainless steel suction biopsy curette (with attached suction syringe) has a scraping tip, gets a deep biopsy but cannot sample the entire endometrium.

The contraindications to endometrial biopsy include:

1. Viable intrauterine pregnancy.
2. Relative contraindications:

    A. Cervix or pelvic infection.
    B. Severe cervical stenosis.
    C. Cervix cancer obstructing the endocervical canal.
    D. Endocervical — lower uterine segment myomas.
    E. Coagulation defects.
    F. Extremely apprehensive patient who will not stay still.
    G. Technical difficulty — vaginal stenosis, previous endometrial ablation.

A review of endometrial biopsies in women with abnormal bleeding showed a relatively modest accuracy in diagnosing endometrial hyperplasia, therefore further investigation may have to be done, especially if symptoms persist.[41]

Technology

Adequate tissue can be obtained by endometrial biopsy in about 90% of cases. It is more reliable if the pathology affects the entire endometrium rather than one area.[42] Prophylactic antibiotics are not required. The operator requires instruction which is not supplied with the biopsy instruments and in order to get a sufficient and representative specimen for histologic examination. In addition, the operator can get an approximate idea of the endometrial tissue volume.

The most commonly used device is the soft plastic Pipelle type which is sterile and disposable. It is a flexible outer sheath 3.1 mm in diameter. The tissue is aspirated through a 2.4 mm side opening at the tip (Fig. 1). The Pipelle is introduced to the top of the endometrial cavity. The postmenopausal uterus may only be 6 cm or less in length. The premenopausal uterus would be about 8 cm in length. An enlarged cavity due to myomas, endometrial carcinoma or relative stenosis of the cervix distending the uterine cavity may sound to 10 cm.

There is a small risk of perforation (0.1% to 1.3%), especially if there is cervical stenosis requiring dilatation or a thin uterine wall due to postmenopausal atrophy or endometrial carcinoma invasion. The central solid core piston is pulled down to create suction in the sheath which is completely rotated slowly and downward to the internal os. Ideally, 4 sampling rotations are done.[42,43]

The Pipelle was developed in Paris, France, in 1984 and "has now become the sampler of choice to detect endometrial adenocarcinoma in an outpatient setting". In 1996, the Tao Brush™ device was approved by the FDA.[43] The accuracy of endometrial biopsy in detecting cancer is about 90%.[39] The Pipelle type of endometrial biopsy is the main instrument used. If symptoms persist consider a fractional curettage. An additional diagnostic procedure is hysteroscopy to identify a focal lesion and inspect the endocervical canal. With transvaginal ultrasound, normal postmenopausal thickness is 4 mm or less but it is variable and non-specific. The Tao Brush™ vinyl sheath endometrial sampler is 9 French diameter, a length of 26 cm and a brush length of 3.5 cm. The brush retrieves material for histologic tissue biopsy and for cytology (Fig. 2). Although not investigated, it is possible that the brush might be better than the Pipelle biopsy for localized type II endometrial cancer.

The sensitivity for the Tao Brush and Pipelle were 95.5% and 86% respectively while the specificity was 100% for both.[44] The authors of UpToDate wrote "In our experience, the Pipelle provides a larger sample for histological sample analysis than the endometrial brush; we prefer the Pipelle for this reason."[45]

The Tao Brush for endometrial biopsy for identifying carcinoma in 633 cases was reported to have 100% sensitivity and 96% specificity. It was considered to be reliable for endometrial sampling.[46] For women with clinical indications for endometrial biopsy, the Tao Brush instrument offered a 95% sensitivity for detecting endometrial cancer, while the Pipelle biopsy had 86% sensitivity. Both had 100% specificity, positive predictive value of 100% and negative predictive value of 98%. When both biopsy instruments were used at the same office visit the positive and negative predictive value for detecting or excluding endometrial cancer was 100%.[44]

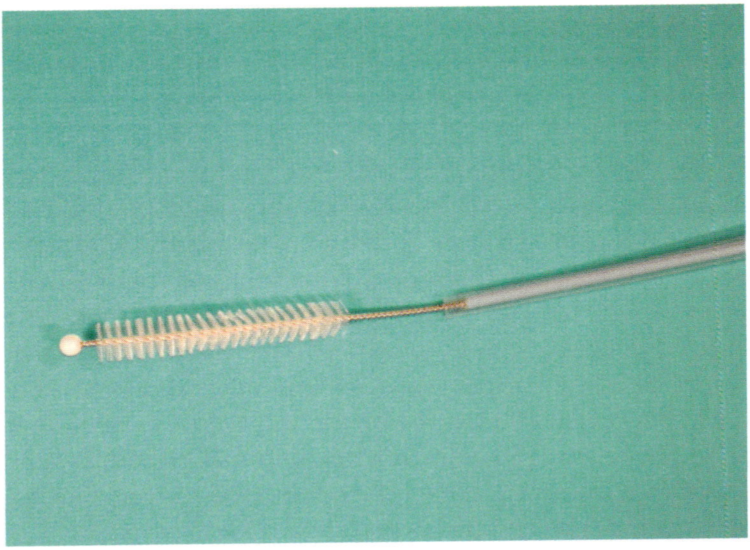

Fig. 2 The Tao Brush™ endometrial sampler retrieves tissue and cytology. The brush length is 3.5 cm. The narrow twisted stainless steel core can be slightly bent to sample the cornual angles.

Both the Tao Brush and the Pipelle endometrial biopsy samplers found five cases of centrally located adenocarcinoma, ranging from 0.4 cm to 3 cm. However, the Tao Brush also detected an adenocarcinoma near the cornu due to its malleable double-braided sterile steel core was bent so that rotation could reach the lateral cornual angles for global sampling. The Pipelle being made of polyethylene tubing, is non-maleable and can sample only the central uterine cavity. Both samplers missed a microscopic focus of adenocarcinoma (*in situ*) in a 0.7 cm polyp and a large 10 cm leiomyosarcoma of firm consistency.[43]

Dilatation and curettage (D&C) of the uterus is considered for:

1. Non-diagnostic endometrial biopsy with high risk of endometrial carcinoma.
2. Insufficient tissue with endometrial biopsy.
3. Endometrial biopsy report of hyperplasia to rule out carcinoma.

4. Cervix stenosis or other technical problem.
5. When hysteroscopy is to be done, to be certain of removing a polyp and a small local endometrial abnormality.

Women with recurrent episodes of postmenopausal bleeding should be investigated with transvaginal ultrasound and hysteroscopy to exclude endometrial disease and ovarian neoplasm. Although there is normal variation of thickness of endometrium on transvaginal ultrasound according to age, ethnic group and possibly body mass, if endometrial thickness is more than 4 mm (or 3 mm if more than five years since the last period) consider endometrial biopsy and hysteroscopy.[47] A review of hysteroscopy in the diagnosis of endometrial cancer and hyperplasia in women with abnormal bleeding found that hysteroscopy accuracy is high for endometrial cancer, especially in postmenopausal women but only moderate for hyperplasia.[48]

REFERENCES

1. Altchek A, Clues to tumors: new concepts of symptoms, signs, syndromes, paraneoplastic syndromes and predisposition to ovarian cancer, in *Diagnosis and Management of Ovarian Disorders*, Altchek A, Deligdisch L, Kase N (eds.), Publ Academic Press — Elsevier Science, San Diego, pp. 231–269, 2003.
2. Legare R, Genetics and gynecologic cancer, in *Precis. An Update in Obstetrics and Gynecology. Oncology*, 3rd edn., The American College of Obstetricans and Gynecologists, Washington DC, pp. 10–20, 2008.
3. Chen LM, Yang KY, Little SE, *et al.*, Gynecologic cancer prevention in Lynch syndrome/hereditary nonpolyposis colorectal cancer families, *Obstet Gynecol* **110**:18–25, 2007.
4. Hoskins WJ, How should women with a genetic predisposition for cancer be managed? *Obstet Gynecol* **110**:5–6, 2007.
5. Lancaster JM, Powell CB, Kauff ND, *et al.*, Society of Gynecologic Oncologists Education Committee statement on risk assessment for inherited gynecologic cancer predispositions, *Gynecol Oncol* **107**:159–162, 2007.

6. Altchek A, Prevention of ovarian serous epithelial cancer, in *Diagnosis and Management of Ovarian Disorders*, 2nd edn., Altchek A, Deligdisch L, Nathan K (eds.), Publ Academic Press — Elsevier Science, San Diego, pp. 516–544, 2003.
7. Walker JL, Cancer prevention and screening in women, in *Precis, An Update in Obstetrics and Gynecology. Oncology*, 3rd edn., The American College of Obstetricans and Gynecologists, Washington DC, pp. 3–9, 2008.
8. Genetics of Breast and Ovarian Cancer (PDQ®) Health Professional Version National Cancer Institutes of Health; *www.caner.gov*, last modified 18/12/2007.
9. Kurman RJ, Visvanathan K, Roden R, *et al.*, Early detection and treatment of ovarian cancer: shifting from early stage to minimal volume of disease based on a new model of carcinogenesis, *Am J Obstet Gynecol* **198**:351–356, 2008.
10. Goff B, Muntz H, Ovarian cancer, recognizing early symptoms can make a difference, *Contemp Obstet Gynecol* **53**:26, 2008.
11. Barber HK, Symptoms, signs and diagnosis, in *Ovarian Carcinoma, Etiology, Diagnosis and Treatment*, 3rd edn., Springer–Verlag, New York, pp. 87–91, 1993.
12. Vine MF, Ness RB, Calingaert B, *et al.*, Types and duration of symptoms prior to diagnosis of invasive or borderline ovarian tumors, *Gynecol Oncol* **83**:466–472, 2001.
13. Lee HR, Lenno VA, Camilteri M, *et al.*, Paraneoplastic gastrointestinal motor dysfunction: clinical and laboratory characteristics, *J Gastroenterol* **96**:373–379, 2001.
14. Goff B, Mandel L, Drescher C, *et al.*, Development of an ovarian cancer symptom index. Possibilities for earlier detection, *Cancer* **109**: 221–227, 2007.
15. Wynn M, Chang S, Peipins L, Temporal patterns of conditions and symptoms potentially associated with ovarian cancer, *J Womens Health (Larchmt)* **16**:971–986, 2007.
16. Markman M, Correspondence, *Cancer* **109**:221–227, 2007.
17. Chi DS, Kauff WD, Cancer of the Ovary, Peritoneum and Fallopian Tube, in *Precis. An Update in Obstetrics and Gynecology. Oncology*, 3rd edn., The American College of Obstetricans and Gynecologists, Washington DC, pp. 88–100, 2008.

18. Sunde JS, Kaplan KJ, Rose GS, Fallopian tube cancer, in *Clinical Gynecologic Oncology*, 7th edn., DiSaia PJ, Creasman TW (eds.), Mosby–Elsevier Philadelphia, pp. 398–410, 2007.
19. Copeland LJ, Epithelial ovarian cancer, in *Clinical Gynecologic Oncology*, 7th edn. DiSaia PJ, Creasman TW (eds.), Mosby–Elsevier Philadelphia, pp. 313–365, 2007.
20. Deligdisch L, Penault-Llorca F, Schlosshauer P, *et al.*, Stage I ovarian carcinoma: different clinical pathologic patterns, *Fertil Steril* **88**:906–910, 2007.
21. Dearking AC, Aletti GD, McGree ME, *et al.*, How relevant are ACOG and SGO guidelines for referral of adnexal mass? *Obstet Gynecol* **110**:841–848, 2007.
22. Altchek A, Deligdisch L, Penault-Llorca F, Speculation and deductive reasoning about ovarian epithelial carcinogenesis and new horizons, in *Diagnosis and Management of Ovarian Disorders*, 2nd edn., Altchek A, Deligdisch L, Kase N (eds.), Publ Academic Press — Elsevier, New York, pp. 305–323, 2003.
23. Hermsen B, Powelly S, Berkof J, *et al.*, Serum CA125 in relation to adnexal dysplasia and cancer in women at hereditary high risk of ovarian cancer, *J Clin Oncol* **25**:1383–1389, 2003.
24. Milam A, Milam M, Iyer R, Detection of early stage ovarian cancer by FDG-PET-CT in a patient with BRCA2-positive breast cancer, *J Clin Oncol* **25**:5657–5668, 2007.
25. Takekuma M, Maeda M, Ozawa T, *et al.*, Positron emission tomography with 18F-fluoro-2-deoxyglucose for the detection of recurrent ovarian cancer, *Int J Clin Oncol* **10**:177–181, 2005.
26. Barton CA, Hacker NF, Clark S, *et al.*, DNA methylation changes in ovarian cancer: implications for early diagnosis, prognosis and treatment, *Gynecol Oncol* **109**:129–139, 2008.
27. Lee CJ, Ariztia EV, Fishman D, Conventional and proteomic technologies for the detection of early stage malignancies: markers for ovarian cancer, *Crit Rev Clin Lab Sci* **44**:87–114, 2007.
28. Legge F, Ferrandina G, Scambia G, From bio-molecular and technology innovations to clinical practice: focus on ovarian cancer, *Ann Oncol* **17**:46–48, 2006.
29. Tchagang AB, Tewfik AH, DeRycke MS, *et al.*, Early detection of ovarian cancer using group biomarkers, *Mol Cancer Ther* 7:27–37, 2008.

30. Philip R, Murrthy S, Krakover J, *et al.*, Shared immunoproteome for ovarian cancer diagnostics and immunotherapy: potential theranostic approach to cancer, *J Proteome Res* **6**:2509–2517, 2007.
31. Munkarah A, Chatterjee M, Tainsky M, Update on ovarian cancer screening, *Curr Opin Obstet Gynecol* **19**:22–26, 2007.
32. Wouters BG, Proteomics: methodologies and applications in oncology, *Semin Radiat Oncol* **18**:115–125, 2008.
33. Agarwal R, Whang DH, Alvero AB, *et al.*, Macrophage migration inhibitory factor expression in ovarian cancer, *Am J Obstet Gynecol* **196**:3481–3485, 2007.
34. Bignotti E, Tassi R, Calza S, *et al.*, Differential gene expression profiles between tumor biopsies and short-term primary cultures of ovarian serous carcinomas: identification of novel, molecular biomarkers for early diagnosis and therapy, *Gynecol Oncol* **103**:405–416, 2006.
35. Preston DL, Cullings H, Suyama A, *et al.*, Solid cancer incidence in atomic bomb survivors exposed *in utero* or as young children, *J Natl Cancer Inst* **100**:428–436, 2008.
36. Rose PG, Cancer of the uterine corpus, in *Precis. An Update in Obstetrics and Gynecology. Oncology*, 3rd edn., The American College of Obstetricans and Gynecologists, Washington DC, pp. 74–78, 2008.
37. National Cancer Institute. Endometrial Cancer Screening (PDQ^{R}) Health Professional Version, last modified April 3rd, 2008.
38. Lu KH, Dinh M, Kohlmann W, *et al.*, Gynecologic cancer as a "sentinel cancer" for women with hereditary nonpolyposis colorectal cancer syndrome, *Obstet Gynecol* **105**:569–574, 2005.
39. Creasman WT, Adenocarcinoma of the uterus, in *Clinical Gynecologic Oncology*, 7th edn., DiSaia PJ, Creasman TW (eds.), Mosby–Elsevier Philadelphia, pp. 147–184, 2007.
40. Schmeler KM, Lynch HT, Chen LM *et al.*, Prophylactic surgery to reduce the risk of gynecologic cancers in the Lynch syndrome, *N Engl J Med* **354**:261–269, 2006.
41. Clark TJ, Mann CH, Shah N, *et al.*, Accuracy of outpatient endometrial biopsy in the diagnosis of endometrial cancer: a systematic quantitative review, *BJOG* **109**:313–321, 2002.
42. Guido RS, Stovall DW, Endometrial sampling procedures, in *UpToDate*, Rose BD (ed.), UpToDate, Waltham, MA, *http://www.uptodate.com*, 2008.

43. Yang GC, Wan L, Del Priore G, Factors influencing the detection of uterine cancer by suction curettage and endometrial brushing, *J Reprod Med* **47**:1005–1010, 2002.
44. Del Priore G, Williams R, Harbatkin CB *et al.*, Endometrial brush biopsy for the diagnosis of endometrial cancer, *J Reprod Med* **46**:439–443, 2001.
45. Feldman S, Evaluation of the endometrium for malignant or premalignant disease, in *UpToDate*, Rose BD (ed.), UpToDate, Waltham, MA, *http://www.uptodate.com*, 2008.
46. Wu HH, Casto BD, Elsheikh TM, Endometrial brush biopsy. An accurate outpatient method of detecting endometrial malignancy, *J Reprod Med* **48**:41–45, 2003.
47. Symonds I, Ultrasound, hysteroscopy and endometrial biopsy in the investigation of endometrial cancer, *Best Practice Res Clin Obstet Gynecol* **15**:381–391, 2001.
48. Clark TJ, Voit D, Gupta JK, *et al.*, Accuracy of hysteroscopy in the diagnosis of endometrial cancer and hyperplasia: a systematic quantitative review, *JAMA* **288**:1610–1621, 2002.

CHAPTER 7

CYTOLOGY FOR EARLY DIAGNOSIS OF GYNECOLOGIC CANCER

Maoxin Wu

INTRODUCTION

Many cancers in general are still non-curable unless they are detected early. Gynecological cancers, especially cervical squamous carcinoma has been largely reduced due to wide application of the Papanicolaou (Pap) smear screening program established by Dr. Papanicolaou in the United States. However, cervical cancer remains one of the greatest killers of women worldwide. There is presently no successful screening model for either endometrial or ovarian cancer. This chapter attempts to update the role of cytopathology and its relevant ancillary tests in early detection and management of gynecological cancers.

Core basics in cytology: traditionally, cytotechnologists and cytopathologists are trained to detect abnormal cells and diagnose

Table 1. General Criteria to Differentiate Benign from Malignant Cells

Benign	Malignant
Organized	Disorganized
Low N/C ratio	High N/C ratio
Uniform cells	Pleomorphism
Normal chromasia	Hyperchromasia
Smooth nuclear contour, thin membrane, lack of grooves or inclusions	Irregular nuclear contour, thick membrane, nuclear grooves and inclusions
Small or inconspicuous nucleolus	Prominent, multiple, irregular, macro-nucleoli
Occasional mitotic figures	Abnormal mitotic figures

malignancy and /or pre-malignancy based on cytomorphological features (Table 1).

Although most mature cells appear differently in their cytoplasm and cell membranes based on their differentiation and functions, the nature (good or bad) of a cell is largely determined by the quality of its nucleus and its nuclear contents. Theoretically, a malignancy or pre-malignancy can be diagnosed even if a single malignant or pre-malignant cell is identified. In general, it is not too difficult to differentiate a benign cell from a malignant cell (Fig. 1) on routine cytology. A benign cell generally have small nucleus with finely distributed chromatin and eneveloped by a well defined smooth nuclear membrane. The nuclear to cytoplasmic (N/C) ratio is usually low in a benign cell. In contrast, a malignant cell should have enlarged nucleus with increased nuclear material appearing either in hyperchromatic pattern or abnormal distribution of the chromatin appearing as enlarged in size or increased number of nucleoli and/or chromacenters. The nuclear membrane of a malignant cell can be irregular in contour or increased appearing as nuclear folds or grooves. The N/C ratio of a malignant cell should be increased comparing to its benign counterpart.

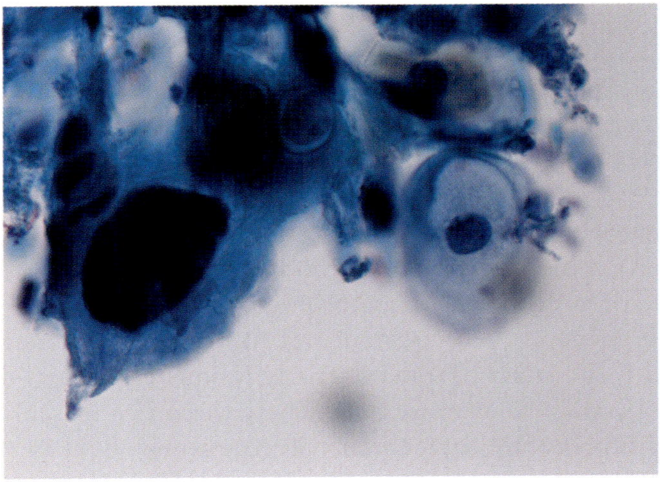

Fig. 1 Comparison of a malignant squamous cell (left) to a benign intermediate squamous cell (right). This malignant cell shows increased N/C ratio with a hyperchromatic nucleus which has irregular nuclear contour and relatively dense cytoplasm which is consistent with squamous differentiation. In contrast, the benign intermediate squamous cell has low N/C ratio and a nucleus with normal chromasia and relatively smooth nuclear membrane. Pap stained ThinPrep slide, original magnification 100×.

The real challenge is to determine the true nature of the malignant potential of a cell that is morphologically falling into the borderline category, so called "atypical" cells, because an atypical cell can be a premalignant cell or a cell with reactive atypia. Despite the fact that it is also difficult for clinicians to deal with a cytopathology report with atypical cells, it is extremely important for all of us (cytopathologists, surgical pathologists and gynecologists) to have a better understanding of this category and develop a better strategy to deal with it in order to improve the efficacy of early detection. It is urgently needed to identify indicators/tests at pathogenic, molecular and/or immunocytochemical levels for triaging these atypical cells of undetermined significance. A good example on such effort is that the role of testing human papilloma virus (HPV) has been shown to be useful in clinical management of patients with cytologically atypical squamous and endocervical cells.

It cannot be over emphasized that early detection of gynecological cancers as of other cancers has to start from (1) patient education and awareness; (2) good sample collection.

1. Patient education and awareness must start at their young age. Behavior modification and good nutrition are all very important for prevention of gynecological cancer. The patient has to understand the importance of routine physical examination even if she is asymptomatic. Early lesions can often be identified by trained professionals. The patient has to seek medical attention before any abnormal symptoms such as pain and bleeding occur.
2. Sampling for cytology is relatively easy and not traumatic to patients.

   (a) Smears can be prepared easily by gynecologists for any gynecological material that potentially contains cellular elements. The material can be scraping, brushing, secretion and fine needle aspiration (FNA) of a lesion or a potentially abnormal area. The material can be directly smeared on a glass slide (Fig. 2(a)); the smeared material can either be fixed with 95% alcohol (either by spray fixation or submerge fixation) for Pap staining or air-dried for diff-quik (DQ) staining.

   (b) Liquid based technology (Figs. 2(b)–(d)) has been widely applied to cytology to enhance the quality of slides, hence better detection of abnormal cells.

   (c) Excess material can be spun down in the cytopathology lab to make a cell block (CB) which can be sectioned and hematoxylin and eosin (H&E) stained for microscopic examination. Sometimes small fragments of tissue can be identified in the CB to assist cytological diagnosis with architectural features in a small scale similar to a surgical biopsy.

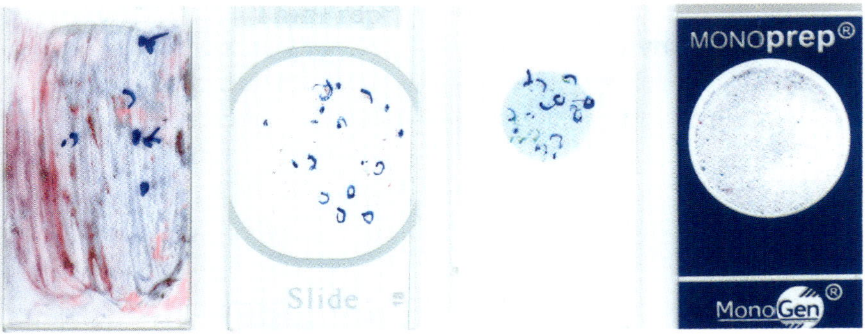

Fig. 2 Gross appearance of four types of Pap slides currently available in the USA. (a) A conventional smear that has been screened by a cytotechnologist noted with blue ink marking areas of abnormality. (b)–(d) are liquid based preparations: Thin Prep (b), SurePath (c) and Monoprep (d). Scaning photograph of representative original slides.

Factors contributing to early detection of gynecological cancers at cytological level are (1) good sampling; (2) good slide preparation; (3) good cell distribution; (4) well trained cytotechnologist and cytopathologist. The common problems encountered in a screening program are sampling error, thick or air-dried smears and rarity of abnormal cells in a background of marked inflammation, blood or necrotic debris. These issues can be minimized as long as the clinicians and the cytopathology team work together.

There are various cancers in the field of gynecology including cancers of vulva, vagina, cervix, uterus, fallopian tubes and ovaries. Despite the diversity of cancer types, as far as cytopathology is concerned, they can be classified as following:

1. Squamous cell carcinomas arising from squamous epithelium including vulva, vagina and cervix.
2. Adenocarcinomas arising from glandular epithelium such as Bartholin's glands, endocervical glands, endometrium, fallopian tube mucosa and ovarian epithelium.

3. Sarcoma arising from muscle and stroma such as leiomyosarcoma and endometrial stromal tumor of the uterus.
4. Malignant mixed mesodermal (Müllerian) tumor (MMMT) comprised of both epithelial and stromal components.
5. Germ cell tumors and sex cord-stromal tumors.

The weight distribution in this chapter will be based on practical application of cytology in relation to early detection of cancer in each area. The role of Pap smear, especially the recent application of liquid-based cytology in conjunction with human papilloma virus (HPV) testing in detecting pre-malignant cervical squamous intraepithelial lesion (SIL) will be emphasized. Current molecular studies relevant to early detection of gynecological cancers will also be updated.

CERVICAL, VAGINAL AND VULVAR NEOPLASMS

Cytology and Liquid Based New Technology

Pap test has served as a successful model in early detection of cervical cancer. Conventional Pap smear has contributed to a significant reduction of cervical cancer mortality among women who are screened regularly. With currently popular liquid based technology and HPV typing, early detection and effective management of cervical cancer can be achieved to a wide extent. Since HPV has been identified as the main cause of cervical cancer, with HPV vaccination, cervical cancer can become a rare disease in the near future in the United States (US). At the present time, cytology with HPV reflex testing still play major role in the field.

Globally, efforts have been demonstrated by the First Asia-Oceania Research Organization on Genital Infections and Neoplasia (AOGIN) Meeting which was held in Malaysia, in July 2005, in which 23 nations including Australia, Japan, Korea, Singapore, India, China and others participated. Based on the proceedings released from this meeting, worldwide, carcinoma of the uterine cervix is still the second most common cancer in women. The incidence is estimated to be approximately 470,600 per year, with almost 80% occurring in the developing world; in North America, cervical cancer is not among the leading seven cancers diagnosed in women, nor among the top seven cancers that result in death; in Central/South America, cervical cancer is the second most frequent cancer diagnosis and cause of death; in Africa, it is the most frequent cancer diagnosis and cause of death; and in Asia, it is second most frequent cancer diagnosis and fourth most frequent cause of death.

Cervical cancer remains a model disease for screening due to its long natural history, ease of sampling and accurate early detection based on cytomorphology. Dramatic reductions in mortality from this neoplasia have been achieved in countries with well-organized detection programs. Nevertheless, the Pap test has low sensitivity, though high specificity for detecting cancer precursors. The large number of women requiring repeated testing and the inability of cytology or HPV testing to identify women at higher risk for disease progression impose greater efforts on the health systems.

Conventional Pap smear has served its purpose well in the past four to five decades. This type of preparation has been largely replaced by liquid based techniques (Fig. 2 and Table 2) in the US. However, conventional Pap smears should still be used, especially in countries where liquid based technology is not available or not affordable.

Three liquid-based Pap tests are approved for use in the US:

Thin Prep (Cytyc, Marlborough, MA)
Sure Path (BD Diagnostics-Tripath, Burlington, NC)
MonoPrep Pap (MonoGen, Lincolnshire, IL)

Liquid-based Pap tests were originally developed to facilitate the computerized screening. In addition to the suitability for automated screening, liquid-based Pap tests alone, when compared to conventional smears, were shown to increase the sensitivity in the detection of epithelial cell abnormality.[1–4] These tests were approved consecutively by the US Food and Drug Administration (FDA): Thin Prep, in 1996; Sure Path, in 1999 and MonoPrep Pap Test (MPPT), in 2006. In the last decade, liquid-based Pap tests have been widely used

Table 2. Comparison of Currently Available Technology for Pap Tests

Code	A	B	C	D
Technique	Conventional	Thin Prep	Sure Path	MonoPrep
Slide type	Thick smear	Thin layer	Thin layer	Thin layer
Technical Base	Direct smearing	Homogenization and Filtering	Density gradient proprietary cell enrichment	Filter aspiration
Advantages	(1) Easy to prepare (2) Inexpensive	(1) Easy to screen (2) Imager system for automated screening	(1) Easy to screen (2) Focal point profiler (3) Molecular test	(1) Easy to screen (2) Fully automated batch-processing instrument (3) End to end bar coding
Disadvantages	Difficult screen	Expensive	Expensive	Expensive

in the US. Regardless of the differences of technology for Pap testing, the cytomorphology and the criteria for making diagnosis should be basically same.

Elements in a Normal Pap

Normal squamous epithelium lining the lower gynecological tract is similar to that of skin except for the absence of surface keratinization. The normal maturation of squamous epithelium proceeds from basal to parabasal to intermediate to superficial (Fig. 3).

- Basal cells are small undifferentiated cells with scanty cytoplasm. These cells are seldom identified in the normal Pap smear except

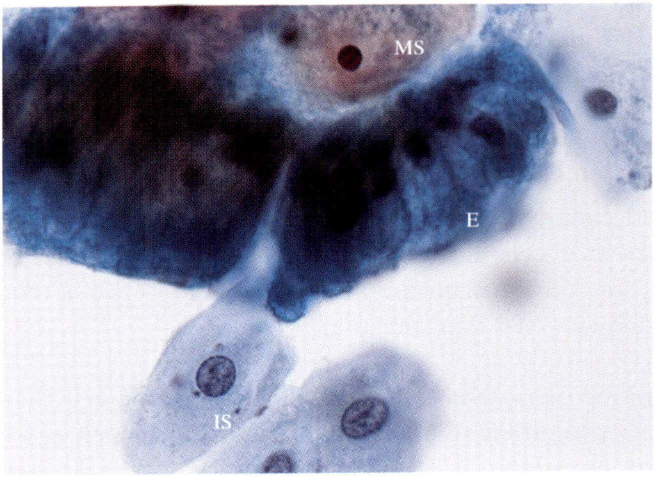

Fig. 3 A typical normal Thin Prep Pap slide from a premenopausal woman in her mid cycle. The slide contains endocervical cells (E), superficial or mature squamous cells (MS) and intermediate squamous cells (IS). Common features for all benign cells are the small nuclear size (superficial mature squamous cells have even smaller, pyknotic nuclei) and a low nuclear to cytoplasmic (N/C) ratio. The appearance of the cytoplasm characterizes the type of cells, such as endocervical cells with columnar foamy cytoplasm, intermediate cells with basophilic cytoplasm due to less cyto-keratin, and superficial squamous cells with orangeophilic cytoplasm due to abundant cytokeratins.

in severe atrophy, in which they are often associated with parabasal cells.

- Parabasal cells start to acquire squamous features such as dense cytoplasm and distinct cell boundaries. The nucleus of a parabasal cell is round to oval, with smooth nuclear membrane contour and finely dispersed chromatin.
- Intermediate cells (Fig. 3) are the cell type more superficial to parabasal cells in the line of squamous maturation. The nucleus of an intermediate cell is used as a key reference for size (about the size of a red blood cell) and chromatin quality (normochromatic). Any squamous cell nucleus that is significantly larger and more hyperchromatic than that of an intermediate cell is likely to be dysplastic. A dysplastic nucleus is also considered to be a premalignant nucleus.
- Superficial cells (Fig. 3), are the most superficial cell type in the normal squamous maturation. This type of squamous cells has already acquired abundant cytokeratin. Thus, the nucleus of a superficial squamous cell has a small, pyknotic or inactive nucleus.
- Normal endocervical glandular cells: as shown in Fig. 3, endocervical glandular cells are columnar cells, each with a small basally located round to oval nucleus and mucin containing cytoplasm. Endocervical cells along with squamous metaplastic cells are indicators for transformation zone and their presence is required for the adequacy of a Pap smear.

Squamous metaplasia begins in a basal reserve cell that has the unique ability to differentiate into either a squamous cell or a glandular cell. Squamous metaplastic cells are hyperplastic reserve cells that acquired squamous cell features such as dense cytoplasm and sharply defined cytoplasmic borders. The nuclear size of an immature squamous metaplastic cell is comparable to that of a parabasal cell. Squamous metaplasia appears to occur in the transformation zone in response to inflammation or other injuries. The pathological significance of an immature squamous metaplasia is that the presence of atypical/dysplastic nuclei in the metaplasia is likely to represent a high-grade squamous lesion. On the other hand, an atypical squamous metaplastic cell may become mature if the causative agent is removed or taken care by immune response. Other types of normal cells such as endometrial (gland and stromal), serous type of fallopian tube mucosa and mixed inflammatory cells may also be seen in a normal Pap slide.

Epithelial Abnormality

Epithelial abnormality refers to nuclear abnormality (meaning that the size and chromatin patterns) is significantly deviated from its normal counterpart or a nucleus that is significantly enlarged or abnormal compared to an indermediate squamous cell. The nuclear abnormality ranges from atypical of undetermined significance, dysplasia (low and high grade) to carcinoma. The efforts for early diagnosis of gynecological cancer should be focused on detecting atypical and dysplastic cells in a screening program.

Squamous dysplasia and squamous carcinoma *in situ* of cervix are all precancerous lesions or carcinomas that involve full thickness of the squamous epithelium before the stage of invasion. Squamous carcinoma *in situ* refers to full thickness replacement by undifferentiated basaloid cells in syncytial arrangement (without any squamous differentiation). Dysplasia of various grades (mild, moderate and severe) is inversely proportional to the degree of squamous differentiation toward the surface epithelium. Since the Pap smear collects surface epithelial cells, cytomorphological features of surface abnormal squamous cells in the Pap test determine the grade of dysplasia. Cervical intraepithelial neoplasm (CIN) was intraduced to emphasize the spectrum of abnormalities and to help standerize the treatment. They were mild dysplasia, CIN 1, moderate dysplasia, CIN 2 and severe dysplasia, CIN 3. In the current Bethesda system,[5] only two (low and high) grades that correspond to the CIN system as CIN 1, low grade and CIN 2/CIN 3, high grade, are used. Compative terminology for cervical carcinoma precursor lesions is present in Table 3 in which the diagnosis "condyloma" should be reserved for surgical pathology report. Current Pap testing report is based on the Bethesda system.

Low grade squamous intraepithelial lesion (LSIL, Fig. 4) corresponds to condyloma (featured by koilocytes) and mild dysplasia

Table 3. Comparative Terminology for Preinvasive Cervical Carcinomatous Lesions

Traditional terms	CIN terms	The Bethesda system
Condyloma	Condyloma	LSIL
Mild dysplasia	1	LSIL
Moderate dysplasia	2	HSIL
Severe dyspalsia	3	HSIL
Carcinoma *in situ*	3	HSIL

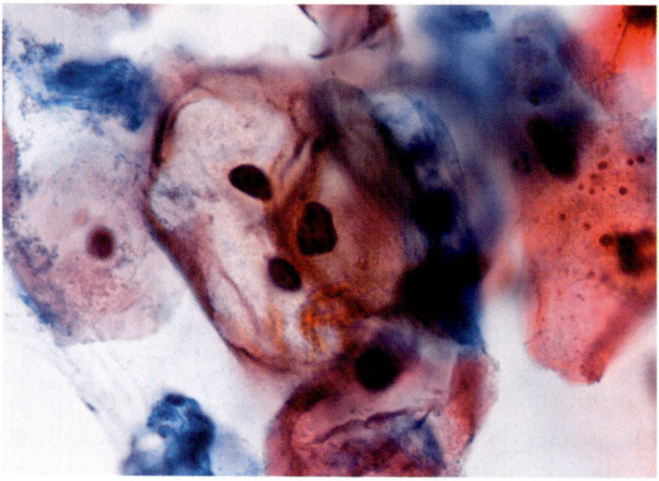

Fig. 4 Koilocytes with enlarged atypical nuclei and large perinuclear cavity-like clearing. Pap stained ThinPrep slide, original magnification 100×.

(large dysplastic nuclei with abundant cytoplasm). The koilocyte is the hallmark of human papilloma virus (HPV) cytopathic effect. A koilocyte is defined as an atypical squamous cell with enlarged hyperchromatic nucleus surrounded by a large clear cavitary space with dense/peripherally placed cytoplasm. Cells represent LSIL may not be koilocytes. Diagnosis of LSIL is based on that an enlarged dysplastic nucleus is located in a large squmous cell with relatively mature cytoplasm with or without cavitary cytopathic effect.

High-grade squamous intraepithelial lesion (HSIL) corresponds to moderate/severe dysplasia (dysplastic nuclei + moderate to scanty cytoplasm) and carcinoma *in situ* (small dysplastic cells in syncytial group, Fig. 5). A single high-grade dysplastic cell (litigation cell) should be recognized and reported as HSIL. The name of the litigation cell is acquired since it can often be missed during routine Pap screening tests especially conventional Pap tests and the hospital or the institution may get sued after the patient is diagnosed with malignancy.

Atypical cells of undetermined significance is a category in which the nucleus of a cell is considerably abnormal compared to its normal counterpart or the nucleus of an intermediate cells but insufficiently so to be dysplastic. For example, a nucleus of an atypical squamous cell of undetermined significance (ASCUS) is about two to three times the area of an intermediate cell nucleus in comparison to four to six times the area of intermediate cell nucleus in squamous dysplasia. Atypical glandular cells of undetermined significance (AGUS) are defined by an atypical nucleus seen in a glandular cell.

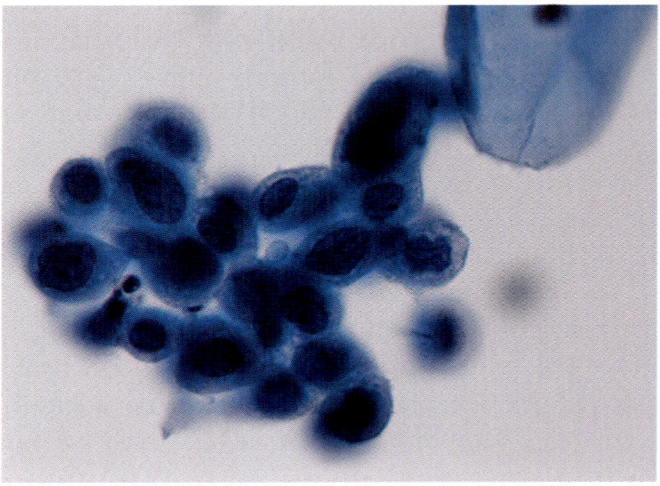

Fig. 5 Cluster of high-grade squamous dysplastic cells with hyperchromatic nuclei, high N/C ratios and irregular nuclear membrane. Pap stained ThinPrep slide, original magnification 100×.

ASCUS or AGUS has acquired a bad reputation for ctopathologists since it is difficult to manage clinically. Thanks to the discovery of the role of HPV in squamous dysplasia and carcinoma, ASCUS with HPV reflex testing has become standard practice which significantly improved the quality of clinical care.

Patients with glandular dysplasia require further evaluation because it may hide serious pathology from all internal genital organs. A study[6] that investigated the prognostic significance of glandular dyskaryosis/AGUS including 26,408 Pap smears revealed that 30 (0.11%) smears were reported as having glandular dyskaryosis; of which; two cases of invasive cervical carcinoma (one squamous cell and one adenocarcinoma); one case with ovarian cancer, eight cases with high grade squamous intraepithelial lesion (HGSIL) and ten cases with other nonmalignant pathology (polyps, hyperplasia) of endometrial origin. These findings reflect a 36.7% positive predictive value for significant squamous and glandular pathology.

Endocervical neoplasia may be first hinted by the presence of abundant endocervical cells. Endocervical adenocarcinoma *in situ* (AIS) is characterized by abnormal glandular arrangements such as microacinar structures and rosettes, comprised of hyperchromatic, crowded and elongated nuclei with coarse chromatin and mitotic figures (Fig. 6). In the author's opinion, one should pay very close attention to these endocervical cells with elongated hyperchromatic nuclei. Once the length of a nucleus exceeds 50% of a normal columnar endocervical cell, AIS should be considered. It is not infrequent that a patient died of endocervical adenocarcinoma and the hospital or the institution that screened the patient's previous Pap smears failed to identify AIS and has been sued. Pap tests are successful mainly in preventing squamous cell carcinoma. Its limited role in cervical adenocarcinoma is probably due to (1) inverted growth pattern of endocervical adenocarcinoma limits an adequate sampling; (2) the lack of early recognition of AIS in Pap tests.

Carcinomas of squamous and glandular types of the cervix are similar to squamous and glandular carcinomas from other parts of the body. There are three distinct types of squamous carcinomas

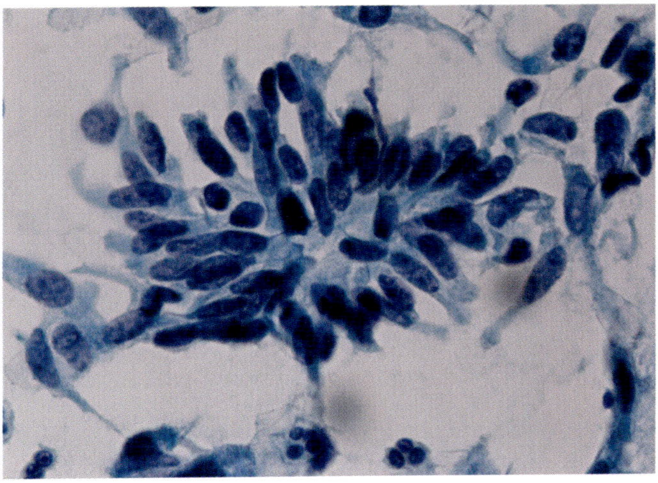

Fig. 6 A cellular smear contains many columnar cells with enlarged elonged nuclei with coarse hyperchromatic chromatin. This represents a case of endocervical adenocarcinoma *in situ* (AIS). Pap stained conventional smear, original magnification 100×.

based on their grades of differentiation from poorly to well: small cell, nonkeratinizing and keratinizing types. Small cell type has small uniform oval shaped cells with scanty basophilic cytoplasm and a relatively large nucleus with coarse chromatin and macronucleolus. Nonkeratininizing type has similar nuclear quality as the small cell type except that the cells are larger and acquired a moderate amount of cyanophilic cytoplasm. The keratinizing type has large pleomorphic keratin producing cells with pyknotic nuclear chromatin and the nucleolus may or may not be seen. Adenocarcinoma shows up as three-dimensional groups of cells which resemble gland formation. The adenocarcinoma cells have less dense chromatin, more prominent nucleoli and vacuolated cytoplasm compared to squamous cells. A common feature for all carcinomas is that the background will be "dirty" (tumor diathesis) with exception of metastatic type.

In the US, Pap test reports are based on the current 2001 Bethesda System (see below).

The 2001 Bethesda System[5]

- Specimen type
  Indicate conventional smear (Pap smear) *vs.* liquid-based preparation *vs.* other
- Specimen adequacy
  - Satisfactory for evaluation
    (describe presence or absence of endocervical/transformation zone component and any other quality indicators, e.g. partially obscuring blood, inflammation, etc.)
  - Unsatisfactory for evaluation (specify reason)
    - Specimen rejected/not processed (specify reason)
    - Specimen processed and examined, but unsatisfactory for evaluation of epithelial abnormality because of (specify reason)
- Interpretation/Result
  - Negative for intraepithelial lesion or malignancy
    (when there is no cellular evidence of neoplasia, state this in the General Categorization above and/or in the Interpretation/Result section of the report, whether or not there are organisms or other non-neoplastic findings)
    - Organisms
      - *Trichomonas vaginalis*
      - Fungal organisms morphologically consistent with *Candida spp*
      - Shift in flora suggestive of bacterial vaginosis
      - Bacteria morphologically consistent with *Actinomyces spp*
      - Cellular changes consistent with Herpes simplex virus
    - Other non-neoplastic findings (optional to report; list not inclusive)
      - Reactive cellular changes associated with:
        - Inflammation (includes typical repair)

- Radiation
- Intrauterine contraceptive device (IUD)

- □ Glandular cells status post-hysterectomy
- □ Atrophy

- Other
    - Endometrial cells (in a woman ≥ 40 years of age) (Specify if "negative for squamous intraepithelial lesion")
- Epithelial cell abnormalities
    - Squamous cell
        - Atypical squamous cells
            - □ Of undetermined significance (ASC-US)
            - □ Cannot exclude HSIL (ASC-H)
        - Low grade squamous intraepithelial lesion (LSIL) Encompassing: HPV/mild dysplasia/CIN 1
        - High grade squamous intraepithelial lesion (HSIL) Encompassing: moderate and severe dysplasia, CIS; CIN 2 and 3
            - □ With features suspicious for invasion (if invasion is suspected)
        - Squamous cell carcinoma
    - Glandular cell
        - Atypical
            - □ Endocervical cells, NOS or specify in comments
            - □ Endometrial cells, NOS or specify in comments
            - □ Glandular cells, NOS or specify in comments
        - Atypical
            - □ Endocervical cells, favor neoplastic
            - □ Glandular cells, favor neoplastic

- Endocervical adenocarcinoma *in situ*
- Adenocarcinoma
    - Endocervical
    - Endometrial
    - Extrauterine
    - Not otherwise specified (NOS)

- Other malignant neoplasms

In routine Pap screening, the majority of patients are negative, meaning there is no evidence of intraepithelial lesion or malignancy. Appearance or cellular composition of a normal Pap may vary depending on the age of a patient and phase of her menstrual cycle. For example, a Pap slide from mid cycle of a young woman shows mostly mature squamous cells due to estrogen effect; a Pap slide from a pregnant woman will show predominantly intermediate cells, heavily glycogenated (navicular cells) mainly because of the influence of progesterone; a normal Pap from a postmenopausal woman is likely to be atrophic with predominantly basal and parabasal cells. The bottom line is that there is no abnormal cell (either premalignant or malignant) present on a given slide.

In contrast to normal, malignant cells presented in Fig. 7 show enlarged nuclei and increased N/C ratios. More specifically, Fig. 7 represents an example of squamous cell carcinoma in paramenopausal woman. Figure 8 shows a three-dimensional group of malignant glandular cells seen in adenocarcinoma. Figure 9 depicts a cellular sample of pleomorphic tumor cells seen in MMMT.

Human Papilloma Virus (HPV)

HPV is a group of double stranded DNA viruses that have the ability to affect host genomes. There are over 100 types identified. Two HPV oncogenes, known as *E6* and *E7*, are able to degrade the proteins of host cellular genes *p53* and *Rb*, thus extending cell proliferation and retarding cell differentiation. In the world-wide, a review of the prevalence of the 11 most common HPV types in HPV-positive

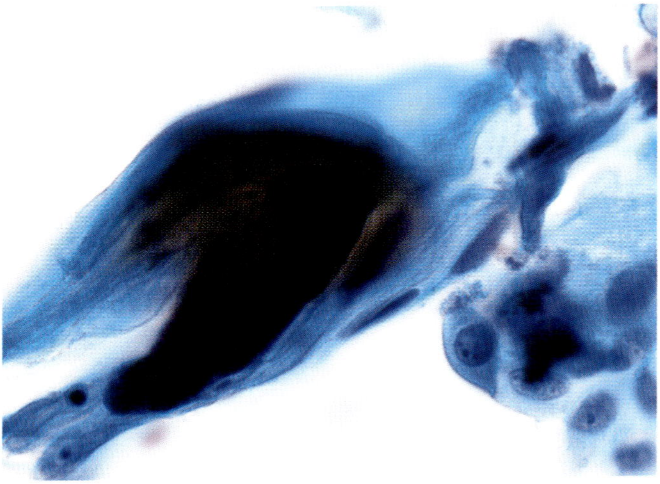

Fig. 7 Large elongated malignant quamous cells with markedly enlarged hyperchromatic nuclei and nuclear pleomorphism present in a background of necrotic debris. This is an example of a nonkeratinizing squamous cell carcinoma seen in a paramenopausal woman. Pap stained ThinPrep slide, original magnification 100×

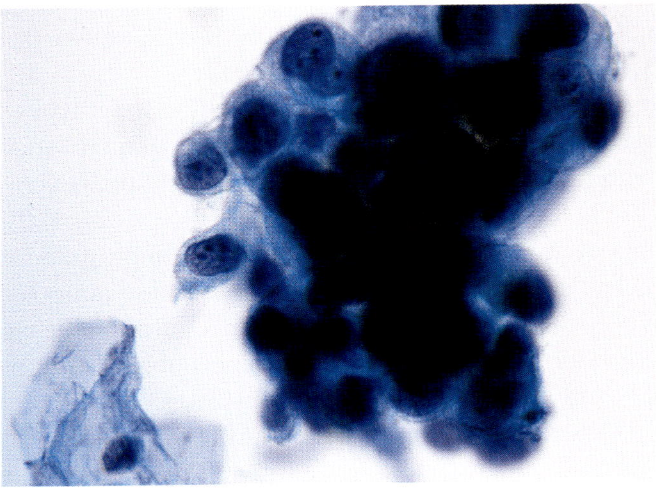

Fig. 8 A three-dimensional cluster of malignant glandular cells with increased N/C ratios, distincted nucleoli and lacy to vacuolated cytoplasm. This is an example of adenocarcinoma of uncertain primary. Pap stained ThinPrep slide, original magnification 100×.

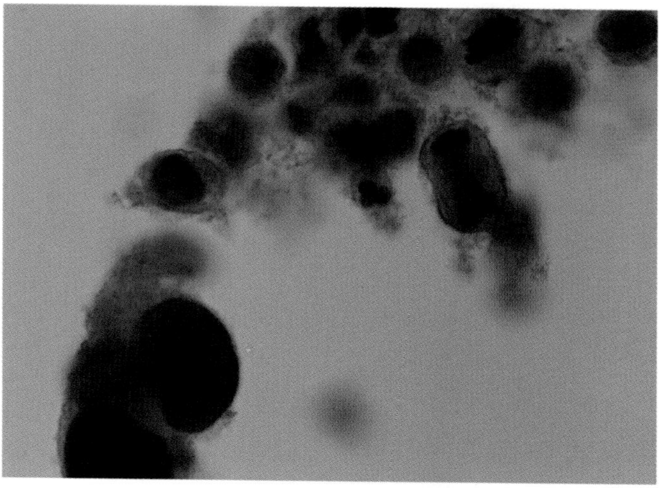

Fig. 9 A biphasic tumor cell population including epithelial tumor cells and stromal type of tumor cells. This shows example of recurrent MMMT seen in Pap test. Pap stained ThinPrep slide, original magnification 100×.

cervical cancer cases ($n = 2855$) indicates that although frequencies varied, HPV 16 followed by HPV 18, were most commonly detected in Africa, Central-South America, South Asia, and North America. HPVs 45, 31, and 33 were also seen globally.[7]

There are many different immunologically distinct types of HPVs, which have been linked to specific conditions: genital cancer (HPVs 16, 18); genital warts (HPVs 6, 11); epidermodysplasia verruciformis EV (HPVs 5, 8); and cutaneous warts (HPVs 1, 2). HPV 16 and HPV 18 appear to be most frequent in cases of high-grade squamous intraepithelial lesions (HSIL) or cases of invasive squamous cell carcinoma (SCC), although the relative incidence of different types varies in different regions.[8] Infection does not inevitably lead to pathological changes and regression occurs in many cases.

HPV DNA testing may be used clinically for (a) screening, either alone or as an adjunct to cytology; (b) triage of patients with uncertain Pap results; (c) monitoring patients post-treatment. Amplification of viral DNA may be through target amplification (PCR) or signal amplification (Hybrid Capture II). HPV testing in combination with Pap cytology has improved negative predictive value (approaches 100%). Such combination results in fewer unnecessary colposcopies. A meta-analysis to assess the accuracy of HPV DNA testing as an alternative to repeat cytology in women who had equivocal results on a previous Pap smear suggests that HC II assay has higher sensitivity and similar specificity compared to the repeat Pap smear (ASCUS as threshold) for CIN 2+ among women in this patient group.[9] However, it is still controversial as to whether HPV testing would be able to replace the Pap testing.

Other efforts aimed to detect precancerous cervical lesions using newly developed rapid biochemical tests that are affordable, accurate, simple to use, and appropriate for low-resource settings are being developed, namely batch test and rapid strip test. The batch test developed by Digene Corporation, US, will use an instant photo signal output. Images of 46 samples will be compared visually on a film with positive and negative controls. The results can be obtained in about two hours. It is suitable for a small clinic or mobile unit. The rapid strip test promises to discriminate between neoplastic transformation and infection by HPV. Arbor Vita Corporation technology detects a biomarker (E6 oncoprotein) which correlates with the neoplastic transformation of cells and cervical cancer. The result may appear in 20 minutes. The ELISA prototype is now being adapted to an immuno-chromatographic strip format capable of detecting common high-risk HPV types. Efforts are focused on improving sensitivity.

Based on a review article written by Cox JT in 2006,[10] HPV tests in combination with Pap tests are 96% to 100% sensitive for detection of cervical intraepithelial neoplasia (CIN 2 or CIN 3) and cancer. However, because HPV infection is common in young women and most commonly transient, the 2006 consensus guidelines were that

1. HPV testing is not recommended as part of primary cervical screening for women younger than 30 years of age.
2. HPV testing is recommended for women of any age for the clarification of ASCUS and as an option for follow-up of women with HPV-positive ASCUS, ASC-H, and or LSIL not found to have CIN 2 or CIN 3.

3. HPV testing is also recommended as an alternative to colposcopy and/or cytology for follow-up of treated cases.

Proper use of HPV testing improves the management of women with cytological abnormalities. In addition, a negative HPV test in combination with a normal Pap test result in women age 30 and older allows the safe extension of the interval between cervical screenings. Thus, when used properly, HPV testing may reduce morbidity and mortality and does so in a cost-effective manner. Presently, routine Pap screening test in combination with reflex high-risk HPV testing becomes a standard practice in the US. Many precancerous lesions are detected and treated in very early stages in patients routinely participating in Pap screening programs. Hopefully, high-risk HPV vaccines will break the cycle even earlier.

HPV virus is not highly immunogenic, regression of HPV being dependent on the immune response, occurring less frequently in immunocompromised patients such as renal transplant recipients. Details of this immune response are not completely understood, but humoral, cellular, and innate immunity may all play a role.

Quadrivalent HPVs 6, 11, 16, 18 vaccine (GARDASIL) comprises virus-like particles produced in recombinant yeast.[11] The vaccine is adsorbed on the Merck proprietary aluminum adjuvant, which strengthens its immunogenicity.

HPV 16/18 vaccine is a prophylactic candidate that contains bivalent viral-like protein particles, L1, adjuvanted by AS04 as an enhancing agent.[12] This vaccine was designed to target HPV types 16 and 18.

CerVax 16 is an experimental therapeutic product which uses E6/E7 proteins (identical to those of HPV16) and a quillaia saponin-based adjuvant capable of promoting both humoral and cell-mediated immunity.[13]

It was recently reported[12,14] that clinical trials have documented the safety, efficacy, and immunogenicity of the quadrivalent and bivalent HPV L1 virus-like particle vaccines. These vaccines have demonstrated greater than 90% efficacy in preventing HPV-related neoplasias of the lower genital tract. The quadrivalent HPV vaccine has been found to be more than 95% efficacious in preventing genital warts. These vaccines have been shown to protect against a wider range of oncogenic HPV types. Nonetheless, women must continue to have routine cervical cytological screening.

Molecular Studies

A number of epigenetic alterations occur during all stages of cervical carcinogenesis in both human papillomavirus and host cellular genomes, which include global DNA hypomethylation, hypermetylation of key tumor suppressor genes, and histone modifications. The reversible nature of epigenetic changes constitutes a target for transcriptional therapies, namely DNA methylation and histone deacetylase inhibitors. To date, studies in patients with cervical cancer have demonstrated the feasibility of reactivating the expression of hypermethylated and silenced tumor suppressor genes as well as the hyperacetylating and inhibitory effect upon histone deacetylase activity in tumor tissues after treatment with demethylating and histone deacetylase inhibitors. In addition, detection of epigenetic changes in cytological smears, serum DNA, and peripheral blood are of potential interest for the development of novel biomolecular markers for early detection, prediction of response, and prognosis.

The realization that genetic and epigenetic alterations are present at the earliest steps of the malignant progression of cervix uteri has led to testing the presence of these abnormalities, such as p16 expression.[15,16] Overexpression of the protein $p16^{Ink4a}$ is typical for the dysplastic and neoplastic epithelium of the cervix. However $p16^{Ink4a}$ negative CINs and carcinomas do exist. All stages of CINs and carcinomas analyzed are heterogeneous with respect to $p16^{Ink4a}$ expression. So $p16^{Ink4a}$ negativity is not a sufficient reason to exclude a patient from the high risk group. Since normal cervical epithelium is negative for $p16^{Ink4a}$, the ratio $p16^{Ink4a}$ positive/$p16^{Ink4a}$ negative samples should increase as the severity of the lesion progresses. Application of immunohisto-/cytochemical test for $p16^{Ink4a}$

may be regarded as a supplementary test for the early diagnosing of cervical cancer.

A large number of studies looking at the methylation status of tumor suppressor genes have uncovered that some genes are found hypermethylated in preinvasive lesions, raising the possibility that testing for methylation of either of these or of a set of these may prove to be a useful screening tool.[17–21] However, there is limited information with respect to the sensitivity and specificity of methylated genes for the identification of women with cervical dysplasia and cancer as well as comparisons of results using different sources of samples, either exfoliated cells or paraffin-embedded biopsy samples. In this regard, a very comprehensive study[22] investigated the methylation profile of 20 genes (*p16*, *p15*, *CCND2*, *RASSF1*, *RARb*, *TWIST1*, *SYK*, *HIC1*, *VHL*, *PRDM2*, *SFN*, *MLH1*, *MGMT*, *APC*, *CDH1*, and *CDH13*) in exfoliates and biopsies of 319 women that participated in a cytology screening study. By logistic regression, the authors determined the best set of candidate genes for employment as disease markers. The key findings are (1) similar detection rate of methylation regardless of sample source; (2) *CDH13*, *DAPK1*, *RARb*, and *TWIST1* were the genes showing a statistically significant increase with lesion severity and *DAPK1*, *RARb*, and *TWIST1*, the best panel of hypermethylated genes; (3) at least one of the three genes was hypermethylated in 57% of samples with CIN 3/CIS and in 74% with invasive cancer, but in only 5% of samples with CIN 1; (4) estimated specificity of the panel was 95% with sensitivity of 74% (95% confidence interval CI 95%, 73%–75%) for invasive carcinoma and 52% (95%, 49%–55%) for CIN 3/CIS. These findings provide preliminary evidence on the potential usefulness of a panel of genes to be tested for hypermethylation in cytology samples; however, additional studies are needed before this epigenetic-based screening test could be adopted. The methylation status of several genes present in the serum or plasma of patients with cervical cancer has been studied with regard to their prognostic significance.[23–25] Together, these data encourage further studies to find a set of methylated genes that would have prognostic significance but that would also serve as surrogate markers of efficacy of epigenetic therapies.

Circulating nucleic acids represent a biomarker that might be used in early detection of cancer, in the follow-up of patients with cancer or as a prognostic factor. Presence of nucleic acids in plasma or serum of patients with cancer has been recognized.[26–32] One study[32] analyzed the effect of tumor and chemotherapy upon the levels of nucleosomes *in vitro*, *in vivo* and in cervical cancer patients and revealed that (1) most of circulating nucleosomes originate from the tumor and that chemotherapy produces an early rise most likely due to tumor apoptosis; (2) nucleosomes are rapidly cleared from circulation; (3) chemotherapy within the therapeutic range of doses has no effect on nucleosome levels in healthy mice and rats. This data suggests that the determination of circulating nucleosomes pre- and post-treatment could be a useful test to predict response to chemotherapy in cancer patients.

ENDOMETRIAL NEOPLASIA

Endometrial Cytology

Endometrial cells are generally detected through Pap tests since direct endometrial sampling is rarely done. However, only the type of endometrial carcinoma that is easily shed from superficial endometrium can be detected by Pap test. Early cytological detection of endometrial carcinoma may be improved by vigorous follow-up of patients with high risk signs or symptoms such as postmenopausal bleeding and direct endometrial sampling whenever an atypical endometrioid glandular cell type is noted on Pap test.

Endometrial glandular cells, stromal cells or both can be identified in a Pap test. Normal endometrial cells can be seen in the first half of the menstrual cycle. Their presence in the second half of the cycle, particularly in women older than 40 years of age or postmenopausal, is considered to be abnormal or a risk factor for endometrial hyperplasia or neoplasia. Especially, when the nucleus is atypical (larger than squamous intermediate cell nucleus and with nucleolus), suspicion for endometrial carcinoma should be higher. Shedding of abnormal or atypical endometrial cells is always abnormal, regardless of its relationship to the menstrual cycle.

Updated Endometrial Carcinogenesis and Molecular Studies

It is generally accepted that there are two types of endometrial carcinomas:

Type I, estrogen dependent, well differentiated endometrial carcinomas.
Type II, ovarian serous adenocarcinoma-like, poorly differentiated type.

In recent decades, progress has been made in defining endometrial precancers. Endometrial intraepithelial neoplasia has been widely accepted as a precancer of type I endometrial cancer, while endometrial glandular dysplasia (endometrial intraepithelial carcinoma, EIC) is a newly described entity as a probable precancer of type II cancer.[33]

Biomarkers of phosphatase and tensin homolog (PTEN), β-catenin, p53, Insulin-like growth factor II mRNA-binding protein 3 (IMP3), N-myc Downstream-regulated Gene 1 (*NDRG1*) are helpful for the early detection of endometrial glandular dysplasia as well as for type II endometrial cancers.[33–37]

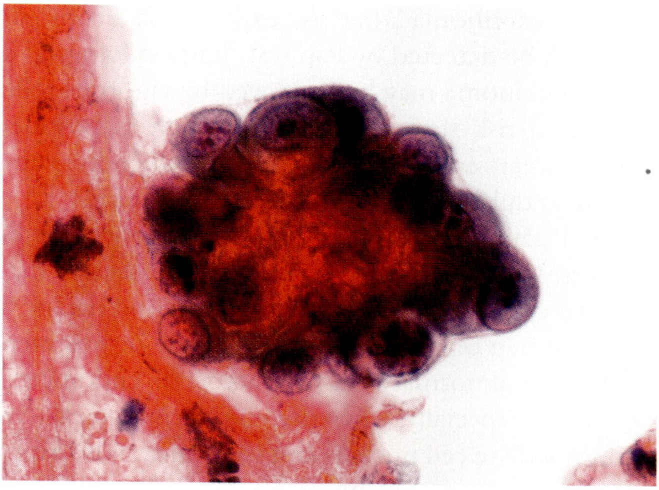

Fig. 10 Endometrial adenocarcinoma appears in cervical Pap test in a flower-like glandular pattern. Pap stained ThinPrep slide, original magnification 100×.

Based on Boruban *et al.*,[38] biomarkers whose expression is altered in cases of endometrial hyperplasia or cancer such as progesterone receptors, insulin-like growth factor I, retinaldehyde dehydrogenase type II, and secreted frizzled-related protein 4, seem to be promising to use as early-stage tumor markers. Mutation of *PTEN* is present in 83% of endometrial adenocarcinoma cases, making it the most frequent early molecular genetic alteration in type I endometrial tumors, which are generally associated with hyperplasia. *p53* gene mutation is not found in endometrial hyperplasia, but researchers have detected this mutation in 20% of cases of endometrial carcinoma and 90% of cases of serous endometrial tumors. Cyclooxygenase-2 is important in tumorigenic transformation of hyperplasia. Expression of cyclooxygenase-2 decreases apoptosis, increases angiogenesis, and is related to invasiveness. Cyclooxygenase-2 expression increases significantly in cases of well-differentiated endometrial adenocarcinoma.

Hepsin is a type II transmembrane serine protease originally identified in the human liver as a cDNA clone. Hepsin was found to be significantly overexpressed in cancer samples compared to matched various tissues such as prostate, renal, ovarian carcinoma. Matsuo *et al.*[39] have examined Hepsin expression and its clinicopathological significance in endometrial cancer. The authors have found that (1) Hepsin expression was significantly higher in endometrial cancer compared to normal endometrium and endometrial hyperplasia; (2) high levels of Hepsin expression were associated with advanced stage ($p < 0.001$), high grade ($p = 0.002$), depth of myometrial invasion ($p < 0.001$), cervical involvement ($p = 0.007$), lymph node metastasis ($p = 0.001$), lympho vascular space (LVS) involvement ($p = 0.006$), ovarian metastasis ($p = 0.002$), and peritoneal cytology ($p = 0.03$) of endometrial cancer. They have concluded that Hepsin protein expression could be an important indication for increased risk for endometrial cancer.

Antibodies to the factor HLDF[40] are shown to be specific markers of apoptosis and permit the estimation of the rate of programmed cell death in the course of a normal menstrual cycle and in pathologic endometrial processes. HLDF expression in the epitheliocytic cytoplasm makes it possible to evaluate apoptosis at early stages, before

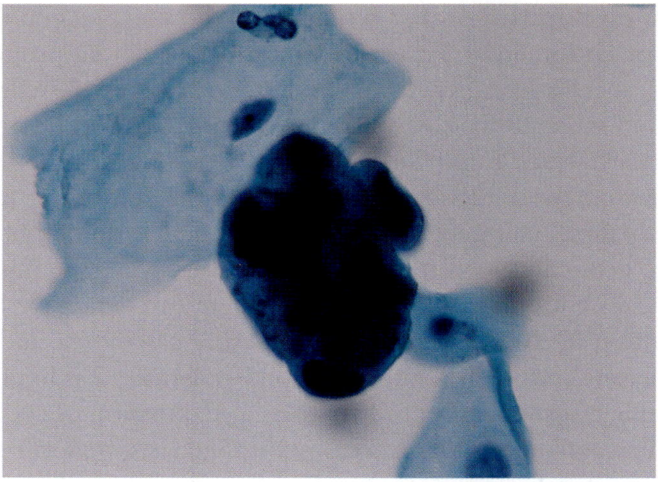

Fig. 11 This is a picture taken from the same patient as that in Fig. 10 with a exception that this slide was process by SurePath preparation. Comparing to the well preserved glandular pattern seen in ThinPrep slide, although the individual nuclear details are clearly visualized, the architecture or tumor seems to be disrupted. Pap stained SurPath slide, original magnification 100×.

the emergence of the first morphological signs and after apoptotic body formation. The study shows increased apoptotic processes at the end of a normal menstrual cycle and during neoplastic cell transformation. Antibodies to the HLDF factor may be used as a new immunohistochemical marker for the differential diagnosis of benign and malignant endometrial processes.

Using color texture analysis, Neofytou *et al.*[41] developed a system for the classification of hysteroscopy images of the endometrium for the early detection of gynecological cancer.

OVARIAN NEOPLASIA

Ovarian and Peritoneal Cytology

Ovarian cancer is the most lethal gynecological cancer. It can arise from any cell type of ovary, including surface epithelial cells, germ cells, granulosa or stromal cells. However, the majority of ovarian cancers arise from the surface epithelium, a single layer of cells that cover the surface of ovary. The lack of a reliable and specific method for the early detection of epithelial ovarian cancer results in diagnosis occurring most commonly at late clinical stages, when treatment is less effective.

Cytology can be used as a tool to detect ovarian cancer by analyzing or examining (1) ovarian cyst fluids via fine needle aspiration; (2) ascites fluid via paracentesis; (3) pre- and post-surgical peritoneal washings.

Benign ovarian cyst fluid generally has low cellularity. An ovarian cyst fluid specimen usually contains foamy macrophages, hemosiderin-laden macrophages in addition to its corresponding benign cyst lining cells such as

1. granulosa cells in follicular cyst;
2. luteinized granulosa cells in luteal cyst;
3. cuboidal or flat serous cells in serous cyst;
4. columnar or flat mucinous cells in mucinous cystadenoma;
5. endometrial cells in endometriosis;
6. squamous cells/anucleated squames in dermoid cyst or mature teratoma.

Malignant counterparts of ovarian cystic lesions would reveal cells with some cytoplasmic features of their benign counterparts but contain malignant nuclei and with high N/C ratios.

Borderline or atypical cystic lesions contain cells falling into the category in between benign and malignant types.

It is generally not too difficult to differentiate clearly benign from definitely malignant cells. It is the borderline or atypical cells that are often not only difficult to deal with both in cytology sign-out and clinical management, but also very important in early detection of ovarian cancers. This author would propose that efforts should be focused on finding molecular or genetic markers that may triage this morphologically difficult group in order to achieve the goal of early detection and early management of ovarian cancers.

Ascites fluid, especially large amount of bloody fluid, is often associated with ovarian malignancy, most frequently metastatic ovarian papillary serous carcinoma in elderly patients (Fig. 12). Serous papillary tissue fragments with borderline nuclear features can also be seen in ascites fluid when borderline papillary tumor involves the surface of the ovary. This kind of atypical cell groups can be confused with reactive/hyperplastic mesothelial cells. In such uncertain situation, immunocytochemical studies with markers such as calretinin, Ca 125, CEA, etc. may be helpful. Malignant acites is often cellular and the sample can be spun down to make cell block (Fig. 13) that can be used for immunocytochemical or molecular studies.

Peritoneal washings are generally associated with gynecological cancer/tumor surgery for the purpose of staging. While positivity for malignant cells is often consistent with metastatic carcinoma, mechanical

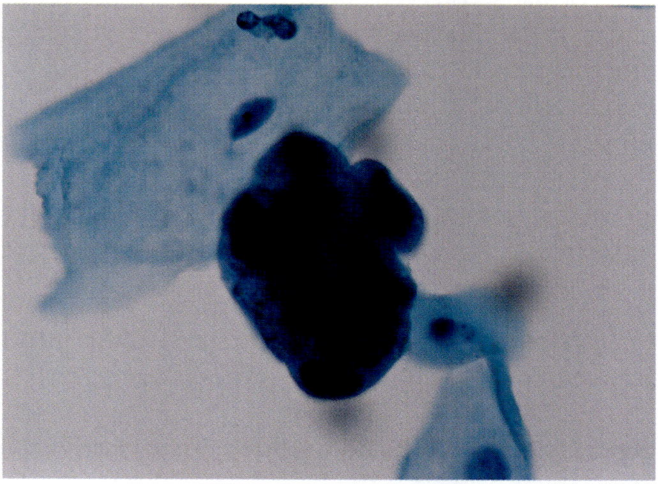

Fig. 12 A three-dimensional cluster of malignant cells with marked nuclear pleomorphism and clear cytoplasm. This is an example of metastatic ovarian serous papillary carcinoma to the peritoneal fluid. Pap stained ThinPrep slide, original magnification 100×.

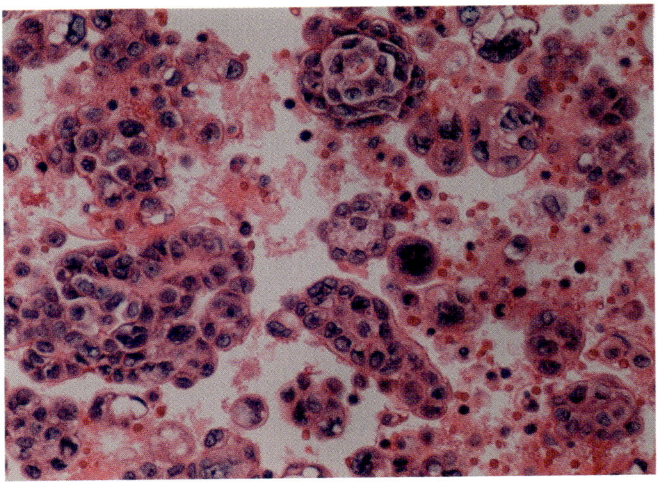

Fig. 13 A cell block slide showing numerous malignant cells that can be potentially used useful for immunocytochemical or malicular studes. Hematoxylin & Eosin stained cell bock slide, original magnification 40×.

seeding can also be seen in less advanced cases. Mechanical seeding refers to (1) rupture of an ovarian tumor (which should be avoided during surgery) and (2) transportation of endometrial tumor cells through the fallopian tubes. In these situations, it is recommended to the cytopathologist to correlate the case with the corresponding surgical pathology. For example, atypical cells in peritoneal washing seen in a patient with superficially invasive endometrial carcinoma as well as free floating tumor cells in the fallopian tube should not be signed out as positive; if an ovarian tumor was ruptured during surgery, cytopathologist should be informed or at least a note should be put on the requisition form. It is also important not to overtreat a patient since some side effects of chemotherapy and/or radiation can be devastating to the patient.

Although efforts have been made over the years in attempts for early detection of ovarian cancer, the results are disappointing so far. Annual surveillance, by trans-vaginal ultrasound scanning and serum Ca 125 measurements in women at increased familial risk of ovarian cancer was shown to be ineffective in detecting tumors at a sufficiently early stage to substantially influence survival in BRCA1/2 carriers.[42,43] While early detection of ovarian cancer continues to be a challenge, further understanding of the pathogenesis of ovarian tumors and maximizing advantages of cytopathology in combination with current molecular technologies may offer some hope for progress.

Updated Ovarian Carcinogenesis and Molecular Studies

Based on Kurman *et al.*[44] a new model of ovarian carcinogenesis based on clinical, pathological, and molecular genetic studies that may enable more targeted screening and therapeutic intervention should be developed in order to detect disease when confined to the ovary (stage I) and thereby prolong survival. The model divides ovarian cancer into types I and II.

Type I tumors are slow growing, generally confined to the ovary at diagnosis and develop from well-established precursor lesions, the so-called borderline tumors. Type I tumors include low-grade micropapillary serous carcinoma, mucinous, endometrioid, and clear cell carcinomas. They are genetically stable and are characterized by mutations in a number of different genes including *KRAS*, *BRAF*, *PTEN*, and *beta-catenin*.

Type II tumors are rapidly growing, highly aggressive neoplasms that lack well-defined precursor lesions; most are detected at an advanced stage at, or soon after, their inception. These include high-grade serous carcinoma, malignant mixed mesodermal tumors (carcinosarcomas), and undifferentiated carcinomas. The type II tumors are characterized by mutation of TP53 and a high level of genetic instability. Screening tests that focus on stage I disease may detect low-grade type Ineoplasms but miss the more aggressive type II tumors, which account for most ovarian carcinomas. Crum *et al.*[45] have studied the fallopian tubes and found a relatively high frequency of early cancer in the fimbria in unselected women with ovarian and peritoneal serous carcinoma, raising the distinct possibility that a significant proportion of these tumors have a fimbrial origin. This finding, if further verified, may alter our strategies in early detection and management of ovarian cancers.

A study[46] of microarray gene expression in serous epithelial ovarian cancer (SEOC) compared with bulk normal ovarian tissue and ovarian surface scrapings revealed that gene expression profiling and sequential statistical analysis of gene subsets can identify new genes and molecular pathways affecting the development of SEOC. The genes of interest are potential targets for future research of SEOC. According to a recent review by Nossov *et al.* proteomics may offer some hope in early detection of ovarian cancer.[47] MicroRNAs (miRNAs), an abundant class of small noncoding RNAs that function as negative gene regulators have also been studied in ovarian cancer.[48] The results indicated that miRNAs may offer new biomarkers and therapeutic targets in epithelial ovarian cancer. Autoantibody profile of ovarian cancer related genes (*TM4SF1*, *C1D*, *TIZ*, *BARD1*, *FXR1*, *OV-189*) may also potentially serve as markers in ovarian cancer detection.[49]

SUMMARY

Cytopathology screening programs have been serving well in early detection of gyneocological cancers, in perticular cervical squamous cell carcinoma. As the field progresses, the pathology and clinical teams have to realize that morphology alone is insufficient to detect gynecological cancers such as ovarian carcinomas in the early stages. Pathogenesis related factors such as HPV in cervical cancer, immunocytochemical studies of tumor markers, and molecular testing of genetic abnormalities will have to merge into the daily practice in addition to cytomorphology.

REFERENCES

1. Lee KR, Ashfaq R, Birdsong GG, *et al.*, Comparison of conventional Papanicolaou smears and a fluid-based, thin-layer system for cervical cancer screening, *Obstet Gynecol* **90**:278–284, 1997.
2. Sherman ME, Mendoza M, Lee KR, *et al.*, Performance of liquid-based, thin-layer cervical cytology: correlation with reference diagnoses and human papillomavirus testing, *Mod Pathol* **11**:837–843, 1998.

3. Bishop JW, Bigner SH, Colgan TJ, *et al.*, Multicenter masked evaluation of AutoCyte PREP thin layers with matched conventional smears, *Acta Cytol* **42**:189–197, 1998.
4. Cibas ES, Alonzo TA, Austin RM, *et al.*, The MonoPrep Pap test for the detection of cervical cancer and its precursors. Part I: results of a multicenter clinical trial, *Am J Clin Pathol* **129**:193–201, 2008.
5. Solomon *et al.*, The 2001 Bethesda system: terminology for Reporting Results of Cervical Cytology, *JAMA* **287**:2114–2119, 2002.
6. Iavazzo C, Vorgias G, Alexiadou A, *et al.*, The histological outcome of glandular dyskaryosis-AGUS — reported in Papanicolaou smears, *J BUON* **13**:97–100, 2008.
7. Muñoz N, Bosch FX, De Sanjosé S, *et al.*, Epidemiologic classification of human papillomavirus types associated with cervical cancer, *N Engl J Med* **348**:518–527, 2003.
8. Clifford GM, Smith JS, Aguado T, *et al.*, Comparison of HPV type distribution in high-grade cervical lesions and cervical cancer: a meta-analysis, *Br J Cancer* **89**:101–105, 2003.
9. Arbyn M, Buntinx F, van Ranst M, *et al.*, Virologic versus cytologic triage of women with equivocal pap smears: a meta-analysis of the accuracy to detect high-grade intraepithelial neoplasia, *J Natl Cancer Inst* **96**:280–293, 2004.
10. Cox JT, Human papilloma virus testing in primary cervical screening and abnormal Papanicolaou management, *Obstet Gynecol Surv* **61**: S15–S25, 2006.
11. Villa LL, Costa RL, Petta CA, *et al.*, Prophylactic quadrivalent human papillomavirus (types 6, 11, 16, and 18) L1 virus-like particle vaccine in young women: a randomised double-blind placebo-controlled multicentre phase II efficacy trial, *Lancet Oncol* **6**:271–278, 2005.
12. Paavonen J, Jenkins D, Bosch FX, *et al.*, HPV PATRICIA study group. Efficacy of a prophylactic adjuvanted bivalent L1 virus-like-particle vaccine against infection with human papillomavirus types 16 and 18 in young women: an interim analysis of a phase III double-blind, randomised controlled trial, *Lancet* **369**:2161–2170, 2007.
13. Pinto LA, Castle PE, Roden RB, *et al.*, HPV-16 VLP vaccine elicits a broadspectrum of cytokine responses in whole blood, *Vaccine* **23**:3555–3564, 2005.
14. Hendrix SL, Assessing human papillomavirus vaccine efficacy and safety, *J Am Osteopath Assoc* **108**:S8–S12, 2008.

15. Nieh S, Chen SF, Chu TY, *et al.*, Is p16(INK4A) expression more useful than human papillomavirus test to determine the outcome of atypical squamous cells of undetermined significance-categorized Pap smear? A comparative analysis using abnormal cervical smears with follow-up biopsies, *Gynecol Oncol* **97**:35–40, 2005.
16. Kalof AN, Evans MF, Simmons-Arnold L, *et al.*, p16INK4A immunoexpression and HPV *in situ* hybridization signal patterns: potential markers of high-grade cervical intraepithelial neoplasia, *Am J Surg Pathol* **29**:674–679, 2005.
17. Feng Q, Balasubramanian A, Hawes SE, *et al.*, Detection of hypermethylated genes in women with and without cervical neoplasia, *J Natl Cancer Inst* **97**:273–282, 2005.
18. Narayan G, Arias-Pulido H, Koul S, *et al.*, Frequent promoter methylation of CDH1, DAPK, RARB, and HIC1 genes in carcinoma of cervix uteri: its relationship to clinical outcome, *Mol Cancer* **2**:24, 2003.
19. Virmani AK, Muller C, Rathi A, *et al.*, Aberrant methylation during cervical carcinogenesis, *Clin Cancer Res* **7**:584–589, 2001.
20. Dong SM, Kim HS, Rha SH, *et al.*, Promoter hypermethylation of multiple genes in carcinoma of the uterine cervix, *Clin Cancer Res* **7**:1982–1986, 2001.
21. Zambrano P, Segura-Pacheco B, Pérez-Cárdenas E, *et al.*, A phase I study of hydralazine to demethylate and reactivate the expression of tumor suppressor genes, *BMC Cancer* **5**:44, 2005.
22. Stroun M, Anker P, Maurice P, *et al.*, Neoplastic characteristics of the DNA found in the plasma of cancer patients, *Oncology* **46**:318–322, 1989.
23. Widschwendter A, Muller HM, Fiegl H, *et al.*, DNA methylation in serum and tumors of cervical cancer patients, *Clin Cancer Res* **10**:565–571, 2004.
24. Widschwendter A, Ivarsson L, Blassnig A, *et al.*, CDH1 and CDH13 methylation in serum is an independent prognostic marker in cervical cancer patients, *Int J Cancer* **109**:163–166, 2004.
25. Yang HJ, Liu VW, Wang Y, *et al.*, Detection of hypermethylated genes in tumor and plasma of cervical cancer patients, *Gynecol Oncol* **93**:435–440, 2003.
26. Sorenson GD, Pribish DM, Valone FH, *et al.*, Soluble normal and mutated DNA sequences from single-copy genes in human blood, *Cancer Epidemiol Biomarkers Prev* **3**:67–71, 1994.

27. Vasioukhin V, Anker P, *et al.*, Point mutations of the N-ras gene in the blood plasma DNA of patients with myelodysplastic syndrome or acute myelogenous leukemia, *Br J Haematol* **86**:774–779, 1994.
28. Anker P, Stroun M, Progress in the knowledge of circulating nucleic acids: plasma RNA is particle-associated. Can it become a general detection marker for a cancer blood test? *Clin Chem* **48**:1210–1211, 2002.
29. Herman JG, Circulating methylated DNA, *Ann NY Acad Sci* **1022**:33–39, 2004.
30. Dulaimi E, Uzzo RG, Greenberg RE, *et al.*, Detection of bladder cancer in urine by a tumor suppressor gene hypermethylation panel, *Clin Cancer Res* **10**:1887–1893, 2004.
31. Wang YC, Lu YP, Tseng RC, *et al.*, Inactivation of hMLH1 and hMSH2 by promoter methylation in primary non-small cell lung tumors and matched sputum samples, *J Clin Invest* **111**:887–895, 2003.
32. Trejo-Becerril C, Pérez-Cárdenas E, Treviño-Cuevas H, *et al.*, Circulating nucleosomes and response to chemotherapy: an *in vitro*, *in vivo* and clinical study on cervical cancer patients, *Int J Cancer* **104**:663–668, 2003.
33. Yi X, Zheng W, Endometrial glandular dysplasia and endometrial intraepithelial neoplasia, *Curr Opin Obstet Gynecol* **20**:20–25, 2008.
34. Norimatsu Y, Miyamoto M, Kobayashi TK, *et al.*, Diagnostic utility of phosphatase and tensin homolog, beta-catenin, and p53 for endometrial carcinoma by thin-layer endometrial preparations, *Cancer* **114**: 155–164, 2008.
35. Chen J, Li S, Yang Z, Lu G, *et al.*, Correlation between NDRG1 and PTEN expression in endometrial carcinoma, *Cancer Sci* **99**:706–710, 2008.
36. Jia L, Liu Y, Yi X, *et al.*, Endometrial glandular dysplasia with frequent p53 gene mutation: a genetic evidence supporting its precancer nature for endometrial serous carcinoma, *Clin Cancer Res* **14**:2263–2269, 2008.
37. Zheng W, Yi X, Fadare O, The oncofetal protein IMP3: a novel biomarker for endometrial serous carcinoma, *Am J Surg Pathol* **32**:304–315, 2008.
38. Boruban MC, Altundag K, Kilic GS, *et al.*, From endometrial hyperplasia to endometrial cancer: insight into the biology and possible medical preventive measures, *Eur J Cancer Prev* **17**:133–138, 2008.
39. Matsuo T, Nakamura K, Takamoto N, *et al.*, Expression of the serine protease hepsin and clinical outcome of human endometrial cancer, *Anticancer Res* **28**:159–164, 2008.

40. Koviazin VA, Shchelokova EE, Kostanian IA, *et al.*, The proapoptotic factor HLDF in the normal, hyperplastic and neoplastic endometrium, *Arkh Pathol* **9**:23–26, 2007.
41. Neofytou MS, Tanos V, Pattichis MS, *et al.*, Color based texture — classification of hysteroscopy images of the endometrium, *EMBS 29th Annual International Conference of the IEEE Volume*, 864–867, 2007.
42. Woodward ER, Sleightholme HV, Considine AM, *et al.*, Annual surveillance by Ca 125 and transvaginal ultrasound for ovarian cancer in both high-risk and population risk women is ineffective, *BJOG* **114**:1500–1509, 2007.
43. Evans GR, Gaarenstroom KN, Stirling D, *et al.*, Screening for familial ovarian cancer: poor survival of BRCA1/2 related cancers, *J Med Genet* April 15, 2008 (in press).
44. Kurman RJ, Visvanathan K, Roden R, *et al.*, Early detection and treatment of ovarian cancer: shifting from early stage to minimal volume of disease based on a new model of carcinogenesis, *Am J Obstet Gynecol* **198**:351–356, 2008.
45. Crum CP, Drapkin R, Kindelberger D, *et al.*, Lessons from BRCA: the tubal fimbria emerges as an origin for pelvic serous cancer, *Clin Med Res* **5**:35–44, 2007.
46. Grisaru D, Hauspy J, Prasad M, *et al.*, Microarray expression identification of differentially expressed genes in serous epithelial ovarian cancer compared with bulk normal ovarian tissue and ovarian surface scrapings, *Oncol Rep* **18**:1347–1356, 2007.
47. Nossov V, Amneus M, Su F, *et al.*, The early detection of ovarian cancer: from traditional methods to proteomics. Can we really do better than serum Ca 125? *Am J Obstet Gynecol* May 9, 2008 (in press).
48. Zhang L, Volinia S, Bonome T, *et al.*, Genomic and epigenetic alterations deregulate microRNA expression in human epithelial ovarian cancer, *Proc Natl Acad Sci USA* **105**:7004–7009, 2008.
49. Yang ZJ, Yang G, Jiang YM, *et al.*, Screening and sero-immunoscreening of ovarian epithelial cancer associative antigen, *Zhonghua Fu Chan Ke Za Zhi* **42**:834–839, 2007.

CHAPTER 8

MOLECULAR AND BIOLOGICAL DIAGNOSIS OF EARLY GYNECOLOGIC CANCERS

Frederique Penault-Llorca

Recently, molecular diagnostic assays have been developed for gynecologic cancer, mostly for ovarian and uterine (cervix or endometrial) cancers. The markers are different for the two types of cancers. For ovarian cancer, the molecular diagnosis is serial and aimed to detect an early lesion of invasive cancer. For uterine cancer, the markers are mainly tissue based and tailored to predict the biological outcome of a preinvasive lesion.

OVARIAN CANCER

The development of useful markers for the detection of ovarian cancer is crucial because of the high mortality associated with the disease and the lack of reliable symptoms, biomarkers and mechanisms of early diagnosis. Effective early diagnosis could change the clinical spectrum of the disease and should have a direct impact on mortality.

There is no recognized model for ovarian cancer screening, nor any clinical test approved for early-stage diagnosis.[1]

To be useful in the clinical setting, a biomarker should be accurate for diagnosis, disease progression monitoring, disease recurrence prediction and treatment response monitoring. On a practical point of view, a biomarker should also be sufficiently non-invasive (i.e. performed on body fluid) and inexpensive to allow widespread applicability. Given that prevalence of ovarian cancer, strategies for early detection must have high sensitivity for early stage disease (> 75%), but must have extremely high specificity (99.6%) to attain a positive predictive value of at least 10%.[2] The current ovarian cancer biomarkers have high sensitivity for clinically diagnosed disease, but very few of them have high sensitivity for early stage disease.

Serum and Urine Biomarkers

Ca 125[3]

Ca 125 is the best performing single biological marker for ovarian cancer. Ca 125, a high molecular weight mucin (MUC 16), was first detected with a radioimmunoassay in patients with advanced ovarian cancer. It is approved only for the use of monitoring disease after treatment. Despite the fact that 80% of women with high stage disease have elevated Ca 125, Ca 125 is elevated in only 50%–60% of women with early stage disease. However, Ca 125 levels can be elevated 10–21 months prior to conventional diagnosis. Ca 125 is also elevated in numerous benign ovarian conditions (particularly in a premenopausal population with endometriosis, adenomyosis and retrograde menstruation) but not on every ovarian neoplasms, thus compromising its sensitivity and specificity. Greater specificity can be achieved by combining Ca 125 and transvaginal sonography (TVS) and/or by monitoring Ca 125 over time.

Ca 125 and Transvaginal Sonography (TVS)

Screening modalities evaluated to date have included TVS and the use of serum tumor marker Ca 125. Using a two-stage strategy, however, a combination of Ca 125 followed by sonography does attain specificity in excess of 99.6%. Specificity of Ca 125 could be further improved by following the trend of Ca 125 with an algorithm that estimates the risk of ovarian cancer.

An algorithm has been developed to calculate the risk of ovarian cancer based on serial Ca 125 values and refers patients at highest risks for TVS. Using this strategy, Jacobs *et al.*[2] randomized 21,962 postmenopausal women over 45 years of age in the UK to a control group or to a screened group. Ca 125 was measured annually for three years. An elevated Ca 125 level > 30 units/mL prompted that TVS and surgery was undertaken if the TVS demonstrated a pelvic mass. Among 10,985 women screened, in which 29 operations were performed to detect six cancers, providing a positive predictive value of 21%. Median survival in the screened group (72.9 months) was significantly greater ($p = 0.0112$) than that in the control group (41.8 months).

Use of the algorithm is currently being evaluated in a trial with 200,000 women in the UK (accrual has been completed) that will critically test the ability of a two-stage screening strategy to improve survival in ovarian cancer. Nevertheless, this approach is still far from perfect. Use of Ca 125 as an initial stage in a two-step screening strategy is limited by the fact that Ca 125 is expressed by only 80% of epithelial ovarian cancers. The sensitivity of such an approach is further reduced due to an inability of TVS to detect a mass that has yet to become appreciable.[4]

Ca 125 in Combination with Other Serum or Urine Markers[1,3,5]

Whatever the outcome, additional serum markers will be required to detect all patients in an initial phase of screening. More than 30 serum markers have been evaluated alone and in combination with Ca 125. Recent candidates include: HE4, mesothelin, M-CSF, osteopontin, kallikrein(s), lysophosphatidic acid (LPA) and soluble EGF receptor. In a study of 89 sera from patients with stage I ovarian cancer, use of three markers in combination (Ca 125, OVX1 and M-CSF) detected

84% of cancers, whereas Ca 125 alone detected 69%. Specificity, however, declined from 99% to 84% with the combination. Sensitivity has been improved by 5%–15%, but specificity has inevitably been reduced.

Mathematical Models

Artificial neural network (ANN) analysis, as a statistical modeling tool, has demonstrated the ability to assimilate information from multiple sources and detect subtle and complex patterns. An ANN-based composite diagnostic index using a panel of four serum markers, Ca 125II, Ca 72-4, Ca 15-3 and lipid-associated sialic acid (LASA), was evaluated for its ability to discriminate malignant from benign pelvic masses. Different sets of population (training and validation sets) i.e. healthy, with benign condition arising from the ovary and with ovarian cancers (including respectively 27 and 38 stage I cancer) malignant pelvic mass were evaluated from four institutions.[6]

ROC analysis confirmed the overall superiority of the ANN-derived composite index over Ca 125 alone ($p = 0.0333$). At a fixed specificity of 98%, the sensitivities for ANN and Ca 125 alone were 71% (37/52) and 46% (24/52) ($p = 0.047$) respectively, for detecting early stage epithelial ovarian cancer, was 71% (30/42) and 43% (18/42) ($p = 0.040$), respectively, for detecting invasive early stage epithelial ovarian cancer.

The combined use of multiple serum tumor markers through ANN improves both sensitivity and specificity for detection of stage I epithelial ovarian cancer. The development of technologies that measure multiple serum markers simultaneously, linked to the creation of statistical methods that enhance sensitivity without sacrificing specificity hold great promise. But none of the test so far is approved for clinical routine.

Genomic Approaches

Loss of Heterozygosity Analysis (LOH)

LOH analyses of solid tumors evaluate multiple regions of gene that are frequently deleted or lost in different types of ovarian tumors.

LOH studies in borderline ovarian tumors (BOT) have shown a LOH rate less than 25% at most of the loci when compared to invasive epithelial cancer (IEOC). However, BOTs demonstrate specific LOH (3p13–14.3 and Xq11.2–q12) suggesting that a large subset of BOTS may not progress to IEOC. LOH analyses has given interesting data for the understanding of ovarian carcinogenesis but is not useful in the clinical setting.

Comparative Genomic Hybridization Analysis (CGH)

This method involves competitive hybridization of tumor and normal reference DNA differentially labeled with distinct fluorescent molecules to normal human metaphase chromosome spreads. Based on the relative intensity of the two fluorescent colors, the region of the chromosome with gain or loss in gene copy number can be identified in a single hybridization. Differences have been shown between high and low stages, as well as BOT and IEOC. However, CGH has no interest in the clinical setting for the moment.

Transcription Profiling (cDNA Arrays)

Transcription or gene expression profiling is a large scale approach for analyzing gene expression data, which have been largely used to identify molecular signatures and to elucidate important aspects of epithelial ovarian cancer (EOC) in order to improve the clinical management of this disease.[7] Despite the high degree of morphological heterogeneity, epithelial ovarian cancer gene expression profiling reflects morphology and biological behaviour. Based on multiple studies, gene expression profiling results can be used to stratify the four different subtypes of EOC, namely serous papillary, mucinous, endometrioid, and clear cell carcinoma, but some overlapping gene expression was also noted. The prediction of the response to platinum-based chemotherapy has been also demonstrated but is not reproducible among different platforms.[8]

Several novel candidate markers for the early detection of EOC have been identified by gene expression profiling and examples that have been validated by ELISA on the protein level in serum from EOC patients and healthy controls. Using gene ontology, genes involved in cell cycle regulation, in the extracellular matrix, and in immunological responses have been identified. They are relevant to epithelial ovarian cancer biology and particular genes potentially can serve as therapeutic targets for small molecules, biologically, and immunologically. Gene ontology studies have permitted the creation of gene signatures. Therefore, a limitation of DNA arrays is that transcriptional difference in the tumor does not completely reflect the protein observed peripherally, since many protein–protein interactions and post-translational modifications may change the protein patterns found in the blood.

This area is still entirely in the domain of research. In fact, cross validation among different platforms and prospective validation in multi-center trials are necessary before microarray technology can move to clinical practice. The potential implications of the results for the clinical management of EOC are enormous.

Proteomics

Proteomics is the study of information flow within the cell and the organism through protein pathways and networks of cellular protein interactions of normal and disease state. Proteomic approaches have been used to define a distinctive pattern of peaks on mass spectroscopy or to identify a limited number of critical markers that can be assayed by more conventional.

Methods

Mass spectrometry allows a high-throughput study such as proteomic analysis of serum or microdissected cells. Matrix assisted laser desorption and ionization (MALDI) with time-of-flight (TOF) detection (MALDI-TOF) and surface-enhanced laser desorption and ionization (SELDI-TOF) are two methods of mass spectrometry currently used in proteomics. In the MALDI technique, the protein samples of interest are immobilized in an energy-absorbing chemical matrix on a chip or a plate and the entire proteome within the range detectable by mass spectrometry undergoes analysis. SELDI is a refinement of MALDI. A selective surface is used to bind a subset of those proteins based on different properties. Both SELDI and MALDI use laser energy to ionize and launch bound peptides (desorption) across a vacuum tube to detector plate. Time of flight is dependent on the mass-to-charge ratio of the peptide (m/z) and the data are recorded as m/z peaks of relative intensities.

As the profile generated by SELDI has generally up to a million data points, bioinformatics algorithms have been developed to recognize important protein patterns.[10,11] Recently, Lopez *et al.*[12] have identified 162 proteins from peptides and protein fragments bound to carrier proteins from the serum samples of ovarian cancer patient. Within this study, three sets of the discriminating carrier-protein bound fragments differentiated samples from patients with ovarian cancer (453) and apparently healthy controls (110) with sensitivities and specificities of up to 93% and 97%, respectively. The proteins are involved in cellular inflammation, differentiation, signaling, apoptosis, transcriptional regulation, and other regulatory mechanisms.

The power of this approach is 4-fold: (a) it is unbiased and does not presuppose any particular disease mechanism, (b) multiple differences — multiple putative disease markers, are often discovered and combinations of markers are likely to be more powerful discriminators than single markers, (c) large numbers of samples (usually blood sera) from appropriate cohorts can be analyzed quickly for discovery and subsequent validation of putative marker sets, and (d) the method does not require *a priori* antibody development for success.

Mass spectrometry has, however, generated controversy centered primarily on two issues: the relative importance of obtaining definitive sequence identification for differentiating masses and the likelihood that peptides or protein fragments, as opposed to intact proteins, can be useful as disease biomarkers.[13] The clinical relevance of the serum peptidome has been vigorously debated. The protein signal peaks used to distinguish between normal and disease have not all been identified. But recent publications have confirmed that specific protein fragments are correlated with disease stages.[14]

A major area of controversy has been the lack of data consistency and reproducibility across the various published studies, although with proper attention to stringent experimental design and protocols, these issues can be addressed in future studies.[15]

Conclusions

Candidate biomarkers for early ovarian cancer have been discovered through empirical development of monoclonal antibodies, studies of gene expression, cloning of gene families and proteomic techniques. Given the heterogeneity of ovarian cancer, it is unlikely that any single marker will be sufficiently sensitive to provide an effective initial screen. Sensitivity of serum assays might be enhanced by utilizing a panel of biomarkers. With the exception of Ca 125, all the assays developed in this chapter need different steps of validation. In the future, the development of clinical trials in proteomics will allow personalized medicine for IEOC. Regular serum screening tests will diagnose cancer long before it is evident clinically, perhaps even before it can be detected radiographically.

CERVICAL CANCER

Human papillomavirus (HPV) is the major cause of cervical cancer, and in the natural history of the disease, persistent HPV infection precedes the appearance of cytological abnormality. Episomal state: briefly, after infecting the host, the virus may exist as an inactive extrachromosomal particle (episome) that is detectable only by DNA testing (latency). This type of infection (subclinical, DNA-only) is extremely common, occurring in up to 50% of sexually active young women. It generally occurs in cells where there is no cytological evidence of disease (normal cytology); 99% of sub-clinical infections are cleared by the body's natural immune process. The virus can become active, viral DNA is transcribed, and viral particles are assembled. The virus begins to replicate independent in the host cell (active infection). This type of infection results in a clinically detectable lesions including abnormal Pap smear, genital wart. Immune response begins on average within three months of productive viral infection. In the rare occurrence that immune response is suppressed, progression to high-grade disease may occur.

When integration occurs, the viral DNA transforms the host DNA. Cofactors, high-risk HPV types, and co-mutagens appear to be necessary for this to occur. The circular HPV episome must break into a linear strand prior to integration into host DNA. This break often occurs at a region of HPV DNA that produces a regulatory product: E2. The E2 product normally serves to control cell-proliferation-inducing genes E6 and E7. In the absence of E2, cell growth is out of control resulting in neoplasm. Only 10%–20% of HPV-infected cases are at risk for progression to neoplasia. These patients will have either a persistent HPV infection or they will have a recurrent infection after a lesion free interval (see Chapters 2, 3 and 7).

New Markers in Cervical Cancer Screening

The study of cervical carcinogenesis has yielded a series of biomarkers that potentially could be used as surrogates for the identification of HPV-related disease of epithelial cells.

These biomarkers are promising for the surveillance of patients with confirmed dysplasia and the need for either continued surveillance after preventive or therapeutic management, or surgery.[16]

HPV Testing

Available assays — molecular methods

Hybrid Capture

HPV testing by Digene Hybrid Capture II (HCII) — The HCII HPV DNA test (Digene Corporation, USA), is the only Food and Drug Administration (FDA) approved test for detecting 13 high-risk HPV. It is widely used to triage patients diagnosed with ASC-US (atypical squamous cells of undetermined significance). The high sensitivity of the HCII assay allows it to be used to triage patients with ASC-US and a negative HCII result into routine yearly screening. However, one limitation of HCII is that it can be performed only on liquid-based cervical cytology samples. Other limitations of this test are that (i) it does not preserve cellular morphology, (ii) analytical sensitivity is 10,000 viral copies/mL (1.0 pg/mL), (iii) cross-reactivity between low and high risk types = 11.7%–22%, (iv) "Blind" Test — result measured by a luminometer. However, there is no ability to confirm whether patient or partner DNA, no ability to confirm that the HPV is responsible for cellular change and, no internal negative patient control.

Tissue Based Assays: *In situ* Hybridization Kits

The commercially available methods for detecting high-risk HPV in paraffin-embedded tissue consist of *in situ* hybridization (ISH). Two ISH kits are developed for research use: the DakoCytomation ISH high-risk probe (Glostrup, Denmark) (the probe consisted of a cocktail directed against high-risk HPV types 16, 18, 31, 33, 35, 39, 45, 52, 56, 58, 59, and 68), and the Ventana INFORM HPV ISH assay (Tucson, Arizona) which uses a nonamplified high-risk HPV probe consisting of a cocktail directed against six HPV types 16, 18, 31, 33, 35, 51 (cross reacting with other high risk HPV 39, 45, 52, 56, 58, and 66, but not with low risk HPV, and a low risk HPV ISH assay (HPV types 6 and 11). ISH assays allow the detection of HPV DNA in tissue and liquid-based cytology samples. Sensitivity is 10–50 copies of target DNA per nucleus. The type of signal (confluent, punctate) may reflect either episomal or integrated form of viral target DNA. The main advantage is the ability to correlate DNA probe results with morphology. The clinical utility is hampered by the manual, labor-intensive nature of the procedure, but the assays have been recently automated by Ventana Medical Systems, Inc.

Surrogate Markers

Proliferation Biomarkers Such as INK4A or p16[17]

The E6 and E7 oncoproteins from high-risk HPV types cause chromosomal abnormalities and genomic instability. In addition, the *E6* gene product mediates degeneration of the p53 tumor suppressor protein, and the *E7* gene product binds to and inactivates the retinoblastoma protein, which results in increased production of the *CDNK2A* gene product, $p16^{Ink4a}$. $p16^{Ink4a}$, a tumor suppressor protein that inhibits cyclin dependent kinases involved in cell cycle control, has been shown to be overexpressed in high-grade dysplasias and cervical carcinomas. In recent years, $p16^{Ink4a}$ has been extensively investigated as a diagnostic aid in various scenarios in gynecologic pathology. Like with all markers, in each of these scenarios, $p16^{Ink4a}$ is neither 100% specific nor sensitive for a given lesion.

Positive $p16^{Ink4a}$ staining can be useful to differentiate between atypical immature squamous metaplasia without CIN and some cases of immature metaplastic squamous epithelium with associated CIN. Low-grade CIN exhibiting $p16^{Ink4a}$ positivity is more likely to progress to high-grade CIN than are $p16^{Ink4a}$ negative lesions. It is possible that $p16^{Ink4a}$ could be used to triage cases of low-grade CIN, which are associated with high-risk HPV and more careful follow up is required. $p16^{Ink4a}$ is expressed in a high percentage of high-grade CIN and expression within the upper two-thirds of the squamous epithelium is a significant indicator of the presence of a high-grade dysplastic lesion. There is poor interobserver reproducibility in the histologic diagnosis of CIN; $p16^{Ink4a}$ immunostaining has been shown to reduce interobserver variability in cervical biopsy specimen interpretation, especially aiding in the identification of small focal areas of high-grade CIN. $p16^{Ink4a}$ is also a value in distinguishing high-grade CIN from mimics such as atrophic squamous epithelium, immature squamous metaplasia, and transitional metaplasia. $p16^{Ink4a}$ may be combined with the proliferation marker MIB1/Ki67. Not surprisingly, most cervical squamous carcinomas also stained with p16, because they contain high-risk HPV. Normal endocervical glands are usually $p16^{Ink4a}$ negative with an occasional case exhibiting focal weak positivity. In contrast, most preneoplastic and neoplastic endocervical glandular lesions, as a result of their association with high-risk HPV, exhibit diffuse $p16^{Ink4a}$ positivity. However, a small number of cervical adenocarcinomas are $p16^{Ink4a}$ negative because they are not associated with high-risk HPV, the relationship between these HPV types and tumor not being as strong for cervical adenocarcinomas as for squamous cell carcinomas.

When compared to molecular tests HCII is considered as a more sensitive test than $p16^{Ink4a}$ for detection of abnormal cytology. HCII has a higher positive predictive value than $p16^{Ink4a}$ for identifying CIN 2/3.[18]

Testing Strategies[19,20]

Testing for carcinogenic HPV was recently introduced into cervical cancer screening. HPV testing has proven to have greater sensitivity than cytologic screening (Papanicolaou smears) for detection of cervical precancer (cervical intraepithelial neoplasia grade 3 (CIN 3) and cervical cancer) and greater reliability.[21,22] HPV testing is now commonly used in the US to triage equivocal cytologic findings for colposcopic referral. Co-testing with HPV and cytology is also approved for routine cervical cancer screening of women aged 30 years or above. Women aged 30 years or older who tested with HPV- and cytology-negative are at extremely low risk for incipient precancer and cancer for over the periods of ten years or more. Therefore, screening intervals in these women can be extended to three years in the US to make co-testing cost-effective.

HPV Persistence

What is the meaning of a Polymerase Chain Reaction (PCR) positive test without cytologic or histologic abnormalities? Does this molecular detection represent an overdiagnosis or does it offer protection against future high-grade cervical epithelial neoplasia or cervical cancer?[16,23]

HPV infection is transient by nature. In a three-years study at a University Health Center: 60% of women tested positive for HPV by PCR. Only 4%–6% had cytologic changes suggestive of HPV infection. After eight months, half had regressed. After 12 months, 70% had regressed. After 24 months, 91% had regressed. The meta-analysis by Koshiol *et al.*[22] reviewed 41 studies on over 22,500 women and this is the first systematic evaluation of the association between HPV persistence and cervical neoplasia. This review confirmed that repeated HPV detection does indicate an increased risk for invasive cervical cancer and its precursors, despite differences in HPV persistence definitions, HPV detection techniques and testing intervals, and other study characteristics. Women who have carcinogenic HPV infection that persists for at least 1 year are at a significantly elevated risk for cervical cancer. HPV persistence was strongly and consistently associated with CIN 2–3/HSIL+. The strength of the association between HPV persistence and cervical neoplasia increased with increasing grade of severity of the cervical disease. This emphasizes the value of HPV persistence as a clinical marker and as an endpoint in clinical trials and suggesting that sequential HPV DNA testing may be useful for cervical cancer screening programs by identifying women who are at high risk for cervical cancer. The FDA approved test "hybrid capture 2 assay" uses all carcinogenic assays as a pool and is probably more sensitive than the HPV genotyping assays based on PCR identifying separated HPV conserved regions. It would be useful to know how the risk for persistent HPV 16 or 18 is different from that of other HPV genotypes. Also, are the results of large studies in favour of HPV testing applicable to liquid-based cytologic testing? Based on the potential for improved sensitivity for liquid-based testing, the gain in specificity for HPV DNA testing may be reduced.

Could HPV Testing Replace PAP Test?

The International Agency Research on Cancer recently published a report based on expert meeting concluding that HPV testing is an acceptable alternative to Pap smears for cervical cancer screening.[24] However, despite its greater sensitivity and overall accuracy, the enthusiasm for using HPV testing in primary screening has been tempered by its somewhat poorer positive predictive value in comparison with cytologic analysis (e.g. 7.0% for HPV testing *vs.* 8.7% for Pap smears, using a threshold of atypical squamous cells of undetermined significance or worse).

What is the Indication of ISH?

ISH techniques allow the detection of integrated versus episomal DNA, which can add an important information concerning the potential of progression of the lesion. This assay should be used to confirm a positive PCR test.

ENDOMETRIAL CANCER

Endometrial carcinoma is one of the most common malignancies of the female genital tract. There are two main clinicopathologic variants of endometrial carcinoma. Type I tumors are usually estrogen-related. In general, they develop in pre- and peri-menopausal women, and co-exist with or are preceded by endometrial hyperplasia. By contrast, type II carcinomas are unrelated to estrogen, are associated with atrophic endometrium, and usually occur at an older age and their precursor is serous intraepithelial carcinoma (SEIC).

Five main molecular genetic alterations have been described in type I endometrial carcinomas (ECI), including microsatellite instability (MI) and mutations of *PTEN, PIK3CA, k-RAS*, and *β-catenin* genes. For type II EC the main genetic alteration is *p53* mutation. These molecular alterations have also been described in atypical endometrial hyperplasia and SEIC.[25]

PTEN[26]

Currently, the most frequently altered gene in ECI is PTEN (phosphatase and tensin homologue). PTEN is a tumor suppressor gene located on 10q23. PTEN plays a significant role not only in inducing cell cycle arrest and programming apoptosis, but also in other aspects of cell physiology, including the regulation of cell adhesion, migration, and differentiation. In most cases, the underlying genetic alteration in cases with lost PTEN expression and function is mutation and, less frequently, LOH without mutation or promoter methylation. Germline mutations in PTEN occur in 85% of patients with Cowden syndrome, an inherited condition associated with increased risk for endometrial carcinoma. Somatic mutations have been reported in approximately 50% of patients with type I endometrial carcinoma and with atypical glandular hyperplasia.

The earliest molecular changes in endometrial ECI carcinogenesis, including PTEN are detected in up to 25%–83% of ECI (50% for PTEN), characterized by loss of expression.[27] Loss of PTEN expression (i.e. PTEN negative glands) tends to be diffuse in endometrial carcinoma but also occurs in morphologically normal endometrial tissue, which suggests that PTEN abnormalities may occur early in sporadic endometrial carcinomas.

The hypothesis that PTEN loss is a biomarker for premalignant clones capable of progressing from hyperplasia to carcinoma came up primarily from the observation that PTEN-loss or PTEN mutations was found in patients with endometrial hyperplasia with increasing degree of histologic severity.[27] In a series of 103 patients with endometrial hyperplasia (EH) who were followed for an average of four years, Baak and colleagues reported that all seven patients who subsequently developed endometrial carcinoma had PTEN-negative hyperplasia. None of the patients with PTEN-normal EH progressed to carcinoma, but only 16% of the 43 PTEN-negative patients progressed.[27]

To assess whether PTEN status could be a helpful tool as a marker of progression to endometrial carcinoma, in endometrial biopsies, additional data were necessary (larger studies with a representative control group). A recent study by Lacey JV *et al.*[29] has shown that loss of PTEN expression in endometrial biopsies was neither associated with nor a sensitive and specific marker of subsequent progression to endometrioid carcinoma. This controlled study evaluated in parallel 138 patients diagnosed with endometrial hyperplasia who develop ECI at least one year later (median, 6 years), and 241 individually matched patients diagnosed with endometrial hyperplasia but who did not progress to ECI during the same follow up.

Conclusion

It seems therefore that PTEN expression in endometrial biopsies is unlikely to be useful in the prediction of progression to endometrial carcinoma. Interestingly, conserved PTEN mutations in matched hyperplasia and carcinoma specimens in some women indicates that PTEN alterations can occur early in and persist during endometrial carcinogenesis. This suggests that PTEN may have other roles in endometrial carcinoma besides influencing which endometrial hyperplasia lesions progress to ECI.

REFERENCES

1. Gagnon A, Bin Y, Discovery and application of protein biomarkers for ovarian cancer, *Curr Opin Obstet Gynecol* **20**:9–13, 2008.
2. Jacobs IJ, Oram DH, Bast RC Jr., Strategies for improving the specificity of screening for ovarian cancer with tumor associated antigens Ca 125, Ca 15-3, and TAG 7263, *Obstet Gynecol* **80**:396–399, 1992.
3. Bast RC Jr., Badgwell D, Lu Z, *et al.*, New tumor markers: Ca 125 and beyond, *Int J Gynecol Cancer* **15**:274–281, 2005.
4. Rosenthal AN, Menon U, Jacobs IJ, Screening for ovarian cancer, *Clin Obstet Gynecol* **49**:433–447, 2006.
5. Tchabo NE, Liel MS, Kohn EC, Applying proteomics in clinical trials: assessing the potential and practical limitations in ovarian cancer, *Am J Pharmacogenomics* **5**:141–148, 2005.
6. Zhang Z, Yu Y, Xu F, *et al.*, Combining multiple serum tumor markers improves detection of stage I epithelial ovarian cancer, *Gynecol Oncol* **107**:526–531, 2007.
7. Mok SC, Elias KM, Wong KK *et al.*, Biomarker discovery in epithelial ovarian cancer by genomic approaches, *Adv Cancer Res* **96**:1–22, 2007.
8. Gevaert O, De Smet F, Van Gorp T, *et al.*, Expression profiling to predict the clinical behaviour of ovarian cancer fails evaluation, *BMC Cancer* **8**:18, 2008.
9. Baggerly KA, Coombes KR, Neeley ES, Run batch effects potentially compromise the usefulness of genomic signatures for ovarian cancer, *J Clin Oncol* **26**:1186–1187, 2008.
10. Petricoin EF, Ardekani AM, Hitt BA, *et al.*, Use of proteomic patterns in serum to identify ovarian cancer, *Lancet* **359**:572–577, 2002.
11. Zhang Z, Bast RC, Jr., Yu Y, *et al.,* Three biomarkers identified from serum proteomic analysis for the detection of early stage ovarian cancer, *Cancer Res* **64**:5882–5890, 2004.
12. Lopez MF, Mikulskis A, Kuzdzal S, *et al.,* A novel, high-throughput workflow for discovery and identification of serum carrier protein-bound

peptide biomarker candidates in ovarian cancer samples, *Clin Chem* **53**:1067–1074, 2007.
13. Baggerly KA, Morris JS, Edmonson SR, *et al.*, Signal in noise: evaluating reported reproducibility of serum proteomic tests for ovarian cancer, *J Natl Cancer Inst* **97**:307–309, 2005.
14. Liotta LA, Petricoin EF, Serum peptidome for cancer detection: spinning biologic trash into diagnostic gold, *J Clin Invest* **116**:26–30, 2006.
15. Diamandis EP, Peptidomics for cancer diagnosis: present and future, *J Proteome Res* **9**:2079–2082, 2006.
16. Castle PE, Invited commentary: is monitoring of human papillomavirus infection for viral persistence ready for use in cervical cancer screening? *Am J Epidemiol* **168**:138–144, 2008.
17. O'Neill CJ, McCluggage WG, p16 expression in the female genital tract and its value in diagnosis, *Adv Anat Pathol* **13**:8–15, 2006.
18. Nassar A, O'Reilly K, Cohen C, *et al.*, Comparison of $p16^{Ink4a}$ and Hybrid Capture 2 human papillomavirus testing as adjunctive tests in liquid-based gynecologic SurePath preparations, *Diagn Cytopathol* **36**:142–148, 2008.
19. Nijhuis ER, Reesink-Peters N, Wisman GB, *et al.*, An overview of innovative techniques to improve cervical cancer screening, *Cell Oncol* **28**:233–246, 2006.
20. Padilla-Paz LA, Emerging technology in cervical cancer screening: status of molecular markers, *Clin Obstet Gynecol* **48**:218–225, 2005.
21. Mayrand MH, Duarte-Franco E, Rodrigues I, *et al.*, Canadian Cervical Cancer Screening Trial Study Group, Human papillomavirus DNA versus Papanicolaou screening tests for cervical cancer, *N Engl J Med* **357**:1579–1588, 2007.
22. Koshiol J, Lindsay L, Pimenta JM, *et al.*, Persistent human papillomavirus infection and cervical neoplasia: a systematic review and meta-analysis, *Am J Epidemiol* **168**:123–137, 2008.
23. Naucler P, Ryd W, Törnberg S, *et al.*, Human papillomavirus and Papanicolaou tests to screen for cervical cancer, *N Engl J Med* **357**:1589–1597, 2007.
24. International Agency for Research on Cancer. Cervix cancer screening, *IARC Handbooks of Cancer Prevention*, Vol 10, IARC Press, Lyon, France, 2005.
25. Silverberg *et al.* (2003). Endometrial cancer in OMS classification of breast and gynecological cancers, IARC, Lyon.

26. Sansal I, Sellers WR, The biology and clinical relevance of the PTEN tumor suppressor pathway, *J Clin Oncol* **22**:2954–2963, 2004.
27. Mutter GL, Lin MC, Fitzgerald JT, *et al.*, Altered PTEN expression as a diagnostic marker for the earliest endometrial precancers, *J Natl Cancer Inst* **92**:924–930, 2000.
28. Baak JP, Van Diermen B, Steinbakk A, *et al.*, Lack of PTEN expression in endometrial intraepithelial neoplasia is correlated with cancer progression, *Hum Pathol* **36**:555–561, 2005.
29. Lacey JV Jr., Mutter GL, Ronnett BM, *et al.*, PTEN expression in endometrial biopsies as a marker of progression to endometrial carcinoma, *Cancer Res* **68**:6014–6020, 2008.

INDEX

2006 consensus guidelines, 249
3 catenins, 170
3p13–14.3, 271
5-fluorouracil, 130, 131

acetowhite, 53, 60, 117
adenocarcinoma, 24, 86, 116, 119–124, 126–129, 132, 133, 140, 144, 233, 243, 246, 277
adenocarcinoma *in situ*, 74, 116, 124–129
mucinous differentiation, 74, 89
adenoid-basal carcinoma, 92
adenoid cystic carcinoma, 92
adenoma malignum, 90
adenomatous hyperplasia, 152
adenomyosis, 162, 165, 268
adenosarcoma, 57, 101
adenosquamous, 120
adenosquamous carcinoma, 86, 91
adjacent dysplasia, 179, 182
adolescent, 115, 116, 123, 124, 131
age, 200, 201, 203, 208, 212–216, 218, 224
aggressive angiomyxoma, 32–34
algorithm, 269
anal intraepithelial neoplasia (AIN), 11
anatomy, 2, 48
androgenic hormone, 151
aneuploidy, 212
angiomyofibroblastoma, 32, 34
anovulatory cycle, 151
antibodies to the HLDF factor, 255, 256
antiestrogenic effect, 161

apoptosis, 273, 280
architectural, 180–182
Arias-Stella, 77–99, 105
artificial neural network (ANN), 270
Ascites fluid, 258
Ashkenazi Jewish women, 184
asymptomatic precursor, 183
atrophic endometrium, 280
atrophy, 71, 102
atypical
  cell, 231
  borderline cystic lesion, 257
  endometrioid epithelium, 190
  glandular cell, 116, 123–129
  hyperplasia, 152, 154, 155, 171
  mitotic figure, 69
  squamous cell, 245
atypical glandular cell of undetermined significance (AGUS), 241
atypical squamous cell – cannot exclude HSIL, 116, 122, 123
atypical squamous cell of undetermined significance (ASCUS), 116, 117, 119, 122, 123, 124, 127, 241, 275
autoantibody profile, 261
autocorrelation procedure, 184
autosomal dominant fashion, 177

Barber, Hugh R. K., 203
Bartholin, 139, 140
Bartholin gland carcinoma, 28
basal cell carcinoma, 20
basaloid, 13, 14, 20
batch test, 249
Bax, 190, 192
BCL-2, 170
benign cell, 230
benign ovarian cyst, 257
beta-catenin, 254, 260
  gene, 280
Bethesda System, 244
biomarker, 268
biomolecular marker, 251
biopsy, 117, 121–123, 125–128, 130–132, 135, 136, 139, 141–144, 202, 209, 214, 216–224
bleeding, 120, 129, 131, 133, 139, 205, 206, 209, 213, 214, 216–219, 221, 224
borderline ovarian tumor (BOT), 194, 195, 271
bowenoid, 134, 137, 139
bowenoid papulosis, 11
Bowen's disease, 134
BRAF, 260
BRCA1, 2, 176, 177, 183, 192, 199–201, 209, 211
BRCA1/2 carrier, 260
breast cancer, 176, 177, 179, 183, 193, 195, 199, 201, 206, 209, 211–213
brush, 126

Ca, 125, 186, 188, 192, 193, 205–210, 258, 268
Ca, 125II, 270
Ca, 15-3, 270
Ca, 72-4, 270
calretinin, 258

carcinogenetic mechanism, 192
carcinoid tumor, 92
carcinoma *in situ*, 66
carcinoma of the vagina, 97
carcinomas of squamous and glandular types of the cervix, 242
carcinosarcoma, 260
CDH13, 252
CDNK2A gene product, 277
CEA, 258
cell adhesion, 280
cell cycle
    arrest, 280
    regulation, 272
cellular, 180, 182
CerVax 16, 250
cervical, 115–122, 124–132, 135, 137, 139
    biopsy, 54
    dysplasia, 178
    squamous carcinoma, 277
cervical cancer, 234
    epidemiology, 66, 72, 86
    grading, 86, 91
    keratinizing, 83
    microinvasion, 82, 97, 103
    non-keratinizing, 83
    papillary, 85
    risk factor, 53, 67, 73
    screening, 278
    sentinel lymph node, 95
    serous carcinoma, 89
    staging, 93, 94, 98
    survival rate, 93
    verrucous, 85
cervical intraepithelial neoplasia (CIN), 66, 68, 116, 117, 119, 120, 122–125, 128–131, 135, 139, 277
    CIN 1, 2, 117, 119, 122–125
    CIN 2/3, 278
    CIN 3, 278
chemotherapy, 53, 67, 175, 195
choriocarcinoma, 106
Chung classification, 101
ciliated, 166, 167
circulating nucleic acid, 253
clear cell carcinoma, 59, 62, 78, 90, 97, 105, 166, 167, 169, 189, 190, 192, 194, 260, 271
clinical, 120, 121, 126–128, 135, 139, 140, 142
    information, 4, 58
cloning of gene families, 274
clustering, 185
colon, 200, 207, 213–218
colorectal, 200, 206, 213–218
color texture analysis, 256
colposcopy, 116, 117, 119, 121, 123–127, 129, 130, 132, 133, 135, 137–139
comparative genomic hybridization analysis (CGH), 271
comparison test, 236
competitive hybridization, 271
complex glandular hyperplasia, 150, 152–155
computed tomography, 211
condyloma, 59, 61, 116, 134, 135, 137, 139, 141
    acuminatum, 10, 12, 60, 108
    planum, 60

condylomatous, 85
cone, 116, 123, 125, 127, 129
biopsy, 55
conization, 116, 121, 125, 128, 129
continuous unopposed, 150, 152
contraindication, 221
Cowden syndrome, 280
cyclin dependent kinase, 277
cyclooxygenase-2, 255
cyst, 206–210
cytobrush, 117, 118, 128
cytology, 115–133, 137, 141
cytopathic effect, 240
cytoreductive surgery, 175

DAPK1, 252
decidualization, 84, 85
deep invagination, 184, 185
dendritic cell, 19
dermatofibrosarcoma protuberans, 32
desorption, 273
diagnosis, 115, 121, 125, 127, 130, 133–136, 138, 139, 142, 268
diethylstilbestrol (DES), 61, 97, 130, 133
differentiated, 132, 134, 135, 137–139, 143, 144, 273
dilatation and curettage, 209, 217–219, 223
discharge, 120, 130, 132, 139
disease biomarker, 273
distension, 203
DNA array, 271, 272
dyspepsia, 203–205
dysplasia, 66, 120, 127, 130, 202, 210, 211
dystrophy, 139

early detection, 201, 202, 205, 211
early lesion of invasive cancer, 267
early onset, 176, 177
early-stage tumor marker, 255
ectopic breast tissue, 3
ectopic prostatic tissue, 106
ectopy, 50
ectropion, 50, 61
efficacy, 250
ELISA, 272
embryonal rhabdomyosarcoma, 31, 57, 99
EMLA cream, 142
endocervical, 116, 118, 119, 121, 123, 125–129
adenocarcinoma *in situ* (AIS), 72, 73, 102, 103, 242, 246
cell, 237
curettage, 54, 121, 123–129
glandular lesion, 277
neoplasia, 242
endogenous hyperestrogenic stimulation, 151
endometrial
carcinogenesis, 254
cytology, 253
glandular dysplasia, 254
hyperplasia, 189, 193, 195, 281

intraepithelial carcinoma, 150, 157–160, 162, 167, 171
intraepithelial neoplasia, 254
polyp, 189
serous adenocarcinoma, 157
stromal, 59
stromal sarcoma, 59
endometrial atypical glandular, 154, 156
biopsy, 151, 156, 167
cancer, 149–151, 155, 157, 160–163, 170, 171
hyperplasia, 150–157, 160, 163, 165, 167, 170, 171
neoplasia, 149–151, 155, 160
polyp, 152, 157, 161–163, 165, 167, 168, 171
endometrial carcinoma (EC), 150, 155, 157, 160–165, 167, 168, 170, 171, 189, 190, 280
early, 162
non-endometrioid, 167, 170, 171
two types, 254
type I, 260, 280
type I, II, 202, 212, 214, 217, 218, 222
type II, 260, 280
villoglandular, 165
endometrioid, 59, 74, 89, 103–105, 189–194, 200, 202, 209, 210, 212, 214, 260, 271
adenocarcinoma, 160, 162, 163, 165, 166, 168, 171
benign, 155
carcinoma, 281
endometrioma, 210
endometriosis, 58, 61, 75, 97, 189–193, 195, 202, 206, 209, 210, 213, 268
depth of stromal invasion, 21, 23, 39, 80, 81, 89
stromal, 59
symptomatic, 190
endometrium, 149–152, 156, 157, 161, 167, 171, 200, 212–218, 220, 221, 224
endophytic, 121, 125, 132, 143
eosinophilic, 157
epidermoid inclusion cyst, 59
episomal state, 274, 276
epithelial
cancer, 177, 180
cell abnormality, 239, 245
hyperplasia, 184
epithelioid trophoblastic tumor, 106
Erb-B2, 212
erythroplasia of Queyrat, 11
estradiol, 151, 161
estrogen, 150, 151, 153–156, 160, 167–169, 280
estrogen dependent, well differentiated endometrial carcinoma, 254
estrogenic stimulation, 149–153, 160
exaggerated placental site, 106

examination, 118–121, 127,
130–133, 135, 140, 200,
205–209, 219, 221
excision, 120, 121, 123, 125, 129,
130–133, 136, 138, 144

fallopian tube, 188, 201, 208
prolapse, 58
fertility drug, 176
five-year survival, 194
flatulence, 203
floret cell, 48, 57
fluorescent molecule, 271
foamy histiocyte, 157
follicular cervicitis, 52, 71, 72
founder, 200

gain, 271
Gartner duct cyst, 59
gastrointestinal, 200, 203, 205,
206
gene
copy, 271
expression, 274
expression profiling, 271
ontology, 272
genetic, 201, 202, 212, 214–216
genital wart, 274
genomic approach, 270
germ cell tumor, 234
germline mutation, 280
giant condyloma (Buschke-
Löwenstein), 11, 20, 85
glandular, 116, 121, 123–130
cell, 245
dysplasia, 242
glassy cell carcinoma, 86, 91
global, 218, 223

Goff, Barbara, 203
grade 3 nuclei, 164
granulation tissue, 58
granuloma inguinale, 19
guideline, 115, 116, 122, 124
gynecologic cancer, 267

hazard, 219
HE4, 269
Hepsin, 255
HER2, 170
hereditary, 200, 201, 212, 213,
215, 216, 218
colorectal cancer, 177
risk, 176, 177
hereditary nonpolyposis
colorectal cancer, 200,
213–217
high-grade serous carcinoma, 260
high grade squamous intraepithelial
lesion (HSIL), 116, 117,
119, 120, 123, 125, 127,
128, 241, 245
HIV, 3, 19, 68
HIV/AIDS, 19, 53, 67, 68
hormonal risk factor, 156
hormone replacement therapy,
149, 171
host cellular gene, 246
human papilloma virus (HPV),
10, 13, 18, 37, 53, 59, 60,
62, 66, 73, 83, 87, 89, 102,
116, 122, 128–131, 134,
136–139, 231, 246, 274
16 or 18, 279
16/18 vaccine, 250
capsid protein, 62, 63, 107,
109

DNA, 116, 119, 123, 127, 131
DNA testing, 248
E2, 62, 65, 275
E6, 62, 63, 65, 109, 246, 275
E7, 62, 63, 65, 109, 246, 275
E7 gene product, 277
episome, 63
genome, 62
high risk, 16, 18, 31, 33, 35, 39, 45, 52, 56, 58, 59, 65, 68, 275, 276
immune-evasive mechanism, 64
immunogenic, regression of, 250
L1, 62, 65, 107
L2, 62, 109
low risk, 65, 276
oncogene, 246
persistence, 279
"persistent" infection, 67
quadrivalent HPVs 6, 11, 16, 18 vaccine (GARDASIL), 250
reflex high-risk testing, 250
sequential DNA testing, 279
subtype, 65
type, 65, 248
types 6 and 11, 276
typing, 234
vaccine, 107
Hybrid Capture II (HCII), 275
hyperestrogenism, 189, 192
hyperkeratosis, 56
hypermethylation, 252
hyperovulation, 176
hyperplasia, 121, 127, 137, 139, 209, 210, 213, 217, 218, 221, 223, 224, 281
hysterectomy, 56, 200, 201, 214, 215, 217, 220
hysteroscopy, 202, 217, 218, 222, 224
image, 256

identical twin sisters, 178
imiquiniod, 136
immature squamous metaplasia, 277
immune system, 19
immunodeficiency, 53
immunogenicity, 250
immunosuppression, 53, 67
implant, 194
incessant ovulation, 176
incidence, 115, 120, 123, 127–129, 134, 136–139
incidental dysplasia, 179, 182
inclusion cyst, 179, 180, 184, 185, 187
infertility, 189, 192, 193, 201, 203, 209, 210
inflammatory atypia, 102
epidemiology, 66, 72, 86
grading, 86, 91
keratinizing, 83
inheritance, 201
in situ hybridization (ISH), 276, 280
inspecific inherited gene, 176
inspect, 140, 141
insulin-like growth factor I, 255

insulin-like growth factor II
mRNA-binding protein, 3, 254
integration, 275, 276
intermediate cell, 238
intermediate squamous cell, 237
intraepithelial, 116, 117, 119, 120, 122, 124, 128–131, 134, 136, 138, 139, 144
neoplasia, 150, 152, 155–157, 160, 162, 163, 165, 169
invasive, 117, 119–131, 134, 136–138, 140, 143, 144, 177–179, 186, 188, 194
investigation, 205, 211, 217, 219, 221

kallikrein(s), 269
keratinizing type, 243
Keyes, 132, 135, 142, 143
Ki67, 183, 185–187
koilocyte, 10, 60, 64, 71, 240
K-ras, 160, 170, 212
KRAS, 260
k-RAS, 280
kraurosis vulvae, 7

laparoscopic technique, 183
laparoscopy, 186
large cell neuroendocrine carcinoma, 92
large loop excision of transformation zone (LLETZ), 55
leiomyosarcoma, 101
leukoplakia, 7
lichen sclerosus, 7, 8, 19, 135, 137, 139, 143, 144
lichen simplex chronicus (LSC), 9, 10, 20
lipid-associated sialic acid (LASA), 270
liquid based technology, 234, 235
litigation cell, 241
lobular endocervical glandular hyperplasia, 90
loop, 116, 120, 121, 123, 125
loop electrosurgical excision procedure (LEEP), 55
loss, 271
loss of heterozygosity (LOH) analysis, 270
low-grade micropapillary serous carcinoma, 260
low-grade serous papillary adenocarcinoma, 194
low-grade squamous intraepithelial lesion (LSIL), 116, 120, 122, 123, 127. 239, 245
low-stage ovarian cancer, 183
Lugol's, 30, 32
lymphoepithelioma-like carcinoma, 92
Lynch syndrome, 200, 213, 215, 216
lysophosphatidic acid, 269

malignant
cell, 230
counterpart of ovarian cystic, 257
fibrous histiocytoma, 33
melanoma, 27, 29, 30, 40, 100
transformation, 64
malignant mixed mesodermal (Müllerian) tumor (MMMT), 57, 59, 166, 168, 234, 246, 260

mammary-like gland, 3, 26
management, 116, 121, 122, 124, 125, 127, 131, 136
masses, 209
mass spectrometry, 273
mass spectroscopy, 272
matrix assisted laser desorption and ionization (MALDI), 272
M-CSF, 269
mechanical seeding, 259
melanoma, 133, 140
mesonephric
 duct, 48, 52, 59
 hyperplasia, 52, 90
 remnant, 91
mesothelin, 269
metaphase chromosome, 271
metaplasia, 71, 153, 156, 157, 164, 166, 167
metastatic tumor, 36, 42
methylation, 252
Mib-1, 128, 170
microarray
 gene expression, 261
 technology, 272
microglandular hyperplasia, 51, 57, 76, 85, 99, 103
 adenocarcinoma, 87
 carcinoma, 79
microinvasive
 adenocarcinoma, 87
 carcinoma, 79
micropapillary variant, 194
MicroRNA (miRNA), 261
microsatellite instability (MI), 170, 280
mild dysplasia, 239
minimal deviation adenocarcinoma, 90, 103
mitotic figure, 69, 73
mixed, 117, 137
MLH 1, 212, 215
Mmp-9, 190, 192
moderate dysplasia, 239
molecular
 diagnostic assay, 267
 signature, 271
 study, 251
monoclonal
 antibody, 274
 proliferation, 152
MonoPrep Pap, 235
Monsel's solution, 54
morphometric assessment, 180
mosaicism, 53
MSH 1, 2, 200, 215
MSH 2, 6, 200, 215
mucinous, 157, 166, 167, 189, 193, 194, 260, 271
 metaplasia, 157
multifocal, 124, 127, 128, 130, 134–137, 139, 140
mutation, 176, 177, 183, 184, 186, 188, 192, 195, 199–202, 208, 209, 212, 215
 of *PTEN*, 255
 of *TP53*, 260
mycosis fungoides, 27, 40
myometrium, 219

Nabothian cyst, 51, 59
neoplasm, 117, 120, 127, 132, 140, 141, 275
neovagina, 144
Neu, 170
neural network, 181, 182
neuroendocrine tumor, 92

N-myc downstream-regulated gene, 1, 254
non-hereditary risk, 176
nonkeratinizing, 243
nuclear
profile, 180, 181
texture, 182–184
nulliparous, 213

obesity, 149, 151, 160, 167, 171, 212, 213, 218, 219
oral contraceptive, 176, 201, 213
osteopontin, 269
ovarian
cancer, 175–178, 182, 183, 186, 188–190, 192, 193, 195, 199–206, 208–211, 213, 215–217, 256, 267
cyst, 179, 189
dysplasia, 177, 178, 180, 182, 188, 192, 195
endometriosis, 190, 192
epithelial injury, 176
occult cancer, 183
preinvasive cancer, 192
screening, 175, 182, 193, 268
serous adenocarcinoma-like, poorly differentiated type, 254
serous cystadenocarcinoma, 179
OVX1, 269

p16, 128, 251, 276, 277
p53, 19, 134, 135, 157, 159, 160, 170, 183, 185–188, 190, 192, 212, 246, 254
gene mutation, 255, 280
tumor suppressor protein, 277
Paget disease, 25, 27, 40, 140
pain, 204, 205, 209, 210, 220
Papanicolaou (Pap) smear, 115, 117–119, 123, 126, 128, 130, 131, 141, 234, 235, 237, 274, 278, 279
routine screening, 246
papillary carcinoma, 157, 165–168
parabasal cell, 238
parakeratosis, 11, 13, 18, 56, 60
paraneoplastic syndrome, 194, 203, 205
parity, 201
pathology report, 96
patient education, 232
pelvic
endometriosis, 189
pain, 189, 193
perforation, 219, 220, 222
perianal intraepithelial neoplasia (PAIN), 11
peri-menopausal, 280
peritoneal, 201, 207–209, 219
tumor, 189
washing, 258
peritoneum, 179, 189, 194
personalized medicine, 274
Peutz-Jeghers syndrome, 91
phenotype, 184, 188, 192
phosphatase and tensin homolog, 254
PIK3CA, 280
Pipelle, 217, 219–223
pixel, 184
placental site nodule, 105
platinum-based chemotherapy, 271

polyclonal benign hyperplasia, 155
polycystic ovarian disease, 151, 163
polymerase chain reaction (PCR), 278
polyp, 128, 133, 217, 218, 220, 223, 224
endocervical, 57
fibroepithelial, 57
mesodermal stromal, 57
pseudosarcomatous, 57
positive emission tomography, 211
postmenopausal, 115, 123, 129, 130, 135, 138, 140
bleeding, 151, 171
postoperative spindle cell nodule, 58
precancer
lesion, 150, 152, 157, 171
of type I EC, 254
of type II EC, 254
precursor, 150, 152, 157, 160, 177–179, 183, 188, 192–195
pregnancy, 84
preneoplastic, 183, 186
prepubertal
vulval fibroma, 33
vulval fibrous hyperplasia, 35
progesterone, 150–152, 154, 156, 157, 166, 168
receptor, 151, 156, 168, 255
progestin, 176, 212, 213
proliferation biomarker
INK4A, 276
prolonged estrogenic stimulation, 149
prone, 184, 188
prophylactic
oophorectomy, 178, 183–186, 188, 192
salpingo-oophorectomy, 188
proteomics, 261, 272
proteomic technique, 274
Psammoma body, 167, 188
PTEN, 190–192, 202, 212, 260, 280, 281
mutation, 281
tumor suppressor gene, 155, 170
punctuation, 53

radiation, 78
radical vulvectomy, 6
radioimmunoassay, 268
rapid strip test, 249
RARb, 252
Rb, 246
reactive atypia, 71
rectovaginal septum, 49, 58, 97
recurrence, 130, 136
reliability, 218
retinaldehyde dehydrogenase type II, 255
retinoblastoma protein, 277
rhabdomyosarcoma, 100, 133
risk, 115, 116, 118–120, 122–125, 127–129, 131, 134, 136, 138, 139, 143, 144, 199–203, 207, 208, 212, 213–219, 222, 223
reduction, 203, 208

safety, 250
salpingo-oophorectomy, 200, 201, 203, 208, 209, 215

sample collection, 232
sampling, 200, 216, 217, 222, 223
sarcoma, 234
sarcoma botryoides, 31, 99, 133
screening, 116–120, 122, 124, 127, 131, 137, 138, 200, 202, 203, 207, 208, 211, 213
    program, 182, 193, 195
secreted frizzled-related protein 4, 255
secretion, 150
secretory carcinoma, 165
sensitivity, 117, 119, 123, 128, 235, 270
serous, 199, 201–203, 205, 206, 208, 209, 211, 212, 214
serous carcinoma, 157, 166, 167, 168, 172
serous epithelial ovarian cancer (SEOC), 261
serous intraepithelial carcinoma (SEIC), 280
serous papillary, 258, 271
    adenocarcinoma, 189, 194
    carcinoma, 177, 179, 185, 190, 192, 194, 195
serum Ca, 125, 259
severe dysplasia, 239
sex cord-stromal tumor, 234
    with annular tubule, 91
sexual gonadal maldevelopment, 151
signaling, 273
silent, 186, 188, 189, 193
simple glandular hyperplasia, 152
simplex, 134, 137–139, 144
skene gland carcinoma, 29
small cell, 243
small cell carcinoma, 92, 106
smoking, 53, 67
soluble EGF receptor, 269
specificity, 117, 119, 202, 211, 217, 222, 235, 270
specimen, 202, 209, 219, 221
    adequacy, 244
squamocolumnar junction, 50, 63, 64
squamoid morule, 153, 155
squamous, 116, 117, 119–122, 124–128, 130–132, 136, 137–141, 143, 144
squamous carcinoma *in situ*, 239
squamous cell carcinoma, 18, 71, 79, 233, 245, 246
    subtype, 20
    verrucous, 20
squamous differentiation, 166
    metaplasia, 153, 156, 157, 164, 166, 167
squamous dysplasia, 239
squamous hyperplasia, 9, 19
squamous intraepithelial lesion (SIL), 66, 68, 70, 80–82, 102
squamous metaplasia, 51, 53, 57, 76, 102, 238, 277
squamous papilloma, 57
stage I, 202, 207, 209
stage I epithelial ovarian cancer, 270
stain, 210
sterilization, 201
stratification, 178, 180, 182, 188
stromal decidual reaction, 156
subclinical, 274
superficial cell, 238

superficial endocervical AIS, 128
superficial or mature squamous cell, 237
supplementary test, 252
suppression, 176
Sure Path, 235
surface-enhanced laser desorption and ionization (SELDI), 273
surface papillomatosis, 184
surveillance, 200, 216
suspicion, 203, 217
symptom, 120, 121, 130–132, 135, 139, 144, 203–205, 209, 212, 214, 221, 222
systemic screening, 175

tamoxifen, 160–162, 171, 212, 213, 218
Tao Brush™, 222, 223
targeted screening, 260
technology, 221
terminology, 65, 72
The American College of Obstetricians and Gynecologists, 116, 124, 125
thick, 207, 214, 217, 218
Thin Prep, 117, 235
time-of-flight (TOF), 272
Toker cell, 26
toluidine, 135, 141, 143
topography, 210
TP53, 202
trachelectomy, 56
transcription, 271
  regulation, 273
transformation zone, 50, 60, 83
transvaginal sonography, 268
transvaginal ultrasound scanning, 259
treatment, 121, 125, 131, 136–139, 144
tri-dimensional, 183, 184
trophoblastic tumor, 106
tubal, 157, 166, 201, 209, 218
tubo-endometrioid metaplasia, 75, 76
tumor marker, 182, 183, 185, 192–195
tunnel cluster, 51
Turner's syndrome, 151
TWIST1, 252

ultrasound, 194, 202, 205, 207, 208, 213, 214, 216–218, 222, 224
undifferentiated, 134, 137, 144
undifferentiated carcinoma, 260
unifocal, 135, 138, 139
upper gastrointestinal symptom, 189
urethral carcinoma, 36, 37
uterine cancer, 267
uterine serous papillary carcinoma, 157

Vabra, 220
vaccination, 107, 126, 136
vaginal, 115, 120, 127, 129–134, 136, 137
  adenosis, 48, 61, 98
  bleeding, 151, 163, 171, 189, 193
  vault, 48, 58

vaginal intraepithelial neoplasia (VAIN), 66, 129–132, 135, 139
verrucous, 132, 135, 140
virus-like particle, 107
visual inspection of the cervix with acetic acid, 117
vulva
    assessment of margins, 6
    excisional biopsy, 5
    incisional biopsy, 5
    self-examination, 3
vulvar cancer
    epidemiology, 18
    etiology, 18
    precursor lesion, 13
    risk factor, 3
    sentinel lymph node, 24
    staging, 21, 22, 29, 30, 37
    superficially invasive, 21
    survival rate, 23
    warty (condylomatous), 13, 14, 20, 85
vulvar dermatoses, 6
vulvar intraepithelial neoplasia (VIN), 8, 11
    basaloid, 39
    bowenoid, 13
    classic, 13
    differentiated, 13, 15
    grading, 17, 24
    pagetoid, 27, 41
    simplex, 13, 15, 19
    type, 18
    undifferentiated, 13
    usual, 13

Xq11.2–q12, 271